STROUD'S DIGEST ON THE DISEASES OF BIRDS

by

ROBERT STROUD

An alphabetically arranged compendium consisting of a complete report of the researches of the author and a digest of the extant knowledge of this subject, written from the point of view of the practical canary breeder.

Illustrated by the Author

Photography: HARRY LACEY

Distributed in the U.S.A. by T.F.H. Publications, Inc., 211 West Sylvania Avenue, P.O. Box 27, Neptune City, N.J. 07753; in England by T.F.H. (Gt. Britain) Ltd., 13 Nutley Lane, Reigate, Surrey; in Canada to the book store and library trade by Clarke, Irwin & Company, Clarwin House, 791 St. Clair Avenue West, Toronto 10, Ontario; in Canada to the pet trade by Rolf C. Hagen Ltd., 3225 Sartelon Street, Montreal 382, Quebec; in Southeast Asia by Y.W. Ong, 9 Lorong 36 Geylang, Singapore 14; in Australia and the south Pacific by Pet Imports Pty. Ltd., P.O. Box 149, Brookvale 2100, N.S.W., Australia. Published by T.F.H. Publications, Inc. Ltd., The British Crown Colony of Hong Kong.

ISBN 0-87666-435-4

DEDICATION

TO ALL OF MY FRIENDS

Who by their kindness or encouragement have aided in making this work possible, and who form a group so large as to prohibit the singling out of any select few for special mention, may they enjoy all of the good things life has to offer; may its sorrows touch them lightly; may it deal with them as they have dealt with me. It is my deepest regret that I cannot mention each of them here and give full credit for their invaluable service.

To them this volume is appreciatively dedicated.

ROBERT STROUD
Leavenworth, Kansas
June 1, 1939

INTRODUCTION

Purpose

Since my former work, DISEASES OF CANARIES, was hastily executed and badly garbled in the hands of the publisher, and because a number of important investigations have been carried to completion since its publication, I now desire to take another step along the road I entered with its conception—the road leading to a complete description and classification of the diseases and ailments of pet birds and to the development of a practical and effective system of avian therapeutics. With this work I hope to bring that ideal one small step nearer, but no one realizes so well as I how far short of my goal I have fallen. The road stretches into the dim future, far beyond the possible accomplishments of any single lifetime, but if in this book I have been able to point the direction and inspire others to carry on from the point where I have left off, I shall consider my efforts worth while.

I have tried, and I hope not without some measure of success, to bring for the first time to the poultryman, the veterinarian, the veterinary student, the zoologist, the aviculturist, the pet dealer, and particularly to the breeders of canaries and other pet birds, a comprehensive treatise on this subject—a book which will supply instant, accurate, and practical information essential to the diagnosis, control and treatment of bird diseases.

The amount of pioneer work required to this end might well have dismayed one better fitted for the undertaking than I, since I have had to carry the multiple handicaps of lack of training, lack of the equipment and reagents essential to carrying forward independent research, and very limited opportunities for keeping myself informed. If I have been able to make a presentable showing, most of the credit belongs to a series of fortuitous occurrences—maybe **happy hunches** would be a better way of expressing it—which have enabled me to jump to correct conclusion far in advance of sound proof, to often hit upon effective treatments for diseases in advance of their accurate identification, rather than to any personal virtue.

By employing the alphabetical arrangement of my material, aided by hundreds of cross references, I have tried to cover my subject in a manner which would enable the reader to find any information he happened to want at the time he wanted it. To this end, symptoms, lesions, organs, organisms, drugs, and foods have all been given their places in the main vocabulary, making it possible to start from a single observed symptom or lesion and quickly trace down the disease and learn all there is to know about it. Unfortunately, in many cases, that is all too little. But I hope, as a practical handbook, the work will not be entirely without value.

A second object of this work is to make available for the first time the complete results of my observations and researches. Under such heading as ASPERGILLOSIS; AVIAN DIPHTHERIA; FOWL CHOLERA; HEMORRHAGIC SEPTICEMIA; B PARATYPHOSUS B INFECTION; APOPLECTIFORM SEPTICEMIA; BORIC ACID AND BORATE; POTASSIUM CHLORATE; TUBERCULOSIS; etc., I have discussed in some detail my discoveries in avian therapeutics and their underlying principles. And I have offered suggestions for the application of those principles to the diseases of man and animals. Their soundness and universal applicability have been demonstrated by hundreds of clinical tests that have been carried out under my direction upon a range of subjects including half-ounce fire finches and two-hundred-pound hogs. It is not only my hope that this material in the hands of bird breeders, poultrymen, and stockmen may eventually lead to the complete eradication of a number of serious bird and animal diseases; but, in the hands of competent investigators, that it may open up new avenues for an attack upon some of the more stubborn diseases of man which have, up until this time, resisted all attacks.

I have given little space to the subject of vaccines and biologics, for without belittling the outstanding accomplishments in this field, I am of the opinion that the true conquest of disease lies elsewhere —in the field of chemico-therapeutics. Treatment with serums and vaccines can be justified only because of our ignorance of chemical reagents and reactions, and where the use of such measures has retarded the search for and prevented the use of chemical therapeutic agents the harm done, in my opinion, greatly outweighs any good we have ever received from the use of biologics.

Presentation

I make no pretense of literary style. In my presentation of the general characteristics, symptoms, morbid changes, and etiologies of the various diseases, it has been my purpose to make my discussions as clear, concise, and scientifically accurate as my modest abilities permit. This has created the necessity for the employment of a great many technical terms with which the average breeder is certain to be unfamiliar. So, in the interest of clarity, I have made a point of defining each of these terms the first time I have employed it. I do not think that the ordinary breeder who begins at the beginning and reads this book from cover to cover will have any difficulty in following my train of thoughts or understanding the technical matters I have been forced to present in correct technical form. In my opinion, most men of science have a supreme contempt for the intelligence of the average man. When writing for the general public, they act as if they were writing for a class of morons, and their work usually sinks to a level that makes the average man wonder if that is not the true classification of the writers.

I have tried to put the discussion of such subjects as treatments, drugs, control measure, dosages, etc., into language no ten-year-old child could fail to understand, and in order to make the work of maximum value to the breeders devoid of special education, I have indulged in many repetitions and illustrations that would be out of place in a strictly scientific treatise and which my more erudite readers may consider in bad form. I would rather be accused of literary atrocity than of putting my material in an obscure form beyond the grasp of my most humble readers; however, I have never found anything in the realm of science which I believed was beyond the grasp of ordinary persons, providing the writer knew enough of his subject to explain it in understandable terms.

To avoid dryness and heaviness, so common to scientific tomes, so frightening to the average reader, I have tried to lighten and enliven the text wherever possible with notes and personal experiences recounted in the language of the bird room and poultry yard, rather than in that of the laboratory and lecture room. I hope that I have produced a work which will be acceptable to veterinarians and veterinary schools, for Heaven knows they need it, but it has been the problems of the practical birdman and poultryman, rather than those of the scientific student, which have received my first and most earnest consideration. For this reason, and in order to keep the work within reasonable length, I have omitted complete technical descriptions of the organisms and parasites associated with bird diseases, but wherever possible I have illustrated their most striking characteristics. The technical student interested in such material is most respectfully referred to the excellent works to be mentioned presently.

Illustrations

All of the illustrations used in this book are from pen-and-ink drawings made by the author; all those not otherwise credited are original or made from memory from sources long since forgotten. I know that some of the drawings, particularly those in the front part of the book and in those cases where I have drawn birds or organs from memory, are very crude. But the only excuse I have to offer is the statement that this is my first attempt at pen-and-ink illustrating; I have not always been familiar with the best technique for bringing out the features I wished to illustrate, but I believe that in most cases I have made myself clear. In many cases where I have made use of pictures by others, the originals were in half-tones, often in color, and their translation into black-and-white ink drawings of necessity left much to be desired.

Indebtedness

It is not possible for the student, regardless of how careful he may be, to draw a hard and fast line between the thoughts and information he has received from his textbooks and general reading and those that have resulted from his own observations and thought processes. In presenting on paper the picture he carries in his mind he is apt to lose sight of the origin of its component parts. This is especially true in a case like my own, where the period of study has extended over a period of a great many years and the writing has had to be done without the benefit of notes or extensive reference material, almost entirely from memory. Therefore, while I have given credit in the text wherever I have consciously used the material of others, there may be places where I have failed to give due credit, simply because the source of my information had been forgotten. In any such cases I hereby offer my most humble apologies.

I wish to make particular mention of "Diseases of Domesticated Birds," Ward and Gallagher, 1927, and "Principles of Microbiology," Moore, 1912, both published by Macmillan Company. These were the textbooks from which I obtained my first rudimentary knowledge of avian bacteriology; their comprehensive bibliographies were the sources of much of my collateral reading. I am certain that I could never overestimate my indebtedness to either of these fine works, nor could I recommend them too highly to the scientific student.

I am also indebted to the extensive literature of the Bureau of Animal Industry and the Hygienic Laboratory, as well as to that of the various state experimental stations which have done extensive work on the diseases of poultry.

In making comparisons between avian and human physiology and pathology, I have made free use of "Loomis's Practical Medicine," and of various physicians of my acquaintance. The properties of drugs have been checked against the U. S. Pharmacopeia, 1905; Merk's Index, 1907; and Blumgarten's Materia Medica, 1929.

I also wish to acknowledge the assistance I received from Thomas Robinson, A. G. Voss, Asa Camball and George Sturm, whose work as proofreaders did so much to knock the kinks out of my atrocious spelling and grammar.

In presenting this work to my fellow bird breeders and to the world in general, I make no pretense of offering a complete digest of the extant knowledge of bird diseases. For while I have been forced to make large drafts against that knowledge in discussing diseases in general and those particular bird diseases with which I have had no personal experience—we all stand on the shoulders of dead men—it has been my purpose to make use of the researches of others only in those cases where they throw light upon some particular problem which has come to my attention. I have tried to make this book a personal digest, and have tried to sift and interpret the findings of others in the light of my own experience. And at least ninety per cent of the material used is the result of my own observations and researches.

All of the treatments offered without qualification are original with me. Where qualifying phrases such as "suggested," "has been employed," "has been recommended," etc., are used, the treatment is one of general knowledge which may have come to me from many sources; but in all other cases where due credit is not given, the treatment is original. And, of course, I accept full responsibility for every statement and suggestion the work contains.

ROBERT STROUD
Leavenworth, Kansas
June 1, 1939

STROUD'S DIGEST ON THE DISEASES OF BIRDS

by
ROBERT STROUD

A

AIR SACS. Unlike that of mammals, the respiratory system of birds has, in addition to the lungs, a large number of air sacs widely distributed throughout the body, air cavities in the principal bones, and a complex system of tubes which carry air from the lungs and bronchi to almost all parts of the body structure, including the quills of the feathers. The membranes of these sacs and tubes are formed from two thin layers of tissue—a mucous layer in contact with the air, a serous surface in contact with the body structure and organs. Some of the smaller tubes are composed of ring-like segments, each of which is formed by a single cell. Some of the smallest of these tubes have a diameter not exceeding eight microns. (A micron is 1/1000 of a millimeter or about 1/25000 of an inch. The average diameter of the red cells from human blood is also eight microns.)

The part that this system of sacs and tubes plays in respiration can hardly be overestimated. There are cases on record of birds breathing through a broken wing bone while their heads were entirely submerged in water, thus escaping drowning. I have known cases of pneumonia in which less than one per cent of the lung tissue was capable of functioning at the time of death, which only occurred after some of the larger air sacs had become filled with a serous exudate.

AIR TUBE RUPTURE. In young birds that are not being properly cared for, in birds that have suffered injuries, in birds suffering from acute infectious diseases involving the respiratory tract, the skin will sometimes be found filled with air. The neck, back, abdomen, or almost any part of the body, or the whole body for that matter, may be puffed up like a balloon—giving the bird a grotesque appearance and making its movements both awkward and

1

difficult. This condition is caused by a rupture of one of the air sacs or air tubes.

Baby chicks and caged nestlings receiving an inadequate supply of vitamin D, the sunshine vitamin, are often afflicted with this condition. It is also seen among birds in the last stages of the bronchial form of Avian diphtheria.

In nutritional cases and cases due to injuries, the air should be drawn off several times per day by puncturing the skin. The injury cases will usually recover without other treatment. The nutritional cases require a corrected diet, which should contain plenty of green food and an ample supply of the sunshine vitamin. The appearance of this condition in young birds is always evidence that they have been improperly cared for.

Where air sacs or air tubes are ruptured as the result of acute infection, the air may be drawn off to add to the bird's comfort, but hope for its recovery rests upon the ability of its owner to cure the infection.

AMMONIAC. From Northern India and Persia come round, irregular-sized, yellow tears of a gum resin called **Ammoniac.** This substance contains volatile oil, resinotannol, salicylic acid and ferulic acid. It has a sweetish-bitter taste; is partly soluble in water, alcohol, and vinegar; and is used in medicine as a **diuretic** (a drug that increases the secretion of urine) and a **diaphoretic** (a drug that causes sweating).*

Ammoniac preparation. To each ounce of a mixture of three parts dilute acetic acid—containing 6% CH_3COOH—with one part of pure grain alcohol add 15 grains of powdered ammoniac; mix in a glass beaker; heat almost to boiling; pour the hot solution into a bottle and stopper tightly; shake at frequent intervals for several hours; let stand overnight; and then filter through cotton and store in tightly stoppered bottles.

For colds, chronic catarrh of the respiratory tract, and asthmatic conditions in general in canaries and other small birds, this treatment is one of the very best we have. The beneficial results are probably due to the secretion of salicylates by the serous and mucous surfaces of the respiratory tract. The dosage for a bird the size of a canary is from three to ten drops to each ounce of drinking water. This may be given for one week, but it should then be discontinued for several days, after which it may, if nec-

---

* **Note:** Diaphoretics, of course, do not cause birds to sweat through the skin, since their skins have no sweat glands. Such drugs do act upon the secreting glands of their respiratory mucosa, however.

essary, again be given for a week. Most cases in which this preparation is of value will respond to less than a week's treatment, however. So far as I am aware, I was the first to suggest the use of this preparation in the treatment of bird ailments.

AMMONIUM BENZOATE. This is the ammonium salt of benzoic acid and is used in medicine as an **antiseptic, diuretic, antipyretic** and **alterative.***

Ammonium benzoate is used in the treatment of asthmatic conditions, bronchitis, and gastro-intestinal disorders. The dose for a canary is from $\frac{1}{8}$ to $\frac{1}{4}$ grain to the ounce of drinking water. The solution should be mixed fresh daily. The drug, because it loses ammonia when exposed to warmth and air, should be kept in tightly stoppered bottles and in a cool place.

AMMONIUM CHLORIDE, NH_4CL. This is the ammonium salt of hydrochloric acid. It comes as a white powder or colorless crystals having a cool, saline taste and acts as a heart stimulant, expectorant (a drug that causes spitting), and an antineuralgent (a drug that relieves the pain of neuralgia). It is secreted by the respiratory mucosa and is used in human medicine in the treatment of bronchial infections, congestion of the liver, muscular rheumatism, neuralgia and chronic glandular enlargements. It is a constituent of many cough syrups.

Preparation. Add 4 parts of ammonium chloride crystals to a small amount of media consisting of equal parts of peppermint water and sugar syrup; add sufficient media to make up to 100 parts; let stand until the crystals are dissolved, warming and shaking if necessary. The dose for a canary is one to three drops to the ounce of drinking water.

This salt acts by increasing the secretions of the mucous surfaces of the respiratory tract, thus tending to wash away bacterial accumulations and aiding in the removal of purulent exudates by rendering them more fluid.

I have recently used this preparation in the treatment of a number of birds suffering from common colds, and other respira-

* **Note:** An **antiseptic** is a substance which arrests the growth of bacteria, not necessarily killing them; an **antipyretic** is a drug which reduces fevers; an **alterative** is a drug that has a beneficial effect upon the general health for which no logical reason can be assigned. It is a tonic without any known tonic elements in its composition. The use of this word is a monument to our ignorance, for as our knowledge increases we are able to place drugs that were once considered alteratives in other classifications. This is illustrated by the iodides, which were once considered the most important of the alteratives, but which we now know produce their effects by stimulating the endocrine glands.

tory conditions attended by asthmatic symptoms with very satisfactory results. In several cases asthmatic conditions of long standing cleared up after short periods of treatment; in other cases the symptoms were greatly ameliorated; colds cleared up quickly, sometimes as the result of treatment for a single day.

ANTISEPTICS. Antiseptics, as has already been said, are substances having the power of inhibiting the growth of bacteria without necessarily killing them. Thousands of antiseptics are known, but only those having some particular properties of value in the bird room can be discussed in this work, and only a few of those in this section.

ANTISEPTICS FOR THE EYES. Only such substances as have a high germ-killing power and are at the same time nonirritating to the most delicate tissues can be employed as antiseptics for the eyes. The substances here suggested for such use should be employed only in the strengths indicated. It must be remembered that chemical injury of the eye tissue is almost certain to result in permanent blindness.

Boric acid. This substance has long been employed as a human eyewash. It is used in solutions of from 1 to 4 per cent. Many writers have recommended it as an eyewash for birds, since it is mild, soothing, and cannot injure the eyes. Boric acid is of rather low germ-killing power, however, and I have found it of no value in the mildest cases of conjunctivitis.

Argyrol. This is a silver-protein preparation which is widely used in human medicine as an antiseptic for mucous surfaces. It is rather powerful, long lasting, and nonirritating. Of the various strengths in which this preparation comes, I find the ten per cent solution very satisfactory for use on birds. It is safe and effective, but it is one substance that I always hate to use, for it stains the feathers so badly. I have used it with good results in some cases of conjunctivitis, but have found it even more valuable for treating infections of the nasal cavities.

Silver nitrate. This is a powerful caustic, in the pure state, and is used for burning off warts, moles and similar blemishes, but in dilute solution it is one of the most effective antiseptics we have. A small amount of alcohol added to the solution greatly increases that effectiveness. A solution containing 2 per cent silver nitrate, 5 per cent alcohol, and 5 per cent glycerine is not only safe to use in the eyes, it is one of the very best preparations we have for such use.

Sodium perborate. This is an oxidation product of borax. It is widely employed in human medicine as a specific for Vincent's angina (**trench mouth,** a disease of the gums), and as a contraceptive; it is also used as bath salt for the purpose of lowering blood pressure. A solution of sodium perborate in water gives off bubbles of oxygen, which have an antiseptic and oxidizing reaction. I have found this substance of great value for the treatment of diphtheric lesions of the eyes and for many other purposes, of which more will be said presently.

For the treatment of diphtheric lesion, whether of the eyes or other parts, sodium perborate is used as a saturated solution.*

Yellow oxide of mercury. This substance is used in the preparation of a number of ointments for various purposes. I have found that an ophthalmic (for the eye) ointment containing 2 per cent of yellow oxide of mercury is one of the most valuable preparations we have for the treatment of conjunctivitis and other inflammations of the eyes. It can be obtained put up in tubes having long slender nozzles, by means of which the ointment can be introduced into the eyes without fouling the surrounding feathers. In the treatment of conjunctivitis a small amount of the ointment is placed under the eyelids, and the surplus which oozes out when the eye is closed is either wiped away or rubbed into the surrounding tissues, depending on whether or not the surrounding tissues are swollen and inflamed. Like most mercury salts, the yellow oxide combines great germ-killing power with unusual penetration, which accounts for the efficacy of this preparation.

ANTISEPTICS FOR THE HANDS. Contagious diseases in caged birds are usually carried from cage to cage on the hands of their attendant. In one case to come to my attention a highly contagious disease was introduced into a large flock of canaries by their owner shaking hands with a gentleman who had called to ask her advice concerning a disease in his flock. After he had gone she handled one of her own birds without first washing her hands. At the appearance of the first symptom, realizing what she was up against, she wired me; but before wire and air mail services could get effective treatment to her, half of her flock had been lost. Be careful!

---

* **Note:** A **Saturated solution** is one that contains as much of the given substance as will dissolve in a given solvent at the prevailing temperature—and it is made by adding more of the substance than the solvent can dissolve, which is best applied to the eyes by dipping a piece of cotton lint in the solution and then holding the moist cotton against the bird's eye for a few moments. The bird will not like this treatment, but he may live and see because of it. It will not injure the eyes.

When dealing with an epizootic * that has gained a foothold in your plant, be doubly careful!

From the heading of this section, I might be expected to give a list of various antiseptics which can be used effectively for sterilizing the hands. That was my original intention, but investigation convinced me that the list would be so large as to be confusing. There are literally hundreds of antiseptics and disinfectants which may be employed for sterilizing the hands. I shall outline two ways of making the hands safe, and the breeder who employs either, along with the other suggestions given, can be sure that he is not spreading disease every time he tends his birds.

Where running water is available, the most convenient method of cleaning the hands is to drop a little liquid soap into one palm, spread it quickly over both hands and then rinse the hands in running water. A good liquid soap may be prepared by dissolving a bar of "Life Buoy" soap in a quart of water and adding one ounce of cresolis to the solution.

Where running water is not available, a good plan is to have two pails or basins sitting in a convenient place in the bird room. In one have a 3 per cent solution of cresolis; in the other have clean water. The hands are dipped into the cresolis solution and then rinsed in the clean water. The operator who has to keep his hands sterile will find that rubbing them night and morning with olive oil will do much toward preventing chapping and cracking of the skin.

It is advisable to tend all well birds first; next, to tend the exposed birds, and to tend the sick birds last. That way, by thoroughly washing the hands before the first birds are tended and again after tending the sick, all danger of spreading the disease is removed; and it will not be necessary to wash the hands so often as it would have been had the birds been tended in a haphazard manner. See AVIAN DIPHTHERIA.

ANTISEPTICS FOR INTERNAL USE. Scientists have found thousands of things that will kill or inhibit the growth of germs outside of the body; very few things that will kill them or inhibit their growth once they have gained entrance to the blood stream, and in this section I shall list briefly a few such substances which are of actual or potential value in bird medicine. Most of these substances are discussed more fully in connection with the diseases in which their use is indicated.

---

* **Note:** An **Epizootic** is an epidemic occurring among creatures other than man.

"Anthorquinone" violet base (du Pont's). This is a fat-soluble organic dye manufactured by E. I. du Pont de Nemours & Company, Wilmington, Delaware, and, as the name indicates, it is a coal-tar product distantly related chemically to the drug quinine. During some recent experiments in color feeding I discovered that this dye is an absolute specific for acute, generalized aspergillosis in baby canaries. For dosage and other directions see ASPERGILLOSIS.

Oxidizing Antiseptics. There are a number of rather powerful oxidizing agents that are seldom employed for internal human medication, but which are of great value in the treatment of bird infections. How these substances act to bring about their cures is not fully understood. It is known that most of them will destroy germs outside of the body, if used in sufficient concentration, but if employed outside of the body in the same strengths in which they are administered internally, few of them would show any germ-killing power whatever. From this fact it has been argued by certain members of the medical and veterinary professions that these substances cannot act as antiseptics within the body. On the other hand, these substances have the power of bringing about chemical changes in organic substances with which they come in contact, particularly proteins, and they do destroy most protein poisons; some, the chlorates and permanganates, are often used in human medicine for the first-aid treatment of snake bites, in which cases they are injected directly into the fresh wounds and do destroy a large part of the poison before it has a chance to become circulated through the body. It must be noted, however, that when taken internally in large doses by humans, these substances destroy the red cells of the blood and cause poisoning by reacting chemically with the iron in the blood. These same oxidizing reactions will destroy most of the known bacterial toxins; unless they can be assumed to have some selective action that has never been demonstrated, however, they cannot, according to the accepted medical theory, be administered safely in doses sufficiently large to have any effect upon a bacterial toxin diffused throughout the body. That is the medical theory. The observed facts are that when administered to birds in the correct doses in certain diseases, these substances are responsible for the most remarkable and spectacular cures ever observed. It was the discovery of this fact that led to the development of STROUD'S SPECIFIC FOR AVIAN SEPTICEMIAS and started me out on a systematic

study of the diseases of birds.   See POTASSIUM CHLORATE;
PERMANGANATES; PEROXIDE OF HYDROGEN; SODIUM
PERBORATE;   APOPLECTIFORM   SEPTICEMIA;   CANARY
TYPHOID: AVIAN DIPHTHERIA; PERITONITIS; FOWL CHOL-
ERA; PSITTACOSIS; HEMORRHAGIC SEPTICEMIA.

Salicylates. These substances are powerful antiseptics and
are known to be secreted by the kidneys and serous and mucous
surfaces. They are known to act as antiseptics in the digestive and
uro-genital tracts and are thought to act as antiseptics in the respiratory tract and the joints. See AMMONIAC; SODIUM SAL-
ICYLATE; SALOL.

Other internal antiseptics. There is a very fast-growing list
of complex organic compounds of remarkable curative powers and
considerable selectiveness.   Many of these substances are dyestuffs or substances closely related to the organic dyes.   Instead
of discussing these substances here, I shall simply list them and
supply their cross references: chinosol, see CHINOSOL; ASPER-
GILLOSIS; methylene blue, see METHYLENE BLUE; NEPHRI-
TIS; urotropin, see NEPHRITIS.   Also see SULFANILAMIDE,
SULFATHIOZOL.

APOPLECTIFORM SEPTICEMIA * and EGG-FOOD POISONING.
This disease, first studied as a disease of poultry by Norgaard and
Mohler, Bureau of Animal Industry, 1902, has been known to bird
breeders by its symptoms for more than two hundred years. Almost every book ever written on the care of pet birds makes mention of this condition, but it was not until 1929 that the disease in
pet birds was shown to be identical with the disease of poultry.
And, even today, it probably causes the death of more pet birds
than all other diseases combined. Canaries by the thousands are
killed by it every year, and certain varieties of parrots are so susceptible that it is almost impossible to keep them in captivity.
Still it is generally the least understood of all our bird diseases.

While Norgaard and Mohler made a thorough study of the
organism found in the poultry outbreak, they made no investigation of the source of the infection or the cause of the symptoms.
They did, however, make the pertinent observation that the flock
in which they found the disease had been fed on hatchery-clear
eggs.

---

* **Note:** The name **Apoplectiform,** which means **Like apoplexy** was chosen
for this disease because of certain apoplexy-like symptoms. A **Septicemia,**
of course, is any disease in which the causative organism is present in the
blood stream.

The organism they found was a Gram positive, nonmotile, nonencapsulated streptococcus of a rather low order of virulence.*

Symptoms of apoplectiform septicemia. Practically all books on canaries and other cage birds mention two common diseases— the first, usually called **Going light** or **Gastro-enteritis**, is characterized by digestive symptoms and great emaciation, and is primarily a disease of young birds, weanlings that have been separated from their parents but have not yet learned to live on a seed diet or completed the baby moult; the second, generally called **Fits**, is characterized by paroxysms of wild aimless flight and certain paralytic symptoms and is most often met with in birds that have completed the baby moult. It has been the opinion of writers on canaries and parrots that these two conditions were of nutritional origin. Overfeeding has been unanimously credited with being the cause of fits; underfeeding, particularly putting birds on an all-seed diet at too early an age, has been thought to be responsible for the development of gastro-enteritis.

Acute hemorrhagic form. A bird, apparently in the very best of health—if a male, he may be singing at the time, if a female, she may be building her nest or feeding her young—suddenly, usually upon hearing a loud noise or receiving some sudden fright, goes into a violent fit, a paroxysm of wild, aimless flight, battering itself against the wires of the cage or the walls of the room. Then it falls to the floor, unconscious. Sometimes the bird is dead when it hits the floor, but in many cases it is only stunned and soon gets up and goes on about its business as if nothing had happened. If one of these birds is observed closely before the fit, it will be noticed that he is highly nervous. A bird that is normally finger-tame may become so nervous that it will jump with fright when the owner approaches its cage. One odd feature about these fits is the fact that should a fit be set off by some particular noise, that same noise will throw the bird into a fit every time it occurs for as long as the illness lasts. I once saw a case where the bird was thrown into a fit every day by the noon whistle. Most affected birds, however, do not survive more than two or three of these paroxysms. Sometimes a bird will come out of a fit with one leg or one wing paralyzed. Paralysis of the wings is most common in canaries, while in parrots the feet are usually affected. Many

---

* **Note:** The **streptococci** are organism of a class that grows in long chains; **Gram positive** refers to the reaction of the organism to a special staining process invented by a man named Gram; **nonmotile**, of course, means that organisms so designated have no powers of locomotion.

persons have ascribed these deaths and cases of paralysis to head injuries received during the wild flight.

As far back as 1922 I had come to doubt many of these views. I had noticed that cases of fits and of gastro-enteritis often occurred in birds of the same age, caged together.   It was hard to believe that one bird was getting too much to eat and another not enough. I had also observed that in every case where a bird died in a fit a major hemorrhage could be found somewhere in its body—often in the thoracic or abdominal cavities, the air sacs, the air cavities in the bones, and particularly in the spaces in the parietal and occipital bones.*   See Figure 1.   In some few cases hemorrhages

APOPLECTIFORM SEPTICEMIA

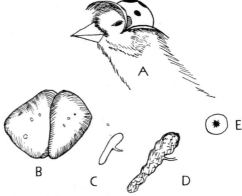

A. The head of a canary, with skull exposed, showing hemorrhagic spots. Each spot represents a different hemorrhage into the air cavities in the skull.
B. The liver from the same canary. Notice the necrotic spots. These are light, dull-yellow in color. Such spots are not observed in all cases.
C. Spleen from a healthy canary.
D. Greatly enlarged spleen from the canary whose head is shown at A. Notice how the organ is elongated and lumpy in appearance, which is characteristic of this disease in those cases where the illness has lasted for a week or more.
E. Section of the spleen shown at D.

Figure 1. Lesions Met With in Apoplectiform Septicemia and Food Poisoning in Canaries.

Free-hand drawings by Robert Stroud

were found in the subarachnoid spaces and between the base of the brain and the sphenoids (the bones that form the floor of the skull).   See Figure 2.

Gastro-enteritic form.   There are no points of similarity between the symptoms of this form of the disease and those of the form just discussed.   The bird suffering from fits often remains in good flesh, and between the attacks it carries on all of its normal functions; but in the form we are now discussing the bird is noticeably ill from the start.   It suffers from digestive disorders, has a greenish diarrhea, carries a subnormal temperature which

---

* **Note:** The **perietal** and **occipital** bones form the crown and back of the skull.

may fall to as low as 100 to 101 degrees F.,* as the fatal termination of the illness is approached. The appetite remains good, but the bird prefers soft food, which it attacks with great vigor. If fed on seed alone, it will spend most of its time over the seed cup, shelling seed, but it will swallow very few of the seeds shelled. Birds suffering from this form of the disease are usually found

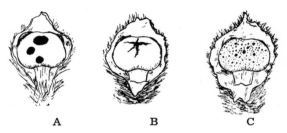

A   B   C

Figure 2
A. This crude, rather bug-eyed sketch illustrates the type of head lesions found in the condition under discussion.
B. This shows the form taken by hemorrhages resulting from blow on the head. In the case illustrated the bird flew into an obstruction.
C. This sketch illustrates the type of head lesions often found in cases of peracute hemorrhagic septicemia (Fowl Cholera), as recently observed in an outbreak in wild sparrows.

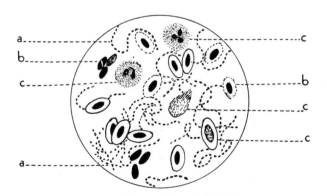

APOPLECTIFORM SEPTICEMIA

Figure 3. Blood from a Young Canary Suffering from Apoplectiform Septicemia.

a a   Streptococci.
b b   Shadow cells.
c c c c   Various kinds of Leucocytes. (See BLOOD.)
Magnification about 600X.

Free-hand drawings by Robert Stroud

* **Note:** The normal temperature of a healthy canary is 107.5 degrees F.

dead over the seed or food cup. It was probably this feature of
the illness that created the impression that these birds were suffering from malnutrition.

There is always great emaciation. The duration of the illness
may vary from five to fifteen days. Death occurs in a convulsion,
and there are no spontaneous recoveries.

The appearance of the abdomen in both forms of this disease
is very characteristic. It is always enlarged, usually red or purple
in color, and has a corrugated appearance caused by the intestines,
particularly the duodenum, showing through the abdominal wall.
This appearance of the abdomen is not so characteristic that it can
of itself be accepted as diagnostic, but in a flock where fits or gastro-enteritis symptoms have made their appearance, it may be
employed for separating the sick from the well, if that is desirable.

Morbid anatomy. The morbid changes found in the two forms
of apoplectiform septicemia differ in degree rather than kind.
Their development depends a great deal more upon the duration
of the illness than upon the form taken by the attack; however,
since the gastro-enteritic form is the one in which there is a slow
steady progress from the onset of the first symptoms to the fatal
termination, it is the form in which the changes are apt to be the
most extensive. If the illness has lasted for several days, the following changes will be found at the autopsy:

Inflammation of the intestines, especially of the duodenum;
enlargement of the liver, which may contain dull-yellow, necrotic
spots of a leathery texture and consistency, if the duration of the
illness has been rather long—Figure 1. Hemorrhages, Figure 1,
into the various body and bone cavities have already been mentioned. In the gastro-enteritic form of the disease the fatal hemorrhage is usually into the thoracic cavity, and this is the only
hemorrhage found. In fits, each fit that the bird has survived has
left its mark in the form of its own particular hemorrhage—and
the difference in the appearance of these hemorrhagic spots is
sufficient to enable the examiner to tell the order of their occurrence. The spot caused by the most recent hemorrhage will be
bright red in color; the others will be darker according to their
age, excepting that those which occurred a week or two before
death will show yellowish brown borders where absorption has
taken place. The hemorrhages into the skull spaces are most easily
observed, for when the skin is removed from the head they stand
out as dark spots. See Figure 1. They are differentiated from
hemorrhages resulting from head injuries by the fact that the spots

caused by hemorrhages resulting from disease are usually round or oval in shape; hemorrhagic spots resulting from head injuries are of irregular outline. See Figure 2.

The most constant lesion of this disease, the one found in all cases, regardless of the form or duration of the illness, is a characteristic enlargement of the spleen. The extent of the enlargement does depend upon the duration of the illness, and the organ may be from two to five or even seven times normal size; it is elongated rather than swollen and is of lumpy, irregular outline; its color varies from dark red to deep purple; and the whole organ has a mottled appearance which is very characteristic, and which is caused by hyperemic engorgement of the normally invisible capillaries. Running lengthwise through the center of the organ is a thick black core, which is best seen if the organ is slightly hardened by immersion in absolute alcohol for a few moments before sectioning. Figure 1 shows the relative sizes and appearances of spleens from a normal canary and from a canary that died after a two weeks' illness with apoplectiform septicemia. (E), Figure 1, gives an idea of the appearance of a section through the thickest part of the spleen shown at (D). The coagulum is made up of shadow cell, red cells, degenerated spleen cell, and leucocytes. An unusually large number of cell nuclei are observed in smears made from this coagulum—these are undoubtedly red cells in the last stage of degeneration. See Figure 4.

Etiology. As mentioned above, the streptococcus of apoplectiform septicemia—Figures 3 and 5—was first isolated from chickens in 1902; it was not until 1931, however, that the infection in canaries and other cage birds was shown by the writer to be identical with

APOPLECTIFORM SEPTICEMIA

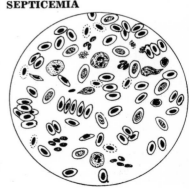

Figure 4. Blood of a Canary that Died from Egg-Food Poisoning

Notice the leucocytes and shadow cells and the large number of free nuclei.

Free-hand drawing by Robert Stroud

the disease in poultry.* At that time, while I was engaged in the study of avian diphtheria, some of my birds died of fits, others developed gastro-enteritic symptoms.

Now, naturally, because of the work being carried on, these birds were kept under the best possible sanitary conditions, and the correctness of their diet was guarded with extreme care. I was puzzled and curious. Post-mortem examinations were made as a matter of routine, and, because the identical changes in the spleens of birds that had died from two distinct sets of symptoms

Figure 5   **APOPLECTIFORM SEPTICEMIA**

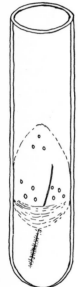

STREPTOCOCCUS OF APOPLECTIFORM
SEPTICEMIA

Agar culture showing pearly, dewdrop-like colonies above the condensation water and a faint, feathery growth along the needle path.

Free-hand drawing by Robert Stroud

further excited my curiosity, I made cultures from the blood and organs of all of the birds that died and from the blood of all those suspected of being sick. (The suspicion of illness was based upon abdominal inspection.) A few days later I was astonished to find identical growths in all the different sets of tubes.

This observation opened up a new line of investigation that has been going on in a more or less desultory manner ever since, and which has established the following facts:

---

* **Note:** The original experiments were started in 1929, and an account of my findings was first published in the "Roller Canary Journal" of the issue of March, 1931. The results of subsequent experiments were published in "American Canary and Cage-Bird Life," August, 1933.

(1) That the disease in canaries, parrots, finches, sparrows, and probably other pet birds is often due to a streptococcus identical in cultural characteristics with that described by Norgaard and Mohler, Bulletin 36, Bureau of Animal Industry, 1902.

(2) That the symptoms of the gastro-enteritic form of this disease, which usually attacks young birds only, are in every case due to the growth of the organism within the body.

(3) That the convulsions, which are such a prominent symptom of the hemorrhagic form of this disease, are the result of an internal hemorrhage; that the duration of the wild flight corresponds with the duration of the internal bleeding (proved by the fact that the birds that are not dead when they hit the floor do not die of that particular attack); that the symptoms of the acute hemorrhagic form of this disease do not depend upon the growth of the organism within the body; that birds more than four months old were usually immune to inoculation with the causative organism; but that these same birds sometimes developed hemorrhagic symptoms and died, though their blood remained sterile. When this fact was established it opened up another line of inquiry, a search for a toxin.

(4) That the symptoms of the hemorrhagic form of apoplectiform septicemia could be caused by a toxin produced outside of the body. I found that by sprinkling the granulated yolks of hard-boiled eggs with cultures of the organism, permitting the material to dry for 24 hours, sterilizing it at 100 C., for periods of from one up to twelve hours, and then feeding the sterilized material to canaries, all of the symptoms and lesions of the hemorrhagic form of this disease could be reproduced. A great many tests of toxic materials, spread over a period of two years, convinced me that this condition is in reality one of food poisoning.*

(5) That the causative organism is in reality a food poisoning organism usually associated with stale eggs and of such a low order of virulence that it cannot cause disease in adult birds, but that the poison could kill birds of any age if the dosage

---

* **Note:** The conclusions expressed in this paragraph do not necessarily apply to the disease in parrots. These birds are not fed on animal protein, so it is not likely that they could pick up the toxin from external sources. It is possible that they are susceptible to infection by the causative organism, which might be picked up through stale and contaminated drinking water. It is worth noting that only young and newly trapped parrots are susceptible to the disease—once the birds are acclimated to domesticity, the condition disappears.

was large enough. I found no difficulty in isolating this organism from various samples of food containing stale egg material or from the dregs of drinking cups of birds fed on egg food. I found that if a cage containing twenty birds was unattended on three successive days during warm weather, until the birds had drunk their drinkers dry, some of the birds were certain to develop fits and that most of them would show the characteristic spleen lesions. I believe that this results from the birds' habit of washing their beaks in the drinking cups after eating soft foods. My first clue to the part played by egg material in the development of this condition came as a result of my search for the cause of the outbreak which occurred in 1929, which prompted my study of this condition. I found that the source of the trouble was a cod-liver oil emulsion I was feeding my birds. I made melted-agar cultures from the emulsion and seeded new cultures from all types of colonies resembling those found on agar slants seeded from the blood of sick or dead birds. The result was that I isolated an organism that could not be distinguished from that found in the birds. Egg had been used as the emulsifying agent in the preparation of this oil.

Unfortunately, through lack of the necessary equipment, I have been prevented from making any attempt to isolate the toxin. So far as I have been able to learn, it is produced only in egg material. I haven't the least idea whether it is a true bacterial toxin or a protein cleavage product.*

In the September, 1938, issue of the "American Canary Magazine" and in several other magazines devoted to canaries, appeared an article entitled "Leukemia of Canaries," by A. J. Durant and H. C. McDougle, Veterinary Department, University of Missouri, in which. lesions identical with those I have observed in chronic cases of food poisoning are described. They based their diagnosis upon the enlargement of the liver and spleen and microscopic examination of the blood.† The lesions described could have easily

---

* **Note:** Recent experiments, carried out during the current year, 1938, and since the above was written, have shown that several distinct forms of micrococci other than the streptococcus mentioned above are capable of producing changes in egg material which cause it to become toxic and produce all of the symptoms and lesions described under this heading, which convinces me that the toxin involved is a protein cleavage product that may be produced in egg material by a number of the organisms responsible for decay. So it seems that the designation of this condition as a septicemia is an error, but, since the streptococcus is sometimes found in the blood of young canaries, I have not seen fit to rewrite the section.
† **Note:** A reproduction of their evidence will be found under the heading LEUKEMIA.

been produced by the bird receiving the egg toxin in sublethal doses over a long period of time.

Microscopic studies of the blood were not made during my early work with this disease, for the simple reason that the equipment was not available to me. For information concerning the morphology of the organisms with which I was working, I was dependent upon the reports of men to whom I submitted materials for examination. In recent cases I have found blood pictures identical with the one shown in the photomicrograph illustrating their article. They do not give the results of their blood counts, but I have found cases in which the proportion of red to white cells in the blood had been reduced from a ratio of 125:1 to 100:1, which is the normal proportions of these cells, to from 8:1 to 6:1. The latter proportion is not uncommon in cases of long standing. Such blood shows a large number of shadow cells and free nuclei.

The transverse enlargement of the spleen in proportion to its longitudinal enlargement in the Durant-McDougle case was much greater than that observed in any of my cases, of which there has probably been between two and three hundred scattered over a period of eighteen years. The width of the spleen in their case was about one-third of its length. In my cases the width of the spleen was usually about one-fifth of its length, though in some instances the width of the spleen was not more than one-seventh to one-ninth of its length.

Treatment. Remove the source of the toxin or infection; see that the birds have plenty of clean, fresh drinking water; discard any protein food that may be suspected of being stale, paying particular attention to any food known to contain or suspected of containing egg material. If possible, add one teaspoonful of STROUD'S SALTS NO. 1 or sodium perborate to each quart of drinking water for a day or two—prolonged treatment is neither necessary nor desirable. Treatment for a single day is usually sufficient to cleanse the birds' systems of toxin, and, if the source of the trouble is removed, that is all that is required; if the source of the poison is not removed, little can be expected from any line of drug treatment. In case my treatment is not available, fair results may be obtained by using commercial peroxide of hydrogen in the drinking water in the proportion of 1:9.

By catching the bird during the fit and holding its head under a stream of cold, running water, the internal bleeding may be stopped and the bird saved for the time being.* Birds suffering from severe convulsions have been saved from death by injecting into the crop ten drops of a 2 per cent solution of STROUD'S SALTS NO. 1, or ten drops of a 0.75 per cent solution of peroxide of hydrogen. †

Since the paralysis of the legs and wings following a fit is the result of a blood clot pressing on a motor center or motor nerve, the condition will cure itself as soon as the clot has had a chance to absorb, providing, of course, that the bird does not die in a subsequent convulsion. This absorption requires from three to four months for a bird the size of a canary and from six months to a year for a parrot. The average time required for a similar absorption to take place in a human adult is about two years, though in both birds and man, the time required for such a clot to absorb depends considerably on the location and size of the clot.

ARGYROL. See ANTISEPTIC FOR THE EYES.

ARTERIES. See CIRCULATION.

ASPERGILLOSIS. This disease, as the name indicates, is an infection with a pathogenic (**pathogenic** refers to the power to cause disease) fungus of the genus aspergillus. The most common offender is A **fumigatus** (the spore heads of this variety are green or brown), though A **niger** and A **flavus** (first of which is the black mold that appears on wheat bread, the other is white) have also been known to cause disease in man, animals and birds—the illnesses caused by these organisms, however, are much less severe than that caused by A **fumigatus.**

The most common form of avian aspergillosis is a pulmonary or generalized mycosis (**mycosis** is the term applied to the pathological lesions caused by mould growing in living tissue) of young birds known as **Brooder pneumonia.** The disease, which has been studied principally as an infection of baby chicks, kills thousands of young birds yearly. No species appear to be immune. It has

---

* **Note:** The suggestion to pour cold water over the head of a bird having a fit is over two hundred years old, which illustrates the fact that practical breeders often arrive at sound practices, even when they are reasoning from unsound theories.

† **Note**: The dose, "ten drops," suggested in the text is for a bird the size of a canary. Larger birds would require proportionally larger doses; thus, the dose for a chicken would be from two to four teaspoonfuls of the solutions mentioned. A 0.75 per cent solution of peroxide of hydrogen can be prepared by mixing commercial peroxide with water in the ratio of 1:3. A 2 per cent solution of STROUD'S SALTS NO. 1 can be made by adding four grains—a good-sized pinch is about four grains—of the salt to half an ounce of water.

been observed by Walker in young ostriches,† and by me as a highly fatal disease of baby canaries and sparrows—which about covers the field so far as size is concerned. Judging from my own experience, fully half of the baby canaries that die in the nests are victims of this infection—and the old birds get blamed for starving their young.

The source of infection is always mouldy or dusty food—though the word **food** as used here must be construed to include the litter of baby chicks. Dust from canary seed, corn, wheat, rye, and many other grains and seed is rich in the spores of this fungus. When these spores find their way into the body they sometimes find lodgment in the tissue, where their growth sets up a disease process. In Europe there are many pigeon raisers who feed the young birds by hand—by mouth, rather—by chewing up the food and forcing it into the young birds in much the same manner as their parents would feed them. Many persons engaged in this work die of aspergillus pneumomycosis, resulting from spores of aspergillus being inhaled as the grain is taken into the mouth. Cows fed on mouldy hay also develop aspergillus pneumomycosis. While birds and mammals of all species appear to be susceptible, mature individuals display a very high resistance to this infection, though once the disease is established in the system, a fatal termination can be expected.

Because of its prevalence, early appearance, similarity of symptoms, and high mortality, brooder pneumonia is often confused with bacillary white diarrhea. The latter disease, however, makes its appearance from the first to the fourth day of life, and practically never runs an acute course in birds infected after the sixth day, while brooder pneumonia cannot make its appearance before the third day of life and may appear during the third week or even later.

Symptoms. The bird, dull and listless, feathers ruffled, stands with both feet on the ground, head drawn back, eyes closed. Later the head may hang between the feet; if the lungs and upper air passages are extensively involved, the head may be thrust forward, and the breathing gasping in character. As the disease progresses there is short, rapid, open-mouthed breathing and a diarrhea of gummy consistency, which fouls the feathers and plugs the vent. The bird becomes very weak and greatly emaciated and soon falls to the ground and dies in a coma.

In canary chicks the infective material always gains entrance

---

† **Note:** Walker, Union of South Africa, Department of Agriculture, 1915.

to the body by way of the digestive tract. The disease may make
its appearance at any time after the ingestion of infective material,
but it usually appears within about five hours. Baby canaries are
most susceptible between the third and fifteenth days of life; though
their resistance is considerable by the tenth day, and each succeeding day increases it. Cooking the mouldy food for one hour does
not always devitalize all of the spores. I have boiled mouldy corn
in a closed water bath that reached a temperature of more than
100 degrees C., for two hours and still had it kill every young
canary to which it was given.

The young canary is hungry and cries for food, opens its mouth
to take the food offered by its parents, but the food taken can be
swallowed only with extreme difficulty, if at all, and after a few
efforts the young bird drops to the bottom of the nest, exhausted—
its neck stretched out as far as possible, its beak open, its body
racked convulsively with the labor of breathing. In a few cases,
however, and these are usually birds that become infected after
the tenth day—the chicks are able to take food until the very last
and are found dead with their crops full. The difficult breathing
just described is the most uniform and easily recognized symptom
of this disease in young canaries; it is always the first symptom
noticed and grows more pronounced as the illness progresses.
Death follows the onset of the symptoms by from six to forty-eight
hours; and it is only chicks that are over a week old at the time
of infection which live for the longer period. In these cases the
mouth fluid becomes thick and viscid; a gummy deposit forms on
the edges of the bill; patches, first white, later a dirty yellowish-
brown in color, form in the back of the mouth, particularly around
the openings of the esophagus and trachea. Prior to some experiments to be described shortly, no treatment of this condition was
possible.

Old canaries show a very high resistance to this infection.
Parent birds will live and thrive on the same material that kills
all of the babies. Time after time I have seen old canaries that
were fed on stale, mouldy food develop digestive disorders, as a
result of irritating poisons present in such material, and then recover as soon as they were placed on a clean wholesome diet. Not
all, but a great many, of the cases discussed under the heading
NESTLING DIARRHEA are the result of aspergillus infection of
the digestive tract of the baby birds, yet it is very seldom that
their mothers contract the aspergillus infection, even though they
are often made very ill from the poisons taken into their systems.
These observations have convinced me that old canaries are almost

entirely immune to aspergillus infection by way of the digestive tract. And in all cases of aspergillosis in adult canaries to come to my attention, the lesions were confined more or less closely to the respiratory tract, and they were of such a nature as to leave no doubt about the locations of the primary lesions. One very interesting case occurred in my bird room.

Twelve badly neglected birds were shipped to me. They were all sick on arrival. The seed in the box they came in was of the very poorest grade—stale, mouldy, and full of dust, unfit for any bird to eat. Naturally, aspergillosis was suspected. The birds were placed in clean cages; given plenty of clean, wholesome, dust-free seed; given plenty of fresh green food and direct sunlight; and they were placed on the potassium iodide treatment for three months. At the end of that time they were all apparently recovered. Some of these birds were sold; others were used in diphtheria experiments; one pair that had recovered from the diphtheria was kept for breeding; but during the second season they both went out of condition. The male would sing and carry on all normal functions, but every slight change in the weather seemed to upset him. He suffered more or less from some obscure digestive disturbance. The female, though she seemed in perfect condition in all other respects, lost the use of one wing. It was at first thought that she had injured her wing in some unnoticed accident. When six months had passed without improvement in her condition, she was killed and examined.

The metacarpus, ulna, and radius (bones of the lower wing. See SKELETON) of the crippled wing and the ulna of the supposedly normal wing were found to be tumefied to an almost unbelievable extent. The internal pressure had warped and split the bone surfaces. Large tumor-like masses were found in both shoulders, just above the point where the air tube enters the humerus (the upper bone of the wing). Several of these masses were as large as BB shot, yet they were actually expansions of the air tubes caused by the internal growth of the mould and the accumulation of tissue debris resulting from that growth. Aspergillus fumigatus was easily identified in smears from the honeycombed bones.

The artery supplying the crippled wing, which for a considerable time, undoubtedly, had been plugged at the point where it entered the disease process, was distended to at least ten times its normal diameter and badly varicosed through its length. No other lesions were found. The body was well nourished, and all of the vital organs were normal.

Sometime later the male was killed for examination. His abdominal air sacs were found to be badly infected. Several of them were filled with exudate, and their adjoining walls were obliterated; all of the peritonial membranes were clouded.*

Morbid anatomy. As explained above, the mould may develop in any part of the body to which it finds access. It may spread over a large part of the respiratory surfaces, entirely fill air sacs, plug tubes, and even burst and honeycomb bones. When growing on a mucous surface, the fungus forms a false membrane of a dull-white, greenish, or brownish color—new growths are white; growths that have reached the spore-forming stage are greenish; older growths are brownish in color. Sometimes nodules may be found in the lungs, though as a general rule this is not the case. More often the infection is diffused throughout these organs and sets up an extensive pneumonic consolidation.

Nodules somewhat similar to those caused by tuberculosis are sometimes found in the submucous tissue, but the general anatomical pictures of the two diseases are so dissimilar that it is impossible to confuse them.

The organs in contact with the air sacs and air tubes may become infected—and in such cases, the fungus may gain entrance to the blood stream and set up foci of infection in various parts of the body; then necrotic spots may be found in any organ, though the kidneys are most apt to be involved.

In older birds, where the air tubes and air sacs are involved, diagnosis from post-mortem examination is never difficult; anti-mortem diagnosis, however, is practically impossible. In young birds, where the infection is more generalized and the course of the illness more acute, it may be necessary to resort to cultural methods to arrive at a satisfactory post-mortem diagnosis, since the bird may die before the fruit heads are well developed, but, because the symptoms run a regular course, the condition can usually be recognized during life.

Treatment. Until recently there was no treatment for young birds other than prevention. In man, localized lesions caused by aspergillus fumigatus and aspergillus niger situated in accessible regions—in the ear, the nasal passages, on the cornea of the eye—are sometimes successfully treated by a prolonged series of X-ray exposures. There is no recognized treatment for the generalized infection in man. I am informed by Dr. Zellemayer, of the U. S.

---

* **Note:** When healthy, the serous membranes of the abdominal and thoracic cavities are as transparent as cellophane.

Public Health Service, that the prognosis in such cases is always death.

The only drug that has been widely used in the treatment of mould infections is potassium iodide. It is considered a specific for actinomycosis (a disease caused by one of the "ray" fungi) in cattle, and has been used in the treatment of that disease in man, though I understand that medical opinion is divided as to its value. It seems that the good doctors are in the unenviable situation of having to use an unsatisfactory treatment because they have not been able to work out a better one. Maybe I can do it for them. I wonder if it would do any good.

Whenever there is sound reason for suspecting that the illness of an old bird may be caused by aspergillus infection, or any other mould infection, for that matter, the potassium iodide treatment is indicated.* In most cases, however, the bird will be too far gone by the time the diagnosis is established for this treatment to be of much value. Where a number of birds, kept under identical conditions, are taken sick at about the same time and where those conditions are such as to indicate widespread exposure to aspergillus spores, the presence of this disease in one bird makes the assumption of its presence in the rest advisable. It is then wise to put the whole flock on treatment.

Iodide Treatment.† This consists of adding one drop of a saturated solution of iodide of potassium to each ounce of drinking water for a day or two; then increasing the dose to a drop and a half and two drops by easy stages.‡ This may be continued for two or three weeks—it is best to give it for two weeks the first time; discontinue it for a week; and then repeat and continue the administration for three weeks. This can be kept up for three months, but one week's rest must be allowed after each three weeks' course. Potassium iodide is a dangerous drug. A single large dose will often set up a condition of shock which is followed by collapse,

---

* **Note:** This was sound advice before I discovered the "Anthroquinone" treatment to be described presently. It is still sound, inasmuch as the "Anthroquinone" treatment has not been tested on adult birds. But there is reason for believing that the iodide treatment will soon be abandoned.

† **Note:** Had my primary interest in science been medical rather than chemical, with the generally slipshod looseness of expression of the medical profession, I would call this the **Iodine treatment.** Free iodine is not used in internal medicine, however; Iodides are used, so I think that the word "Iodide" should be employed to describe their use.

‡ **Note:** To measure fractional drops of the iodide solution, place a pint of water in a glass pitcher, then add sixteen drops of the solution—there are sixteen ounces in a pint—at first, and fill the bird's cups from the pitcher. The dose may be increased at the rate of one drop per pint every two days until thirty-two drops, which is two drops to the ounce, are being used.

coma, and death within from a few moments to a few hours; but by gradual dosing it is possible to bring the body to a point of saturation that would surely be fatal if approached too rapidly, but which will destroy many forms of microscopic life within the body. To test the power of this drug to destroy bacteria and other low forms of life, just notice that while you are using it, even in the smallest doses, no scum or slime forms in the drinking cups. See IODIDES.*

In 1931, during one of our psittacosis scares, William C. Dustin, writing in one of the then popular trade journals, reported his experience with a disease of parrots, which he thought to be psittacosis. The disease broke out in a shipment of newly imported parrots. He sent some of the bodies to a laboratory for examination and added chinosol (this is a complex organic dyestuff of high antiseptic properties. It is discussed under its own heading) to the drinking water of the sick birds. Most of the sick recovered. The laboratory reported that the bodies were of birds that had died of aspergillosis pneumomycosis. Mr. Dustin does not give sufficient information in his article to permit the calculation of the chinosol dosage he employed. I have not used chinosol for the treatment of aspergillosis, but I have tried it in certain micrococci infections of the intestinal tract and the kidneys with indifferent results. I have found, however, that a 1:5000 solution of chinosol can be used as drinking water by canaries for several months at a time, without their developing any symptoms of poisoning. See CHINOSOL.

Recently, two other breeders—Fred E. Daw of Oak Park, Illinois, and William Southern of Clifton Hill, Missouri, have suggested the use of mercurochrome in the treatment of aspergillosis of baby canaries. Mr. Daw told me of adding five drops to a commercial mercurochrome solution—he did not say or probably know the strength of the solution—to each ounce of drinking water supplied to the old birds. The babies recovered. Mr. Southern merely asked me to test the drug, suggested that the commercial solution be given directly into the beak in single-drop doses. He wrote: "I can assure that this drug is not poisonous to the babies and that a drop of it administered into the beak will not harm them. If you try it, I think that you will be agreeably surprised by the results."

---

* **Note:** In hot weather, when the birds will naturally be drinking more water than usual, the dosage of iodides must be adjusted accordingly. It must be remembered that drugs may enter into chemical combinations with metals. Always use glass or crockery drinkers for the administration of medicines. Any unco-ordinated movement in a bird taking iodides indicates poisoning.

"Anthroquinone" treatment. During the summer of 1938, I was engaged in some color-feeding experiments with white canaries, the results of which were the development of the first processes from the production of pastel pink and lavender plumage on these birds by feeding them on organic dyestuffs. One of the dyes used in my experiments was "Anthroquinone" Violet Base—manufactured by E. I. du Pont de Nemours & Company, Wilmington, Delaware—which is a fat-soluble, violet dye. During the course of my experiments with this dye, at a time when the weather was very hot and damp, some of the babies developed aspergillosis, from scattered soft food in the bottom of the cage becoming mouldy. The dye was being hand fed to healthy babies, to test its toxicity, by mixing it in the dry food in proportion of from 1:1500 to 1:300. This larger dose amounts to about 1 milligram per day for each gram of body weight for seven-day-old chicks, which would be the equivalent of 2.23 ounces per day for a 145-pound man—a rather heavy dosage. Some of the birds were kept on this dosage for a period of four months without showing any signs of poisoning.

Without any particular hope of worth-while results, but, at the same time, not forgetting the fact that sulfanilamide had been used in dyeing for forty years before anyone thought to test its therapeutic properties, I fed the "Anthroquinone" preparation to the desperately sick babies. At the time I first gave them the dye I did not expect them to live overnight. They remained at the point of death for four days, but on the evening of the fifth day their breathing was easier. The next morning their breathing was normal and they were, for the first time since the onset of the illness, able to take full crops of food. They were weak, starved little creatures, and it took several days of careful nursing to bring them up to par, but they grew up into fine, healthy birds.

Subsequent experiments have demonstrated that it is possible to cure every case of acute, generalized aspergillosis resulting from the infection of baby canaries with the spores of aspergillus fumigatus by the administration of Du Pont's "Anthroquinone" Violet Base in the proportion of one part dye to each 300 parts of food consumed—dry weight.

I claim priority in the discovery of the therapeutic properties of this substance, since I was informed by the manufacturer, Dr. Rose of the Du Pont Technical Laboratories, that they had no information concerning its physiological properties; that all they could say was that the substance was probably harmless in small doses, since it was as pure as any dye made. I believe that the results obtained justify the testing of this substance on other animals and on man.

How "Anthroquinone" Violet brings about the results observed is unknown. The action in no way resembles the specific reaction brought about by the use of oxidizing agents in such diseases as Avian diphtheria, Fowl cholera, Hemorrhagic Septicemia, etc., where complete cure takes place within a matter of a very few hours, and often results from a single dose of the medicine used. The early doses of "Anthroquinone" Violet do nothing more than suspend a fatal issue. No real improvement in the condition of the patient is noticed until the dye has been administered for from three and one-half to four days. This may be partially explained by the fact that "Anthroquinone" Violet is a fat-soluble substance and is not eliminated through the organs of excretion after it is once incorporated into the tissues of the body. It is slowly destroyed within the body, but the process takes many months, which makes it reasonable to believe that the curative effects are dependent upon the amount of fat used and stored during the period of administration, which, of course, is limited by the ability of the system to use and store fat.

Preparation of "Anthroquinone" Violet. Take any good nestling food and sift it through a fine screen to remove all seed hulls and coarse matter which might be injurious to the baby birds, or, if you prefer, make your own nestling food by mixing five parts dry ground bread with five parts of ground rape seed, from which the hulls have been removed, and one part egg-yolk powder, and then adding one-tenth part mineral food or crushed cuttle bone, one-twentieth part table salt, and one-fifth part cod-liver oil. Weigh out forty-nine grams of the food and one gram of the dye; mix thoroughly by rubbing the mixture between the hands until the entire mass takes on a uniform color. Should the dye fail to color the other substances uniformly, add more cod-liver oil and continue to rub the mixture between your hands until the color does become uniform. Weigh out ten grams of this mixture and mix it with fifty grams of the nestling food. Each three hundred parts of this dry mixture will contain one part of the coloring matter. It is administered as a gruel made by masticating it with green food grass, dandelion leaves, chickweed, or cabbage—or by rubbing it up with scraped apple or boiled carrot and thinning it with hot water until it is the consistency desired. Enough food may be mixed at one time for three feedings, but it must be heated to body

Figure 6.   **ASPERGILLUS**

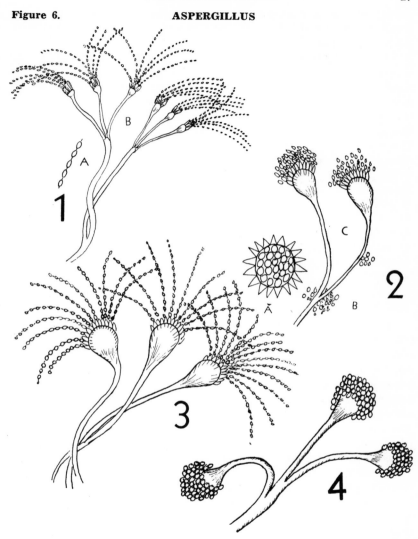

1. A low-growing, fine-textured mould which makes its appearance on neutral agar kept at room temperature—about 90 degrees F.—at the end of three days.   The growth is roughly round, rather dense, and the colonies, which are velvety and thicker in the center than they are at the edges, have a slight tendency to coalesce.   They are at first white, later green, lastly brown.   The color makes its first appearance in the center of the colony and never extends to the outer edge.   The surface of the media is never completely covered.   a, spores;   b, structural features of plant.
2. A high-growing, loose-textured colony which makes its appearance

within 12 hours of seeding and may spread over the entire surface of the media within a few more hours. The stems may reach a height of one-half inch. The growth white, but in old cultures small of yellow material can be seen with the naked eyes. The material appears to be an amorphous secretion of the flower heads. The spores are colorless, of irregular size, and appear to be of two kinds: One of which forms on the stems and joints of the plant; another which forms in the fruit heads. The yellow material appears to be produced by the triangular petals which surround the fruit heads.

a, fruit head as seen from above; b, spores as they appear to be formed on the stems; c, the general appearance of the plant.

3. This form found associated with brooder pneumonia in canaries has not been cultivated. I am hoping to make a thorough study of the organism during the coming summer. Drawn May, 1940.

4. This variety resembles that shown in Fig. 6 No. 2, in its early growth. The threads are white at first, but they soon turn brown or dark gray. The stems are large and branched; the heads and spores are slightly larger than those of Fig. 6 No. 2, the spores are black in color, and are formed on the surface of the heads, and in old growths the clumps attain enormous size. Experiments under way as this is written—June, 1940—indicate that this variety is highly fatal to baby canaries.

Free-hand drawings by Robert Stroud

temperature before it is given to the babies. The babies must be fed at one-hour intervals during the period of daylight and twice between dark and midnight. If the hen refuses to cover them, they must be placed in an incubator and their body temperature maintained at 107½ degrees F.—the incubator temperature will be slightly lower than this figure, for the babies will generate some heat for themselves. In the case of those babies that are unable to swallow the food, it should be mixed very thin, placed in the back of the mouth, and worked down with a blunt match stick.

Prevention. It is much more important to be able to prevent a disease than it is to be able to cure it. Prevention in the case of aspergillus infection consists of using only clean, fresh, dust-free, mould-free seeds and food and in seeing that the floors of the cages, coops or pens are kept clean and dry. It is during warm, moist weather, when fungi will grow on anything, that one must be particularly vigilant.

ASPERGILLUS FUMIGATUS. Fungi of the genus aspergillus are very widely distributed in nature and include most of the common food moulds. The species A fumigatus is one of the most common of the lot, and it is by far the most pathogenic. Most of the green and greenish-white moulds occurring on foods belong to this species. A niger is of common occurrence on bread and is recognized by the black color of its spores. The spores of aspergillus are found in the dusts of practically all grains and seeds. The fungus may be cultivated on potato, rye bread, white bread, plain acid agar and most boiled grains. It grows best at from 35 to 40 degrees C., but grows readily at room temperature. Usually within 24 hours of seeding the growth appears as a white feathery layer on the surface of the medium. As the growth ages it becomes darker, turning first green and then brown.

Morphologically, aspergillus consists of mycelial threads, fruit heads, and spores which radiate from the heads in gracefully curved lines. Figure 6 is a free-hand microscopic drawing of aspergillus fungi grown on agar. It is magnified about four hundred times.

ASTHMA. Ninety-nine out of every hundred books on cage birds, heads its list of diseases with **asthma;** tells all about it and recommends a specific treatment—all in the space of a single paragraph of less than one hundred words. I am sorry, but I do not find the problem quite that simple. The truth is that asthma, as a specific disease of birds, does not exist. What is usually called asthma, for want of a better name, is asthmatic breathing, a wheezing in the throat, which is a symptom of many unrelated conditions.

Asthmatic wheezing may be the result of the constriction of the air passages by the contraction of scar tissue after recovery from an attack of the bronchial form of avian diphtheria; it is usually present as a symptom of aspergillosis and thrush involving the upper air passages or the mouth and throat; it is the most constant and noticeable symptom of such conditions as the bronchial form of avian diphtheria and contagious bronchitis; it is practically always present as a symptom of chronic fowl paralysis. An asthmatic wheezing is also a symptom of avitaminosis A; of a common cold; of streptococcus, staphylococcus, and micrococcus infections of the nasal sinuses; of any catarrhal inflammation of the upper air passages; of gapeworms in the trachea; and I do not know how many other conditions. At the time of this writing I am investigating a condition that appears to me to be caused by some protozoan parasite and in which wheezing is an important symptom, often the only easily noticeable symptom.

Where no history of the asthmatic symptoms of a given case is available, determination of their cause is often next to impossible. And without some knowledge of the cause of the symptoms, intelligent treatment is almost out of the question. All that can be done in such cases is to adopt an experimental line of treatment and hope for the best.

If a bird has had clean food, has lived under generally healthful conditions, has had plenty of exercise and direct sunlight, a sudden onset of asthmatic breathing—assuming that the bird in question has not been exposed to other birds suffering from similar symptoms—will probably mean nothing worse than a common cold or some equally mild irritation of the respiratory mucosa. In such cases, Ammonium Chloride or Ammoniac should be tried first. This failing, the bird should be turned into a large flight for a while. Plenty of fresh green food should be given daily to take care of any possible deficiency in the supply of vitamin A in the diet. Ammonium Benzoate added to the drinking water for a few days may help. Antiseptic preparation such as ARGYROL and NASAL OIL—placed in the nostrils are sometimes of great value in cases of this kind resulting from bacterial infections of the nasal passages. There are still other cases for which no effective treatment can be found. The best the breeder can do is to make a sincere effort to determine the cause of his bird's trouble, and do the best he can toward treating it intelligently. If after a fair trial he finds that there is nothing that can be done for the ailing bird, his best course is to choke it. For, as he shall see before he reaches the end of these pages, there are some cases where the asthmatic bird is the carrier of serious infections.

All birds showing asthmatic symptoms should be isolated and observed, for by such observation the clue to the true cause of the condition may be discovered. Notice whether or not the bird wheezes more during the night than he does during the daytime. See if he sleeps with his head hanging between his feet rather than turned back into his feathers—this is an indication of fowl paralysis. If there is a discharge from the nostrils, it may mean diphtheria, aspergillosis, thrush, or a common cold. There is plenty about some of these chronic conditions that we do not understand. I have always found them more difficult to really do anything with than the serious epizootic diseases which can whip out a flock in a few days; in such case one does at least know what he is dealing with; a diagnosis can be established from the bodies.

AVIAN DIPHTHERIA. In our discussion of Apoplectiform septicemia it was shown how a disease displaying two distinct sets of symptoms had masqueraded for over two hundred years as two distinct diseases to which distinct and mutually exclusive causes had been assigned. In that case, isolation and identification of the causative organism not only cleared up the misunderstanding, but enabled us to discover why the two sets of symptoms were so different. But in this section we are dealing with the hydra-headed chameleon of all bird diseases, and the germ is not so accommodating as to point out the way for us.

Characterization. Avian diphtheria is an acute, contagious, highly fatal disease attacking all species of birds which not only takes different courses in different species, but which takes different courses and produces different lesion in the same species, often in the same outbreak. **Diphtheria, Roup, Canker, Fowl flu, Vent gleet, Septic fever, Shipping fever, Bird scourge, Contagious bronchitis, Contagious pneumonia, Epithelioma contagiosum, Contagious catarrh, Gapes, Bird pox,** and possibly **Psittacosis,** are just a few of the names that have been applied to this disease. Those that the fancier of pet birds uses when it gets into his plant are not intended for polite reading. These names are suggestive of more than the great number of variations which occur in different outbreaks of this disease; they speak volumes for its importance, since men do not invent names for things which concern them little. It has been estimated by the U. S. Department of Agriculture that this one disease costs American poultrymen millions of dollars every year.*

Etiology. As many different causes have been assigned to this disease as there have been names for it, but we now know that the true cause is a filterable virus, an organism so small that it can never be seen under the most powerful direct-vision † microscope, so small that it will pass through the pores of a porcelain filter fine enough to hold back all ordinary bacteria. This knowledge does little toward explaining the different forms taken by this disease, nor does it explain the presence of other pathogenic organism always found associated with it. I shall have more to say about this angle of the matter presently.

More scientific work has been done on the search for the cause of this disease than on all other bird diseases combined. Many of the world's foremost investigators, working in the world's finest laboratories, have devoted their time and energy to the solution of this problem, only to arrive at conflicting results. As stated above, it is now firmly established that the true cause of avian diphtheria is a filterable virus present in the scabs from the bird-pox lesions, and which, for that reason, is called **pox-virus.**

---

* **Note:** Some of the names given such as **gapes** and **fowl flu** and a few others, have no standing in bird literature, yet they are frequently applied to this disease by bird fanciers and poultrymen.

† **Note:** There has recently been invented an electronic microscope which is claimed to have the power to produce pictures having a magnification of 26000 diameters. What may eventually be learned with such an instrument is a question that only the future can answer. The ultimate limits of the direct-vision optical microscope is fixed by the wave lengths of light at about 3500 diameters magnification, which is insufficient to make the filterable viruses visible.

The things that we do not know about pox-virus would fill several very big books, but we do know that a five per cent solution of carbolic acid, a two per cent solution of cresolis, a two per cent solution of potassium permanganate, a two per cent solution of copper sulphate, and a 1:1000 solution of mercuric chloride all fail to destroy its disease-producing power in twenty minutes of exposure; that tincture of iodine fails to kill it in ten minutes; that steam at 100 C. fails to kill it in five minutes but does destroy it in thirty minutes; that the dry scabs can retain their disease-producing power for many years. On the other hand, we know that a two per cent solution of sodium hydroxide and a one per cent solution of alkaline sodium hypochlorite destroy it in a very few moments. The reason for this effectiveness is probably to be found in the power of these two substances to dissolve proteins, to break up the scabs and get at the virus.

Sources of infection. Since avian diphtheria is a specific disease, the primary source of infection is always, directly or indirectly, an infected bird. It is highly contagious and is spread by contact. But it can also be spread by indirect methods. It may be brought into the poultry yard on the shoes of the owner; by free flying birds, by newly purchased stock, by hatching eggs from infected stock, and by birds returned from the shows. It is usually brought into the bird room by newly purchased stock or by birds returned from some pet shop. See ANTISEPTICS FOR THE HANDS.* The wise breeder will make it a point to see that all new or possibly infected stock is quarantined for at least three weeks before admitting it to his bird room. He will see that his hands are clean and that he does not carry the infection into his room or yard on his shoes. And once the disease makes its appearance, he will see that he does not carry it from yard to yard on his shoes or from cage to cage on his hands.†

Another source of infection is used equipment—cages, shipping

---

* **Note:** It is my opinion that some pet shops in this country make a deliberate practice of spreading this disease. When birds are shipped to them, one or two are always returned as being unsatisfactory, and the frequency with which these returned birds develop avian diphtheria and infect the flock can denote only one of two things: That they have been handled with inexcusable carelessness, or that they have been deliberately infected.

† **Note:** A simple method of cleaning the feet when entering the poultry yard, or when passing from yard to yard, is to have at each gate a box containing a whiskbroom, a jug of sodium hypochlorite solution, and a pair of rubbers. The rubbers are slipped on before entering the plant, and at each gate the poultryman stops for a moment and brushes the soles of the rubbers with a little of the hypochlorite solution. Doing this is no great trouble, but it may save him thousands of dollars in disease losses.

boxes, etc. By actual test, contaminated shipping boxes have caused this disease after a year of disuse. In one case to come to my attention, a neglected shipping box placed in the bird room cost the breeder over a thousand dollars' worth of fine birds. It is wise to be careful.

Incubation period. The time between exposure and the development of the first symptoms of disease is known as the **incubation period.** Exactly what happens during this period is not well understood, but it is generally supposed that the causative agent requires a certain length of time in which to multiply up to a point where it is capable of causing the symptoms and lesions of disease. During this period the exposed bird carries the virus of the disease within its body but cannot transmit it to another individual. Transmission is possible only after the end of incubation. The incubation period in avian diphtheria varies greatly. For natural transmission in canaries, sparrows and finches, it is from eight to twenty-one days—the average period is fourteen days. Out of several hundred cases of which I had accurate record of the time of exposure, only one bird developed the disease in eight days—two thirds of the birds showed their first symptoms on the fourteenth and the twentieth days. During this study every bird was examined daily. The incubation period for experimentally inoculated pigeons is from five to six days; for experimentally inoculated chickens it varies from as little as three days to as much as twenty-five days. Birds inoculated with fresh pox scabs develop the disease quicker than do those inoculated with filtered virus. The average period of incubation of avian diphtheria in chickens is twelve days.

Symptoms and course of the disease. The bird carries on all of its usual functions during the period of incubation and for a considerable time thereafter. The male canary sings and mates; the female canary mates, builds her nest, lays her eggs and feeds her young. The first symptom is usually a slight fever. This does not make the bird appear or feel sick—actually it seems to be feeling better than usual. It is very active and the feathers are carried close to the body; the song is loud and ringing. If watched closely, however, it will be observed that the bird stops its activity every little while and pants a little—the wings are held out from the body, indicating that it is too warm—but the general activity remains at a very high pitch. To persons unfamiliar with this disease, the bird seems to be in much better health and spirits than usual. Canary hens that have not been in breeding condition before, often come into condition, build their nests, lay their eggs and hatch them. The males are singing constantly. Then the appetite becomes abnormal and the droppings take on the color and consistency of yellow ochre—the kind that is put up in tubes for the use of school children in their water-color work.

From this point on the symptoms may follow one of three general courses, which, for convenience, I shall refer to as **bronchial, external diphtheric,** and **pox.** * It must be remembered, though, that there is no hard, fast line between these three divisions; they are of necessity more or less arbitrary. They do not cover all of the variations met with in this disease; sometimes they merge, one into the other. Yet, as we shall see, there does seem to be some natural foundation for these divisions. Sometimes an outbreak will run from beginning to end with all cases falling into the one general pattern. In other outbreaks the onset of the epizootic is marked by one form of the disease, its middle course by another, and its ending by still a third. In still other outbreaks, all three forms may be present at the same time or even in the same bird.

Bronchial form. This condition has often been called **Contagious bronchitis, Fowl Flu,** and **Contagious pneumonia.** In this form of the disease the male continues to sing—or, if a hen, the bird continues to carry on its usual functions but the periods of panting become more frequent. The song takes on a softness that it did not have before—the softness of death—and the bird sings at a lower and lower pitch, as well as with less and less volume, until, at last, he is going through the motions of singing without making any sound. Up until this time the bird has not felt sick.† Gradually the fever mounts; the panting spells become more frequent; the breathing more rapid; then the bird is sitting in the bottom of its cage gasping for breath—the respiratory rate reaching 150, 175, 200 per minute and each breath has become a gasping, body-racking convulsion. This stage of the disease may be reached within from three to ten days after the onset of the first symptoms, and it may continue for from a day or two to more than four

---

* **Note:** There is an **internal diphtheric** form of this disease involving lesion in the mouth—but the symptoms are those of the bronchial form. The mouth lesion is not necessary for the development of this form of the disease, however, so I do not consider them a justification for a distinct classification.

† **Note:** Many diseased birds are sold in the stores while in this stage of the disease. Their constant singing and low, soft voices make them especially attractive to the novice fancier.

weeks. The fight for life that some of these little creatures make is really astounding. The bird continues to eat, is, in fact, ravenously hungry, though it can no longer shell and swallow seeds and swallows soft food with difficulty. It will consume really enormous amounts of any food that it can handle. Toward the end of this

Figure 7   **AVIAN DIPHTHERIA**

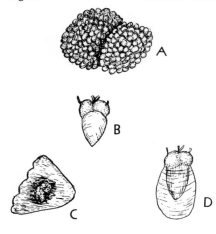

A. Mulberry liver, as found in peracute form of AVIAN DIPHTHERIA.

B. Normal heart.

C. A lung from the same bird. The pneumonic spot in the center of the lung is always gray at the time of death and much thicker than the normal tissue surrounding it.

D. Heart from a bird that has died after a long illness with a bronchial form of the disease, showing advanced pericarditis. Note how the pericardium is distended. It may contain a bloody or gelatinous exudate.

stage the bird develops a very painful diarrhea, and fever-blister-like sores (herpes) appear on the vent and around the eyes. In some cases the droppings turn from yellow to a bright, grass green; they may become bloody towards the last. Death in this form of the disease comes from heart failure or exhaustion.

External diphtheric form. In this form the first symptom one notices is that when the bird stops singing, or whatever it is doing, it rubs its head vigorously against the wires of its cage—a chicken will choose a fence post or the side of a building—as if it itched. Examination will reveal a small sore which may have a hard, brown scab surrounded by a swollen, inflamed area, or which may consist of a thickening of the skin and a destruction of its outer layer. This latter sore oozes a viscid fluid and is covered with a soft, friable, yellow exudate—very much like that which sometimes forms on your own fever sores—which can be easily wiped off, leaving the spot raw. This is the true diphtheric lesion, but the sore with the hard brown scab is the kind usually found during the early stages of the illness. In some cases the sores will look

very much like insect bites. There will be a small dark spot, resembling a wound, surrounded by a wide, reddened and swollen
area. I have often wondered if these lesions were not actually insect bites, mite bites, and if it was not possible that mites might
in some cases carry the disease from cage to cage—I have found
them under conditions where no mite could have possibly existed,
however, though mosquitoes may have been present. The true
diphtheric sores are most common on pigeons; the pseudo-insect-
bite type is the form most commonly met with on canaries. Besides
the three kinds of skin lesions just described, tough, white patches
appear at the corners of the mouth. In some cases and in some
outbreaks a single type of skin lesion will make its appearance
throughout the course of the epizootic, though in other outbreaks
all of these lesions may be present in different birds or in the same
bird.

These sores may appear on any part of the body; though they
are most commonly found on the head and back. They do not seem
to be very painful excepting when they are on the feet. In many
cases one or more of these sores may appear and develop slowly
over a period of from several days to two weeks. The fever mounts
and the breathing becomes more rapid; there is, however, no mouth
breathing in these cases, as a general rule. Then in some cases
the sores will disappear; in other cases they will suddenly take
on renewed activity and spread rapidly over large areas of the
body; but in both instances the bird develops the ravenous appetite and the same painful diarrhea as marks the termination of
the bronchial form of the disease, and dies.

Pox. In this form of diphtheria, so common in chickens and
turkeys, the lesions are largely confined to the unfeathered areas
of the head and neck; they have a wart-like appearance and often
cover the comb and wattle and the soft tissues around the beak
and eyes. These wart-like lesions are not met with in canaries.
Instead, large, hard, lumpy swellings appear on their heads—particularly around the ears, the sides of the jaws, and above the eyes.
When cut open, these swellings do not bleed. They are composed
of a tough, yellow, fibrinous material. I have had no opportunity
to make microscopic studies of these lesions.

The general course of this form of the disease differs little from
that of the two forms just described. There is high fever, abnormal
appetite, rapid breathing, a painful diarrhea, the droppings turning
from ochre-yellow to green, or becoming bloody, just before death.

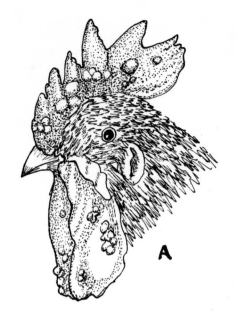

A

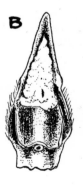

B

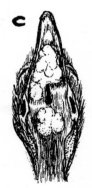

C

THE LESIONS IN POULTRY

A—The head of a rooster showing pox nodules on the comb and wattle.
B and **C**—Diphtheric lesions on the tongue, palate and pharynx of a hen.

—From Moore, Bureau of Animal Industry, 1898.

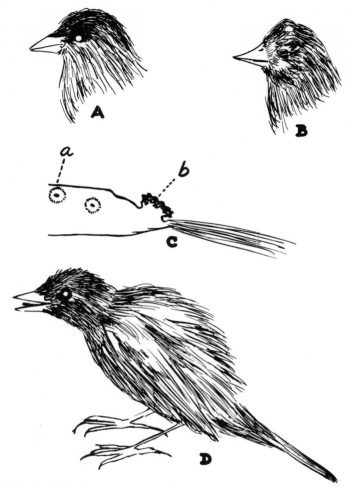

A—Illustrates hard brown scabs surrounded by swollen inflamed area around eyes and beak in the external diphtheric form.

B—In the Pox form of Avian Diphtheria large, hard lumpy swellings appear on the birds' heads as illustrated.

C—a—Sores resembling insect bites (a small dark spot, surrounded by a wide, reddened and swollen area) usually appear in various places on the body at some stage of Avian Diphtheria.
    b—Shows fever—blister-like sores (herpes) on the vent in the bronchial form.

D—Shows bird in early stages of Avian Diphtheria, while usually active it stops frequently and pants with wings held out from the body indicating it is too warm.

See Pages 34, 35 and 36

The swelling may close the bird's eyes, making it impossible for him to find food and water. There is usually no difficulty in breathing. Towards the last, blisters are usually found on the vent and around the eyes. The abdomen in this form of the disease and in the external diphtheric form is usually shrunken and wasted—

Figure 8.   **AVIAN DIPHTHERIA**

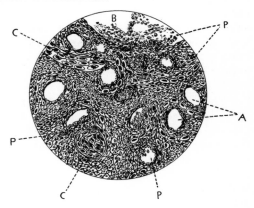

DRAWING OF A SECTION OF THE LUNG OF A CANARY SHOWING LESIONS OF BRONCHIAL PNEUMONIA ASSOCIATED WITH AVIAN DIPHTHERIA.
B. Pus-filled bronchus.
A. Healthy air cells.
C. Capillaries.
P. Pus in bronchus, in interstitial tissue, in air cells.
Proportions of the drawing arrived at by placing a scale of squares on the diaphragm of the eyepiece. Details drawn in free-hand by Robert Stroud.
Magnification about 400×.

the skin over it is withered and wrinkled like that of a withered apple. In the bronchial form of the disease the abdomen is always enlarged and more or less inflamed. A clinical thermometer with a top reading of 113 degrees F., will not record the peak temperatures reached during the febrile phases of the illness, but, before death, the temperature often falls and becomes subnormal, sometimes reaching a low of 96 degrees F. Death in the diphtheric and pox forms of this disease is usually from exhaustion; though in some few cases the birds die suddenly from what appears to be a general toxemia.

There is a peracute form of avian diphtheria in which the bird dies within a few hours of the onset of the first symptoms. The bird is taken sick suddenly, sits with puffed-out feathers, head turned back, sleeping. The breathing is shallow and very rapid. At first, the bird stands on one foot; later, on both feet. No attempt is made to either eat or drink. The abdomen is greatly enlarged and very dark in color. Death occurs in a convulsion within from three to five hours after the onset of the first symptoms.

There are chronic cases which show no well-marked symptoms beyond a subnormal temperature, an abnormal appetite, and ochrecolored droppings. At first the bird seems to be only slightly out of condition. As the illness progresses, the bird becomes very weak and greatly emaciated. It appears to feel cold all the time and loves nothing better than to sleep in the sun or snuggled against an electric light. These birds may live for two months or more. Death is usually from general exhaustion. There are no sores or other diphtheric lesions. Such cases are apt to appear towards the end of the outbreak. Considered individually, these cases can be diagnosed only by inoculating other birds with their excreta, or by caging them with healthy birds—for all birds caged with them will develop characteristic cases of avian diphtheria. Such birds can, and often do, infect an entire flock before the nature of their ailment is suspected, and then are themselves the last to die.

There are other chronic cases which result as the aftermath of an acute attack. In the bronchial form of avian diphtheria, the suborbital sinuses are very apt to become affected, and because they have very poor natural drainage, they often become plugged; then an artificial drainage through the top of the head may establish itself. The bird recovers from the acute attack, but there is this one running sore on the top of the head, and it refuses to heal. Its discharge, a clear viscid fluid, remains infective for about one month. Three months after the recovery, the discharge from this head sore was no longer capable of causing diphtheric lesions. When one of these affected birds was caged with healthy stock, however, some of the latter developed identical sores on their heads. A few died from the nasal infection.

Morbid anatomy. In the bronchial form of avian diphtheria in canaries, death is usually the result of heart failure. The long siege of high temperature and difficult breathing wears the heart muscles to shreds. The least fright or excitement may cause the right ventricle to rupture and discharge its blood into the pericardium. When the thoracic cavity is opened the heart appears greatly enlarged—about the size, shape and color of a kidney bean. Examination reveals that the pericardium (heart sac) is distended out of all proportions, but that the heart, itself, is actually smaller than normal. See Fig. 7, page 35. Often, as previously mentioned, it will be found that the heart wall has given away and permitted blood to escape into the pericardium, but this only accounts for a part of the distention of the pericardium. Even in those cases where the bird dies from exhaustion or asphyxiation, this sac will be found filled with a serous, fibrinous, or gelatinous exudate, or a mixture of all three. There may be a small amount of bloody or cloudy fluid in the peritoneum (lining of the abdominal cavity), though the amount is never large. The duodenum is usually inflamed and may contain dark, hemorrhagic spots. The liver is greatly enlarged and softened, and may show necrotic spots, but its outer envelope and connective tissues remain intact. There are no constant or remarkable changes in the spleen. The pancreas is sometimes a deep purple color. Pneumonic consolidations in the stage of gray hepatization are found in both lungs. The diseased area is located in the center of the organ and may be surrounded by a margin of healthy tissue. The pneumonic spot is always thicker than the unaffected areas and extends straight through the organ from front to back. If separated from the surrounding tissue, the pneumonic tissue will sink in water. B-D, Figure 7 show a heart from a case of the bronchial form of avian diphtheria in comparison with the heart of a normal canary. C, Figure 7 gives a rough idea of the appearance of the pneumonic spot. The contrast in the fresh specimen is much greater than indicated by the drawing, since the healthy tissue is pink and the diseased tissue is gray in color.

From the blood and organs of those birds that die of heart failure before the development of the fatal diarrhea can be obtained in pure culture, an organism which by morphological and cultural characteristics cannot be differentiated from the pneumococcus of Frankel—the cause, or one of the causes, rather, of human pneumonia. This same organism is often found associated with the chronic nasal infections which sometimes follow the acute attack.

After the development of the fatal diarrhea, **B. pasteurella,** the germ of fowl cholera—is practically always found in the blood and organs. The gelatinous exudate mentioned above as being sometimes found in the pericardium is characteristic of diseases involving the presence of organisms of the pasteurella group. See FOWL CHOLERA; HEMORRHAGIC SEPTICEMIA.

In the diphtheric form of the disease the internal lesions are less well marked. The heart usually appears to be normal, though in some cases punctiform (point-like) hemorrhages are found in its wall. There is usually a small amount of dark, bloody, serous exudated in the peritonial cavity. The liver may be much smaller than normal, almost bloodless (the edges are often transparent and colorless) and of a soft, jelly-like consistency. Its envelope is intact, however. Small hemorrhagic spots in the walls of the duodenum are not infrequently observed. There are no pneumonic lesions in the lungs. It is characteristic of this form of the disease that all fat has disappeared from the body and that the visceral organs occupy only about half as much space as they normally occupy in a healthy bird. Death appears to be the result of exhaustion or of general toxemia. B. pasteurella is often found in the blood and organs.

The diphtheric skin lesions have been described. During the latter stages of the illness these will sometimes take on the distinctly diphtheric characteristics (thickened skin; destroyed epidermis; yellow, friable exudate) and great activity, spreading rapidly over a large part of the body. From the discharge of these sores and from the blisters around the eyes and vent there can sometimes be cultivated a streptococcus identical in cultural characteristics with the germ of human erysipelas, **S. pyogenes.**

Changes in the pox form of avian diphtheria do not differ materially from those just described, excepting in the presence of the swellings and the absence of sores. Following the development of the fatal diarrhea, B. pasteurella can usually be found in the blood and organs.

I mentioned in the description of the peracute form of this disease that the abdomen is always greatly enlarged and very dark in color. This is the result of an enlargement of the liver which is so great that when the abdomen is opened the organ literally springs out at the examiner. It is from five to seven times normal size, blue-black in color, and necrotic throughout. The envelope and the interstitial connective tissues are entirely destroyed; the tufts are so greatly enlarged and so broken apart that they stand out individually, like the seed coverings of a black berry or mulberry, giving the organ the appearance of a big rotten mulberry. A point that may be of interest in these cases is the fact that every canary to die of this form of the disease had a history of exposure to a parrot suffering from psittacosis. Birds infected from the ingestion of bits of this liver tissue all developed typical cases of the bronchial form of avian diphtheria. See A, Figure 7.

Sanitation. Since avian diphtheria is one of the most contagious and fatal of the diseases known to birds; since its causative agent is highly resistant to heat, sunlight, drying, disinfectants, and other destructive agents; since the incubation period is long and the onset of the active stage of the illness extremely insidious, marked by the mildest of symptoms, it is one of the most difficult of all bird diseases to control by sanitary measures. It is only in the most rigorous sanitary measures that we dare place any hope whatever, and even these have a good chance of failure.

The danger of carrying the disease from place to place on the hands and feet has been discussed; it is important, however, to stamp it out wherever it happens to be, to make contaminated quarters safe for unexposed birds, and that is not so easy. I have known breeders to remove all birds from their bird rooms, have their house fumigated, or even repainted, and yet fail to make their rooms safe for uninfected birds. I am not talking about stamping out the disease by the kill-and-disinfect method—that is a hopeless waste of time and life. I once killed all exposed birds and washed all used equipment daily in strong disinfectants for a period of more than five months, without being able to stamp out this infection; though as a result of these rigorous methods I was able to keep my losses to a minimum during the period. Even so, there is much that can be accomplished by good sanitation. I have found the following method of great value:

Examine all birds at frequent intervals; remove all well and unexposed birds to new, clean quarters; remove all birds that are known to have been exposed to the disease to other quarters, as far removed from those of the unexposed birds as possible; permit the sick birds to stay where they are or remove them to smaller quarters and clean up the place where they have been housed.

All droppings must be removed and burned or deeply buried with a few pounds of chloride of lime. Dropping boards, floors, perches, food boxes, and all other equipment must be scrubbed with a strong solution of lye (sodium hydroxide) sodium hypochlorite, or strong lye soap—a boiling solution of good yellow soap, containing one ounce of soap to each gallon of water is easy and safe to handle and will remove all infective materials if it is applied thoroughly. For the poultry house it should be kept boiling in a gasoline drum. All equipment should be scrubbed with a stiff fibre or wire brush. The walls as well as the floors should be scrubbed, and the outside as well as the inside of the house looked after. Remember that any place where a bird could have rubbed its head, any place where it could have thrown droppings by whipping its tail, is pretty certain to be contaminated. Fence posts should not be forgotten. And all of this scrubbing must be done twice—the first time to soften the material, the second time to remove it. The yard may be cared for by sprinkling it liberally with chlorinated lime and then turning the surface under. At least several weeks should elapse before birds are again placed on such ground, and there should be at least one good rain between the application of the chlorinated lime and the return of the birds. If possible, it is best to let such ground lay idle for a few weeks; then seed it down and not use it for poultry again for a year.

The bird room must be cleaned with equal care. Once each week, at least, all cages and other equipment must be washed inside and out with a boiling solution of soap and water. The washing must be done twice, through two waters, and every inch of surface must be scrubbed with a stiff brush or a stiff, short whiskbroom, and if your cages are of a construction that permits the hand to enter the inside only through a small door, you had better throw them away and get some with removable bottoms and ends, if you do not want to kiss your birds good-bye. Hot water, soap, and a good stiff brush will make any cage safe, if they are applied thoroughly and twice. I find that this method is preferable to the use of strong disinfectants. As mentioned above, I once fought this disease for five months, during which time I was breathing the fumes of disinfectants daily. I inhaled so much disinfectant that my doctor told me I had infusion in both pleurae, that I was apt to go out like a light at any time. Then I had sense enough to work out the soap and water idea.

Flight rooms must be emptied and cleaned, and the birds from them should be caged separately or in groups as small as possible. This is important because all birds do not take the disease at their first exposure; if subsequent exposures can be avoided you may save yourself a lot of trouble and losses. It is a good idea to re-paint the room—paint over infective material, however, is just a means of preserving the virus for a new outbreak. Clean before you paint.

Examining suspected birds. Note the color of the droppings and rapidity of the breathing. When there is no disease present in the bird plant, a few birds with yellow droppings or breathing more than 86 (the normal respiratory rate of a canary) per minute does not necessarily mean that there is anything seriously wrong, but, with disease on the premises, every bird showing these symptoms must be considered infected. Take each bird in your hand; brush the feathers back over the head and look for sores or swellings; look for blisters around the vent and eyes; look for flea-bite sores on the back of the head, the neck, the back, the abdomen, and along the angle of the jaws. Notice whether the abdomen is enlarged, normal or shrunken. If the breathing is normal, if the droppings are black and white, if no sores of any kind are found, the bird has passed the inspection. If all birds in a given cage or flight pass this inspection and if no cases have originated in that cage or flight within the last twenty-one days, the birds may be considered unexposed; otherwise they are classed as exposed or diseased. The exposed birds should be caged separately, if possible, but the diseased birds can more conveniently be thrown into one hospital flight. They cannot harm each other, and they will thus be easier to care for and treat.

Prevention. In ninety-nine out of every hundred outbreaks of avian diphtheria the disease can be traced to new birds introduced into the flock without proper quarantine. All new stock should be kept separately and fed and tended last for a period of at least three weeks before it is introduced into the poultry yard or bird room. If this simple instruction were followed in all cases, though it won't be, some of the most heartbreaking disappointments the breeder is called upon to face would be avoided.

Treatment. STROUD'S SPECIFIC, which consists of STROUD'S SALTS NO. 1 and STROUD'S EFFERVESCENT BIRD SALTS, was discovered as a result of experiments on avian diphtheria. It was the first specific treatment for this disease ever put on the market, and in the more than ten years that have gone by since its discovery, I have heard of no one discovering another. In many other places throughout these pages you will read of this treatment being recommended for other diseases, but it was for the treatment of this disease that it was originally compounded, and it is in the treatment of this disease that it can be expected to give its best results; and, if properly administered, it acts as an absolute specific and will bring the disease under control from the very first dose. One teaspoonful of the Effervescent Salts is added to each quart of drinking water for the entire flock, sick and well alike—and it must be given in glass or crockery drinkers. For the very sick birds and for birds that for any reason do not appear to be responding to the treatment, the dosage of this preparation is doubled. The Salts No. 1 is fed to the sick birds only, mixed in some soft food that they can and will eat. It is given in the proportion of from one to two teaspoonfuls to each quart of soft food —more may be given if you can get the birds to eat the food. It is essential to get this substance into the birds in fairly large quantities. A little honey may be added to the soft food to kill the taste of the medicine. In some cases I have found it advisable to feed this preparation on bread moistened with milk and sprinkled with powdered sugar and maw seed in order to get the very sick birds to consume it in sufficient quantities.

Where STROUD'S SPECIFIC is unavailable, effervescent sodium sulphate or phosphate, **Sal Hepatica,** Eno, or any of the other mild effervescent salines put up for human use, may be substituted for STROUD'S EFFERVESCENT BIRD SALTS and added to all drinking water in the proportion of one teaspoonful to the quart of water. In choosing the effervescent mixture to use it is best to select one containing citric acid. **Sal Hepatica** and citro-carbonate mixed in equal parts makes a good mixture. The very best grade of Sodium Perborate should be substituted for STROUD'S SALTS NO. 1. For treating poultry, eight grains of potassium chlorate, one-half to one teaspoonful of sodium perborate, or twenty grains of calcium permanganate may be added to each quart of the same water. When treating canaries it is best to give the oxidizing solution for half of each day and the laxative solution for the other half of the day.

Another good general treatment for canaries and cage birds was suggested to me by William Southern, and consists of giving the birds pure, fresh orange juice as drinking water for half of each day (note what I just said about citric acid), and for the remainder of the day a solution of **copperas,** iron "ferro" sulphate for drinking water. The iron solution should contain five grams of copperas to each liter of water, which is about one teaspoonful of the iron salt to each quart of water.

For the treatment of this disease in parrots, see PSITTACOSIS.

The sores should be treated twice daily. A 2 to 4 per cent solution of silver nitrate, 20 per cent argyrol, or a saturated solution of potassium or calcium permanganate, potassium chlorate, sodium perborate, or a 5 per cent solution of sodium hypochlorite may be used. All but the last item can be used on any part of the body, but the hypochlorite might injure the eyes. Sores on the rest of the body are often best treated by burning them with a stick of silver nitrate or by injecting them with a saturated solution of permanganate. If the sores are to be treated by direct application, they must be opened and the antiseptic solution rubbed in with the tip of the finger. In the pox form of the disease I have had good results from cutting the swellings and packing the cuts with powdered permanganate.

In cases displaying bronchial symptoms the sores should be neglected until the general treatment has controlled the general symptoms and relieved the breathing—for any excitement may cause the birds to drop dead of heart failure—and once the general symptoms have disappeared, the sores usually heal quickly of their own accord.

All birds, both sick and well alike, should be kept under the most wholesome conditions possible. In addition to their regular diet of seed or grain they should have all the green food they can eat, a good soft mash, and plenty of black loam constantly before them.*

Don't be like one breeder, laugh at this loam idea without trying it. In browsing through some very old books in the New York library, he ran onto this idea in a book on canaries that had been published in England in the Seventeenth Century. He reprinted the suggestion and poked fun at it, but the dead man he was poking fun at knew more than he, for the suggestion is sound. I do not know what it is, but there is something in clean black loam that is helpful in controlling the intestinal symptoms of this disease and of fowl cholera. And in those cases where the final, fatal diarrhea can be prevented or controlled the birds usually recover. It is not very important whether we know what the loam does or not; what is important is that the birds seem to know all

---

* **Note:** August 11, 1940. Drs. Selman A. Wakeman and H. Boyd Woodruff of the New Jersey Agriculture Experimental Station have just reported the discovery, in fresh field and garden soil, of organisms which destroy germs of the Gram negative group—which includes the organisms of the Pasteurella group—Hemorrhagic septicemia and Fowl Cholera—as well as germs of such human diseases as typhoid, dysentery and cholera. This rather belated confirmation of what the birds seem to have known right along is very gratifying, since it shows that we are not complete morons. In the account of this work to come to my attention, the good doctors do not mention the source of their suggestion, but any bird suffering from intestinal inflammation could have told them all about it, had they taken the trouble to watch him and understand his actions.

* **Note:** A press dispatch from Boston under the date line of November 5, 1941, states in substance that a new drug, found in soil, called **gramicidin**, was on this date discussed before the American College of Surgeons. This drug is said to be the discovery of Dr. Rene Dubose of Rockefeller Institute and to have a potency against GRAM positive bacteria 100,000 times that of sulfanilamide. 0.003 milligrams is said to be sufficient to protect a mouse against 10,000 lethal doses of virulent pneumococci. We are doing pretty well. If we keep on, some day we might have as much sense as a sparrow; but, of course, the good doctor would not mention that fact, nor that the existence of a substance in soil having therapeutic properties was first observed and published by an English canary breeder more than 200 years ago; that it was independently discovered by me in 1920 and first published in this country in Pet Magazine in 1929 and again in 1933 in my book, DISEASES OF CANARIES, on page 126, where I am discussing the treatment of fowl cholera in canaries, appears the following sentences: "In many outbreaks of this disease the only treatment needed is to give the birds a good tonic and plenty of black loam earth. They will eat the earth and seem to find something in it that kills the germs in the bowels." I also mentioned the use of loam or sod on pages 35, 78, and 109 of this same book. I could not isolate the substance for lack of necessary facilities.

about it—how they do go for it. I have seen canaries and sparrows consume more than their own weight of loam in a very few hours; in fact, it was a sparrow that first told me about it.

The chronic cases with head sores, nasal cases, should be treated by injecting the sores with permanganate. Enough of the solution should be injected to turn the surrounding tissue black, but in making the injection, care should be taken not to let the needle slip and penetrate the brain. A single treatment is usually sufficient.

Theory. In keeping with its importance, I have discussed this condition in great detail. Much of what has been said here applies with equal force to many other conditions and will not have to be said again. I have pointed out that while pox virus is undoubtedly the causative agent involved in the formation of the diphtheric lesions, other pathogenic organisms are usually found to be present in the various outbreaks. In some outbreaks several different organisms may be present, but usually each outbreak, and each particular form taken by that outbreak, is associated with some specific organism. It is my opinion that these organisms—they are called **Secondary invaders**—are present in the bird's body or environment in a saprophytic (germs that live on dead matter and do not cause disease are called **saprophytic)** or parasitic state at the time of the outbreak; that the pox virus either causes an increase in their virulence (virulence is the power to cause disease) or breaks down the bird's resistance to such an extent that normally nonvirulent organisms are suddenly able to invade the body and set up a severe and fatal disease. I think that it is more reasonable to believe that the bodily resistance is broken down by the pox virus, rather than that the virulence of the organisms is increased; though there would naturally be some increase in virulence in these organisms, too, since the passage of disease-producing organisms successively through several creatures of the same species always increases the virulence of that strain of organisms for that particular species of bird or animal. I do not believe that the pox virus is ever responsible for the fatal termination of the illness; that, to me, appears to be the result of the secondary invasion for which the virus opens the door.

The experience of stockmen with the spontaneous development of hemorrhagic septicemia in cattle in which the resistance to infection has been lowered by shipping or hard driving, the spontaneous development of pneumonia in man as a result of exposure and hardship, the consistent presence of organisms of the Salmonella group in outbreaks of hog cholera, and the frequency of apparently spontaneous outbreaks of erysipelas in hospitals, particularly among operative cases, are all evidence of the reasonableness of this theory—especially since the four organisms most commonly found associated with diseases of pox-virus origin are identical in morphological and cultural characteristics with those involved in the outbreaks just mentioned. Too, this would account for the fact that lines of treatment designed for destroying the toxins absorbed from the diphtheric lesions produce such almost magical cures. See PSITTACOSIS; HEMORRHAGIC SEPTI-CEMIA.

AVIAN SALMONELLOSIS. Since the organisms of paratyphoid and food poisoning on the one hand and those of the **Salmonella** (Hog Cholera) group on the other are, for all practical purposes, identical, and since the name **paratyphoid** has been much more widely used in bird literature than the newer name, salmonellosis, I prefer to discuss these conditions under the heading B. PARA-TYPHUS B INFECTION.

AVIAN TUBERCULOSIS. This is a rather common disease of poultry and of wild birds kept in zoological gardens. It is not a common disease of pet birds. See TUBERCULOSIS.

BACILLARY WHITE DIARRHEA, B. PULLORUM INFECTION.

Bacillary white diarrhea is an acute, contagious disease of baby chicks caused by **Bacterium pullorum.** Infection by this organism is responsible for chronic, localized lesions in the ovaries of adult hens, and there are rare cases where it has been responsible for typhoid-like septicemias of adult chickens. Other species of birds are not known to be susceptible to the natural disease. Rabbits and guinea pigs are killed by the subcutaneous injection of pure cultures of this organism, and it has been shown to produce a toxin fatal to rabbits.

Etiology. B. pullorum is a long, slender, nonmotile bacterium with slightly rounded ends. It is obtainable in pure culture from the blood and organs of infected chicks. As mentioned, the organism is found in the ovaries of chronically infected hens. It is passed on by the hen to the chick by means of the egg. The disease develops in the chick shortly after it is hatched.*

Symptoms. The onset of the symptoms takes place during the first forty-eight hours of life. At this time the young chicks are very susceptible, and the spread of the disease throughout the brood is very rapid. In some outbreaks the losses run as high as ninety per cent. By the end of the fourth day of life the chicks have developed considerable resistance to the infection. There are usually no new acute cases after the end of the first week. Chronically infected birds, and those that recover from the acute infection, grow up to provide reservoirs for passing the disease along to the next generation.

The sick bird stands with fluffed feathers, drooped wings, the body swaying back and forth, and has a generally dejected appearance. There is some loss of appetite, and the weakened condition of the bird renders it unable to compete with its healthier fellows in the general scramble for food. There is a painful, whitish-colored diarrhea of a gummy consistency, which adheres to the vent and feathers, stopping the opening, and from which the condition takes its name. The chick soon falls into a short period of coma and dies.

Chronically infected hens show no symptoms of illness that

* **Note:** For a complete description of this organism and the disease it causes see "Diseases of Domesticated Birds." Ward and Gallagher, Macmillan Company, 1927.

can be traced to the infection. They are said to be poor layers, however, and some of their eggs have misshapen yolks.

Morbid anatomy. The most characteristic lesion of this disease is the lack of characteristic lesions. Usually the yolk is unabsorbed, though this is not invariably the case. Sometimes there are yellow bands or lacings on the liver; the lungs may show necrotic spots. The only infallible diagnosis for this disease is that established by the presence of the causative organism in the blood and organs.

The only lesions found in the carrier hens are the presence of misshapen yolks in the process of formation.

Prevention. Since there is no known treatment for this disease, either in the acute or chronic form, the only hope of controlling it rests upon preventative measures.* If all carriers could be stamped out and the plant thoroughly disinfected, the disease would naturally disappear. The great difficulty standing in the way of this worthy accomplishment is the fact that chronically infected hens do not wear signs on their backs. To overcome this difficulty a great deal of work has been done on the development of bacteriological tests for the detection of the carrier hens. One of these tests, the **agglutination test,** has received considerable application. It is based upon the fact that blood from an infected bird will cause a suspension of the causative organism to agglutinate.†

Since this is slightly outside of my own personal experience, I am unable to pass judgment on these tests. Some poultry breeders and hatcherymen swear by them; others swear at them; and both cite impressive arrays of alleged facts in support of their various views. The veterinarian who makes his living blood testing is naturally all for them. In several Western states he not only went so far as to make a "racket" out of it, he succeeded in having his "racket" written into laws which were later declared unconstitutional by the United States Supreme Court. The scientific view is that while the tests are not perfect, they do detect a large number of the carrier hens and are, therefore, of value. To which the practical poultryman says: "Hooey! I only have to

---

* **Note:** This fact does not say much to the credit of the veterinary profession, since the disease is purely a septicemia and should not be hard to cure. Given sufficient experimental material, if I could not cure it in a year I would be heartily ashamed of myself. I feel so certain of this that I would be willing to gamble my life on the outcome.

† **Note:** In a positive test the suspended organisms come together and form clumps, leaving the rest of the fluid clear. In appearance the reaction is very similar to that of the coagulation of the casein of milk, but it is brought about by a substance manufactured by the body of the sick bird for the purpose of keeping its blood stream clear of these particular organisms.

have one infected egg in a tray to lose my chicks. If I am going to lose my chicks anyway, why should I spend my good money for a lot of useless falderal?" And the "vets" do not seem to have thought of an answer to that one yet. Of course, strict sanitary measures are relied upon as far as possible to prevent the spread of the disease.

BACILLUS COLI INFECTION. B. coli is a normal inhabitant of the intestines of man, animals and birds. It is not generally capable of causing disease, but it has been found associated with a great variety of lesions in both animals and birds, and strains of this organism isolated from inflammatory lesions have shown considerable virulence. A number of investigators have reported cholera-like epizootics in poultry, pigeons, quail, canaries, and other birds in which B. coli appeared to be the etiological factor. The outbreaks have appeared under circumstances which would naturally have tended towards depressing the birds' powers of resistance— such as close confinement, crowded caging, shipping about, etc.

The most constantly reported lesions are inflammation of the intestines, peritonitis with serous or plastic exudate, and pericarditis with fluid or solid exudate.

The only outbreak of B. coli infection in canaries to come to my attention occurred in the flock of a breeder living in Indiana. Bodies were sent to me for examination, but the presence of B. coli in these bodies could mean nothing, since, regardless of the cause of death, it would have been present as a post-mortem invader. I instructed the lady to take two microscopic slides; place them in the oven of her stove until they were quite hot; permit them to cool there; take one of her sick birds in her hand and paint one of its toes with iodine; clip the toenail back far enough to make it bleed; then lift up the top slide; let the drop of blood fall on the bottom slide; press the slides together; wrap them in clean paper and send them to me. A strain of B. coli virulent enough to cause a serious septicemia of canaries was isolated from the sample of blood she sent to me. The inoculated birds were made very ill, but they did not die. The organism was present in the blood during the illness.

In all of the bodies examined by me the peritonial cavity was completely filled with a grayish-yellow, cheesy exudate which completely covered the abdominal organs and had, by its pressure, completely obliterated the abdominal air sacs.

The disease cleared up as soon as the entire flock was put on a mild saline treatment, which consisted of sodium phosphate and citro-carbonate mixed in equal parts and added to the drinking water in the proportion of one teaspoonful to each quart of water used.

B. PARATYPHOSUS B INFECTION. From many cases of fatal food poisoning and from many typhoid-like diseases in man, animals, and birds have been isolated a number of identical or closely related organisms. Salmon found an organism of this group in hogs infected with cholera and thought it to be the cause of that disease; Nocard found a similar organism in fevered parrots and thought it to be the cause of psittacosis; Moore has described a disease of pigeons in which this organism, or one of this group, was undoubtedly the causative agent. Joest, Gilruth, Pfeiler, Adam, Manning and others have found it in canary epizootic.

In 1929 I found this organism associated with a certain type of pox virus infection in canaries. I observed that different forms taken by the disease were associated with different secondary invaders. See AVIAN DIPHTHERIA. I found several cases of sporadic disease in canaries where this organism appeared to be the causative agent.

Ward and Gallagher, "Disease of Domesticated Birds," page 252, after a study of the German literature on canary diseases, conclude that the great majority of outbreaks of contagious disease in canaries fall into one of two groups: one, those outbreaks caused by a member of the hemorrhagic septicemia group; the other, those

Figure 9.   **B. PARATYPHOSUS B INFECTION**

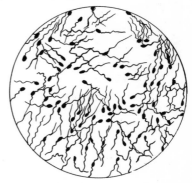

A COVER-GLASS PREPARATION OF B. PARATYPHOSUS B.— After Schweinitz.

Magnification about 1000×.

caused by B. paratyphosus B. This, of course, was their opinion, not mine, since both of these groups of diseases are rather uncommon in America. Friends in England, however, inform me that over there canary paratyphoid is very common and often cleans out an entire bird room within forty-eight hours.

B. paratyphosus B.* Is a short, plump, Gram negative, active motile rod with rounded ends; it has from one to five flagella, which average about seven microns in length. It, or a closely related organism which cannot be differentiated from it, is a normal inhabitant of the intestines of man and a great many animals. It has been found in the blood of a great many animals and birds suffering from septicemia.† Figure 9 shows a cover-glass prepara-

Figure 10.   **B. PARATYPHOSUS B INFECTION**

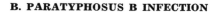

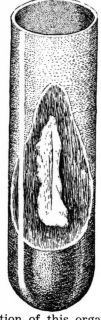

THE GROWTH OF B. PARATYPHOSUS B ON AGAR—After Schweinitz.

tion of this organism after Schweinitz. Figure 10 gives a rough idea of the appearance of its growth on agar media.

Avian paratyphoid. As indicated above, this disease has been observed in pigeons, fowls, pheasants, ducks, geese, canaries, and other birds. There are some differences in the diseases in different species of birds; and sometimes different outbreaks in the same

---

*** Note:** This organism is considered identical with **B. suipestifer,** the germ associated with hog cholera.

† **Note:** For a complete description of B. paratyphosus B, see any standard work on pathogenic bacteria.

species present such marked dissimilarities as to be considered distinct diseases. Moore has reported a disease of pigeons which he called **megrims,** * in which emaciation, a peculiar turning and shaking of the head and occasional paroxysms of wild aimless flight are characteristic symptoms. In this disease the only marked change found at autopsies was a friable exudate in the subarachnoid † spaces over the cerebellum and the posterior portion of the cerebrum.

Zingle has described a disease of pigeons caused by the same organism, or one closely related to it, which is characterized by yellow, knot-like nodules in the breast muscles. In both of these outbreaks the spleen was found to be free from macroscopic (large enough to see with the naked eye) lesions.

In fowls that have died of avian paratyphoid there is usually found an inflammation of the digestive tract, pericarditis, congestion of the liver and kidneys, and an enlargement of the spleen that is much greater than that observed in fowl cholera.

The disease in canaries. In the summer of 1935, a friend sent me six canaries. She wrote that her birds were dying like flies from what appeared to her to be a contagious disease. She described the symptoms as follows:

At first the bird appears to be less active than usual. As the disease progresses the bird sits on the perch with its feathers fluffed out, head turned back, eyes closed. At intervals it shakes its head, sometimes crying out as if in pain. In two cases, after an illness of only a few hours, the birds died in paroxysms of wild aimless flight (undoubtedly caused by internal hemorrhages). In most cases the birds lived for several days and suffered from a painful diarrhea, which was thin and watery at first, but was usually bloody before death. Throughout the course of the illness rapid breathing was a constant symptom. The respiratory rate was well over 150 per minute. Death came in a convulsion in most cases, though some of the birds simply fell from the perch, dead. Most of them continued to eat and drink until shortly before death—some dying over the seed cup.

The two most constant symptoms were the bloody droppings and the unmistakable evidence of severe pains in the head.

* **Note:** Circular 109, Bureau of Animal Industry, 1907.
† **Note:** The **subarachnoid spaces** are spaces between the two inner coverings of the brain—the **arachnoid** and the **pia,** which are called **meninges.** The spaces mentioned are normally filled with fluid.

Morbid anatomy. The six birds arrived dead. The express agent had been thoughtful enough to make a note of the time of each death. All had been dead less than twelve hours and two less than three hours at the time of delivery. They were examined at once.

Rigor mortis was pronounced in all six bodies. The legs were stiffly extended parallel with the tail—evidence of death in a convulsion. The letter had described all of the birds as being greatly emaciated, but the bodies appeared in good flesh. (This apparent discrepancy was caused by the rapid formation of gas in the muscular tissue shortly after death.) The muscles, heart, liver and spleen of those birds that had been dead less than three hours were deep purple in color; in those bodies that had been dead more than three hours these tissues were a rich, bright, cobalt blue.

In three of the six bodies friable exudates similar to those described by Moore in pigeon megrims, were found' covering the back of the brain; in the other three bodies there was found some evidence of inflammation of the meninges, but exudation was slight. In all cases the kidneys were congested and enlarged, the liver enlarged and very fragile, the intestines inflamed. Two of the bodies showed marked pneumonic consolidations in both lungs; the lungs from the other bodies showed numerous small congested areas, which gave them a speckled appearance. A characteristic enlargement of the spleen deserving of a detailed description, was found in all cases.

The color of the spleen, as mentioned above, was deep purple in those cases where the birds had been dead less than three hours and bright cobalt in those cases where the birds had been dead for a longer period. These organs were perfectly cylindrical in shape, with perfectly spherical ends. The surfaces were smooth and glistened with a bright metallic luster. Ignoring color, they had the general appearance of polished-steel roller bearings. All six spleens were about 9.5 mm to 10 mm in length, and they varied in thickness from about 2.5 mm to 6 mm. The internal structure was entirely destroyed. When the capsule was punctured the pulp escaped as a thick, dull-yellowish-brown mass. Unfortunately, neither culture median nor microscopic equipment were at hand at the time.

Etiology. Bacteriological examinations, made by Dr. E. F. Waller, Instructor in Veterinary Pathology, Iowa State College of Agriculture, Ames, Iowa, from other bodies from this same outbreak, revealed the presence of B. parathyphosus B (Salmonella eartrycke) in the blood and organs. This finding, reported to me several months after the outbreak had been controlled and the sick cured, was in accord with my diagnosis, based of necessity upon symptomatic, anatomical and clinical considerations.

Treatment. In the three weeks that elapsed between the beginning of the outbreak and the discovery of an effective treatment something like one hundred birds were lost out of a flock of about one hundred and sixty. Birds of all ages were affected. The treatment I suggested consisted of a slightly alkaline, effervescent saline given in the drinking water of sick and well alike in the proportions of one teaspoonful of the salts to each quart of water. Up until the time the treatment was given no bird had recovered from the illness. There were twenty odd birds sick at the time the treatment was given and new cases were developing at the rate of about ten per day. No new cases developed from the time the first dose of the medicine was given, and within three days all of the sick had recovered from the acute illness, though some of them had seemed to be at the point of death when the treatment was commenced. In all but one case, to be described presently, recovery was complete and permanent.

One bird regained his song but never really became well. Later he developed the symptoms of chronic nephritis and was sent to me for study and treatment. When he failed to respond to treatment, he was killed and examined. The following lesions were found.

Lungs normal; heart smaller than normal, walls inflamed and injected with blood; liver much smaller than normal, greatly softened, its edges transparent and bloodless; duodenum inflamed; anterior lobes of both kidneys in advanced state of chronic fatty degeneration; central lobes of both kidneys showed numerous deep-red necrotic spots; posterior lobes normal. But again it was the spleen in which the principal lesions were found.

This organ was roughly round in shape, 11 mm to 12 mm in diameter, very light dull-yellow in color, and its surface was wrinkled and corrugated, like that of a withered orange. The covering was from 1 mm to 1½ mm in thickness and of a tough, leathery consistency. When the outer covering was removed (it peeled off easily) a number of other layers of increasing smoothness and decreasing thickness were found. It was the same color and consistency throughout. No sign of the original structure remained. The same complete atrophy extended to the splenic vein and splenic artery. They were plugged for a distance of about 4 mm, to the first branch serving normal tissue.

It is my opinion that the pathological changes—probably a complete thrombosis of the splenic artery and partial thrombosis (plugging) of the hepatic (pertaining to the liver) and renal (pertaining to the urinary system) arteries, during the progress of the acute illness had been so extensive that, even though the bird was completely cured of the acute infection, it was impossible for the organs to repair themselves and take up their normal functions.

Source of infection. Considerable thought was given to the question of the possible source of this outbreak. The disease first made its appearance in young birds living in a large flight room, and from there spread throughout the plant. The gentleman of the house is a livestock buyer, dealing principally in hogs. No livestock was ever kept on the premises, but it is possible that hog offal may have been carried into the room on his shoes. It is also possible that mice may have had access to the room. Several of my English friends have told me that over there mice are generally believed to be the carriers of this disease, which seems reasonable, since B. paratyphosus B is known to be the cause of epizootics in mice and rats. No new stock had been purchased or brought into the plant. Careful investigation suggested no source of infection other than those mentioned.

B. PULLORUM. This is the organism responsible for BACILLARY WHITE DIARRHEA—which see.

B. SANGUINARIUM. This is the organism responsible for FOWL TYPHOID—which see.

BALDNESS. There are a number of factors which may be responsible for the loss of feathers from the heads of birds, and the most common of these is the general ignorance and neglect of us who own them. In the hope of combating this general lack of understanding and saving others from some of my own errors, I have divided this discussion into five parts and treated each kind of baldness in some detail.

Congenital baldness. In crested birds, canaries, pigeons, etc., the crest is a direct inheritance from only one parent. The factor in the germ cell that causes the development of the crest is what is known as a **lethal-dominant factor,** which means that when the young bird inherits that factor from one parent it develops a crest, but, when it inherits the same crest-factor from both parents, it dies. Thus, no bird having a crest could have gotten the crest-factor from more than one parent, nor could he pass it on to more than half of his offspring. The factors making up the crest, determining its shape, size, color, etc., are independent of the crest-factor, responsible for the development of the crest. To illustrate: I once bred some crest-bred (**crest-bred** birds are those having one crested parent but no crest) Norwich canaries together for a number of generations. Since all of the birds lacked the crest-factor, no crests were produced. Then I mated one of these birds to a small roller with a very scrubby crest. The crested young developed large, Norwich-type crests, proving that the presence of the crest came from one parent, its shape, size, etc., from the other. This means that the crest-factor and the factor responsible for the kind of crest that develops are contained in different chromosomes.*

Now, each crest is composed of two general factors: One, a rosette of feathers growing out of the top of the head; the other, a bald spot located between the rosette of feathers on the top of the head and the normally placed feathers at the back of the head. These factors are permanently linked; neither can occur without the other; but the factors governing their relative proportions and development are not linked with the crest-gene, and so can be inherited separately. If two crested birds are mated together, about one-fourth of the young will inherit the crest-gene from both parents. These birds will be unable to live. They will either die in the shell or die as the result of ingrown feathers at feathering time. About one-fourth of the young will receive two genes (factors), one from each parent, governing the size of the rosettes, but only one gene for the development of the crest. These birds can live, and they will develop enormous crests, real mop-heads. About one-fourth of them will receive one crest-gene, one rosette-gene, but two bald-spot-genes, and in their development the double force of the bald-spot tendency will crowd the rosettes down over the eyes and leave the top of the head bald, as in "A" Figure 11. The skin of this bald dome is utterly devoid of the kind of cells from which feathers are grown; so it would be as hard to grow feathers on such a head as it would be for you to grow hair on

---

* **Note:** A chromosome is a small rod-like body in the nucleus of the germ cell. It has been demonstrated that these little rods and the still smaller, dot-like bodies of which they are made up, are the carriers of inheritance from one generation to the next. The real carriers are the small objects of which the chromosomes are made, called **genes.** These are so small that they cannot be seen under the most powerful microscopes, but they have been recently photographed by the use of ultra-violet light. Different species of animals have different numbers of chromosomes in their cell nuclei.

the palms of your hands, notwithstanding anything you were told in your youth. The last one-fourth of the babies from our crest-crest mating will fail to receive the crest-gene from either parent. They will have no crests, but they may receive from one or both parents the genes responsible to the development of good crests;

Figure 11.   **BALDNESS**

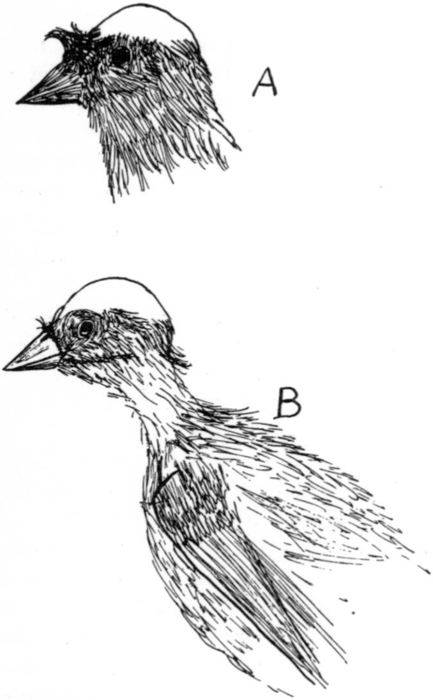

A. A BALD-HEADED CREST. This is a case of congenital baldness. Similar cases result from breeding crest to crest. The crest is restricted to a small area in front of the eyes. No feathers can ever grow on the top of the head.

B. This sketch represents a bird stuck in the moult. The condition can result from overbreeding hens or from a young bird stopping moulting before the head is feathered. Chilling and placing in the training cage at too early an age are the most common causes of this condition in young canaries.

Drawn by Robert Stroud

however, these genes must remain dormant until such time as they are again coupled with a crest-gene, but the birds having them can pass them along to their offspring. These birds are called **crest-bred.**

The perfect line of breeding for crested birds is to mate a crested bird to a crest-bred bird.

When a crested bird is mated to a bird having no crested inheritance, part of the young will receive from the crested parent the crest-gene but will fail to receive, because the other parent does not have them, the genes responsible for a good crest. Sometimes these birds have split crests or crests with naked spots in the center. A continuation of this line of breeding will eventually lead to a strain of bald-headed birds. And these birds, like the ones described above, can never grow feathers on their bald spots.

In the wild state all birds are divided into two general classes, which, for want of better names, we call **yellow** and **buff.** These words have no reference to color; they refer to the distribution of the pigment in the feathers. The **yellow** bird, of which the bright yellow canary and the hen English sparrow are good examples, has the pigmentation carried to the very edges of the feathers. **Buff** birds, of which the dull-yellow canary and the cock sparrow are good examples, have a colorless margin around each feather, though in wild birds, where the males are the **buffs,** this colorless area is often filled in with some bright pigment. The **yellow** bird shows a hard sharp outline; the **buffs** have more of a fluffy appearance. Again look at the sparrows and notice how much fluffier the cock is than the hen. There is a reason for this fluffiness of **buff** birds. That margin around each feather is not just so much feather from which pigment has been omitted; on the contrary, it is an accretion to the amount of feather web. Other things being equal, the **buff** feather is always larger and wider than the **yellow** feather by the amount of its colorless edging. In the wild state these **yellow** and **buff** factors were sex connected, all **yellows** of a given species being of one sex and all **buffs** of that species being of the other sex, but by line breeding this sex connection has been broken down in canaries and some of our other domesticated birds. We have **yellows** and **buffs** of both sexes as a consequence.

Now, when we mate **yellow-yellow,** each chick receives one gene for body size and yellow from each parent, and the development of that chick and its feathers are both restrained by the double dose of these growth-restricting genes.

The result is that where **yellow-yellow** matings are used generation after generation for the purpose of intensifying the coloring of the feathers, the feathers become shorter, narrower and more brittle with each generation. The time comes when we get birds with feathers so thin that they will hardly cover the body and so brittle that they will not stand the wear of these little, energetic creatures' active lives—for, at the same time, the birds have been becoming smaller and more active with each generation, too. Naturally such birds are apt to be half naked between moults.

When we reverse this process we get bigger birds with more, larger and thicker feathers. See LUMPS.

Treatment. The only treatment for the results of incorrect breeding is to change one's breeding methods. Always mate crests to crest-breds, **yellows** to **buffs,** and the difficulties just described will not occur in your flock. There are cases, however, where it is only by violating nature's laws that we can open the door for improvements we wish to bring about. In such cases conduct your mismatings with your eyes open. Know what you are doing and why, and then have the decency to destroy the misfits you produce.

Baldness due to the destruction of feathers. Birds fight, and they lose feathers in the process. They rub their heads on the bars of their cages—some finches have to be kept in cloth-topped cages to keep them from constantly rubbing themselves bald. Lice and mites suck the oil from the feathers, and the lice larva eat the feather webs. Sometimes idiotic breeders—I know because I have done it myself—smear their birds with this or that special "goo" to rid them of lice and mites; or sometimes they dip them in this or that special solution to destroy the mites and lice, ending up by destroying the feathers. Now, it is a general rule of nature that a bird shall moult but once each year. Wing and tail feathers, upon which depends the power of flight, and life and death in the wild state, are replaced whenever they are lost; but body feathers are not, as a rule, replaced until the next moult. And there is nothing that you can do about it without endangering the life and health of your bird. Oh, there are ways to cause a bird to moult; there are ways to stimulate the growth of feathers on a particular spot; and you will learn all about them in these pages. The best treatment for all such cases, however, is to let nature take its course.

There are two exceptions to the rule governing the replacement of body feathers. Babies that have been picked in the nest or before entering the baby moult will grow new feathers at once. When a spot of the feathered area of the skin is burned severely enough to destroy the epidermis without destroying the dermis, the feathers will regrow on that spot as soon as the burn has healed.

Baldness due to exhaustion. High-production egg-laying allows the chicken hen little chance to store up in her body the materials and vitamins necessary for a full growth of feathers. A canary hen that has been forced to raise six or seven nests of babies during the season is in the same situation. Moulting time finds these birds lacking the vitality necessary for the growth of a full coat. They moult their flight feathers and the larger body feathers on their breasts and back, but the rest, the least important of their feathers, they do not change. Soon the old feathers wear out and you have birds looking like "B" Figure 11. If chickens, such birds should be put on free range where they will have a chance to run, chase bugs, dig in clean ground, and bask in the sunshine. The canary hen needs practically the same things. She should be turned into a flight and given a chance to stretch her wings. Plenty of green food and a well-balanced diet that is not too stimulating are essentials. If she has been overstimulated during the breeding season she may insist on keeping on with the breeding. The cure for that is to cage her and place her on a diet of seed and green food for a week or two; then return her to the flight for a week, keeping her on the seed and green food diet. She will soon start to drop her feathers and may then be given a little soft food daily, being careful not to give her any of the richer and more stimulating seeds, like hemp seed. After one moulting season is over, the best thing to do is to place these bald hens in the flight and let them go until the next moulting season, when, if not bred in the meantime, they will grow a nice full coat of feathers.

Baldness due to lack of necessary food. Birds are the recipients of no magical powers; they cannot make something from nothing. If your chicken hen is confined where she can catch no bugs, fed on a straight grain diet—and even that containing no yellow corn— she may grow a full coat of feathers, but if she does, she will never be the same thereafter, for she can only do so by robbing the tissues of her own body. Some of the things she needs for making feathers are contained in grain in such small quantities that she is forced to eat several times the amount of grain she would otherwise require in order to supply the needs of her growing feathers only partially. Is it any wonder that such birds often come out of the moult with ruined digestions and lowered vitality.

The same thing applies to the pet canary to an even greater degree. Thousands of owners of pet canaries, too lazy to take the trouble to learn how to care for their birds, imagine that when they keep his cup full of cheap, stale package seed and throw him a leaf of stale, wilted, half rotten lettuce once in a while they have performed their whole duty.

Birds need some animal protein at every season of the year, and that need is doubly great during the moulting season. The chicken should have free range, if possible, but where this is not possible the difficulty can be overcome by seeing that it has meat and bone scraps, sunflower seed, flax seed or oil cake, and plenty of good fresh cabbage in its diet. A canary should have egg food, a good tonic seed mixture, and plenty of wild greens. During the moulting season the staple seed mixture should contain more canary seed than is necessary at other seasons of the year. This is because the silicon required for feather-making comes largely from this one element of the canary's diet. The bird owner who will take the trouble to supply his bird's needs during the moult will be rewarded by seeing his pet with a coat that will delight the eyes, and what is more, keep the bird warm all winter.

Baldness due to upset moult. It is often very easy to upset the moulting bird and cause the feathers to stop growing. Anything that upsets the correct, balanced functioning of the sex glands and the thyroid is very apt to stop the moult. Hens may be forced into laying by too rich a diet; young roller canaries may be taken out of flight and placed in training before they have finished the baby moult, because the breeder is too anxious to get them into full song; there may be sudden changes in the weather. Any of these things can upset a bird and stop it from moulting. The hens lay all right, but the chances of them producing young of value in the fall is very remote; the young males come into song, but as soon as the baby feathers on their heads and necks wear out they begin to look like turkey buzzards. There is little that one can do about the weather; the breeder can and should discontinue his breeding operation at an early enough date in the summer to permit his birds to moult during the natural moulting season, however, which is always the hottest part of the summer— thus avoiding the chances of the moulting birds running into bad weather.

As for treating these conditions, that is out of the question. Any treatment, with the exception of moving the half-moulted birds to warm quarters, is apt to be harmful. The bird that is **stuck in moult,** which is what this condition is called, can easily be forced into a general moult by keeping it in a room that is too hot; by plying it with certain drug, such as potassium chlorate; by stuffing it on certain foods, such as lettuce and bread and milk. These measures are dangerous to the general health, however, and they may bring about a condition known as **soft moult,** in which the bird continues to drop and grow feathers until it moults itself to death. The best treatment I know of for all such cases is to throw all your half-moulted birds into flight and let them remain there until nature has a chance to correct the difficulty. You will find that most of the birds that failed to have a full moult in the fall will go into a short moult in the spring and replace the missing feathers. See LUMPS; SOFT MOULT; MOULT; FUNGOID SKIN; and FEATHER MITES.

BENZOIC ACID AND BENZOATES. The oldest antiseptic known, benzoic acid, C_6H_5COOH, is present in several natural gums and balsams, such as balsam of Peru, Tolu, etc., and, so far as is known, was first used for the preservation of Egyptian mummies. It is now used in medicine principally as an antiseptic for the lungs and kidneys. Because of its power to cause the urine to take on an acid reaction, it is often given in conjunction with urotropin in the treatment of kidney infections. Because it is partly excreted by the lungs and respiratory mucosa, it is of value in the treatment of infections of the respiratory tract. The sodium and ammonium salts are most frequently used. Sodium benzoate is also used as an antipyretic, particularly in the treatment of fevers resulting from respiratory disorders. The dose for a bird is about 1/16 to ¼ grain to the ounce of drinking water. See AMMONIUM BENZOATE.

BIRD POX. See AVIAN DIPHTHERIA.

BIRD CAGES. See CAGES.

BISMUTH. This metal forms a large number of salts used in medicine principally as antiseptic dressings for wounds, in the treatment of diarrhea and intestinal inflammations, and in treating gastric ulcer. Recently some of the organic salts of bismuth have been employed in the treatment of syphilis; they are administered by intramuscular injection. Many of the bismuth salts are but slightly soluble in water and dilute acids. They are decomposed in the intestines, however, and the metal is thrown down as bismuth oxide—a heavy, white powder, entirely insoluble in gastric juices—which possesses the unique property of adhering to inflamed tissue—thus forming a protective coating over it, which permits healing to proceed unhampered by external irritations. The bismuth salts most frequently employed in the treatment of intestinal disorders are the subnitrate and the subgallate. Since they contain very high percentages of bismuth and are extremely insoluble, they are more apt to give the desired results without producing poisonous effects.

BISMUTH SUBGALLATE. This salt comes on the market as a saffron-yellow powder, insoluble in water. It is prepared for use in the bird room by grinding from four to ten grains of the salt with one hundred grains of sugar. A good way to do this is to place the drug and the sugar on a piece of white paper, place another piece of paper over them, and then roll the mixture with a bottle or rolling pin. The object is to break up the sugar grains and get an even mixture.

I know that many breeders will say: "Oh, why should I take the trouble to do that? I just give the bismuth to my birds as it comes from the drug store." All I can say to that is that maybe if this breeder would take more trouble his birds would have less. The very fact that his birds ever need bismuth is evidence that he is not taking enough trouble with other things, particularly their food. Canaries, finches and parrakeets are very small creatures. It is true that they are not as susceptible to some drugs as we are; it is true that bismuth is not ordinarily a poisonous drug; but it should always be remembered that all drugs are given for the purpose of bringing about certain specific effects. The least dose which will give the desired results is always the correct dose. As for bismuth, many breeders, particularly novices, stuff their birds with it until it is a wonder the poor creatures are able to breathe. At the first sign of bowel-looseness they reach for the bismuth, and in ninety-nine cases out of a hundred there is not a thing wrong with the bird. I have used this drug just once in the last five years. It is of value in the treatment of simple diarrhea, caused by eating spoiled food, and the inflammation of the bowels that is apt to follow overeating after starvation. Weaning canary chicks, which are apt to pick up and swallow anything, and birds that have suffered the hardships and deprivations of long shipments may in some cases be benefited by the judicious administration of bismuth. It is never indicated in those cases of diarrhea which are the result of general diseases, like diphtheria and paratyphoid, however.

BISMUTH SUBNITRATE. Everything that has been said about the subgallate, excepting the color, is equally true of this salt, which comes as a white powder. Some prefer to use one salt, some the other, though their actions are identical.

BLEEDING. Bird blood has very great clotting power. Cut a man's leg off and without the application of methods for stopping the bleeding he will be pretty certain to bleed to death. Under the same circumstances, a bird will not bleed enough to weaken it noticeably. There are very few cases where it is necessary to take any special steps to keep a bird from bleeding to death, excepting in certain special cases where the clotting power of the blood does not come into action. If, instead of cutting the bird's foot off, you should cut off just one claw, the case might be different. There is a channel down the center of a bird's claw, and bird blood in contact with this channel and the smoothly cut claw does not clot readily. The best way to draw blood from a bird for the purpose of examination is by clipping the claw back far enough to just open its channel; the best way to stop the claw from bleeding is to touch it quickly and lightly to the lighted end of a cigarette.

During the moult the quills of the growing feathers are almost bursting with blood, and the blood does not clot readily in contact with the quill. The result is that any injury to the growing quill may result in serious bleeding, which, if it does nothing worse, will foul the other feathers and ruin the bird's appearance. The best way to stop this bleeding is to catch the bird, locate the injured quill and remove it.

In the case of a canary most wounds can be cauterized with a lighted cigarette. Cotton lint causes blood to clot very quickly. I have found that wrapping a little cotton lint around a wound and keeping the bird quiet until the blood hardens is an excellent method of providing the wound with a protective dressing that will remain in place during healing. In those cases where styptics (substances which stop bleeding) are necessary, alum, copper sulphate or iron chloride may be used.

BLEEDING FROM THE BOWELS. See AVIAN DIPHTHERIA; B. PARATYPHOSUS B INFECTION; TAPEWORMS.

BLEEDING, INTERNAL. The symptoms of internal hemorrhage from a ruptured blood vessel is a paroxysm of wild, aimless flight. Internal hemorrhages into the thoracic cavity, skull cavities, subarachnoid spaces, and the cavities in the large bones often indicate apoplectiform septicemia. Hemorrhages into the abdominal cavity may indicate diphtheria in the peracute form or paratyphoid. The two conditions are differentiated under these circumstances by the condition of the liver. Mulberry liver does not occur in paratyphoid.

Bleeding from a mucous surface is indicated by the discharged blood, by the whiteness of the bird's bill and feet, and by great weakness. Blood discharged from the vent may be mixed with the feces and dark in color, in which case it originated in the bowels; or it may be unmixed and bright red in color, in which case it originated in the cloaca or uterus; a pink or reddish color of the urine may indicate bleeding from the kidneys. There is usually little or nothing one can do in such cases.

BLINDNESS. I am not familiar with any general studies of avian eye disease, though I understand such studies have been made. In this section I will have to confine my remarks to dis-

cussions of conditions which have come under my personal observation. I have observed two serious conditions of the eye which are
apparently unrelated to any general infection.

In the first of these there is no inflammation of the tissues
surrounding the eyes. The bird becomes blind as the result of an
opacity located between the cornea * and the iris and directly over
the pupil, to which it gives a milk-white appearance. Sometimes one
eye alone is affected; sometimes both are involved. I have been able
to learn nothing concerning the cause of the condition. It cannot
be considered very contagious, however, because only a few birds
are affected, and the young of affected parents do not develop the
condition as a result of association with their affected progenitors.
On the other hand, I have never known any bird that did not have
a history of exposure to some other bird similarly affected to
develop this condition.

Under the heading FOWL PARALYSIS, at the conclusion of
the discussion of the disease in poultry, there is a rather long
note which quotes from an article by Dr. J. A. Durant. It will
be noticed that Dr. Durant mentions blindness as one of the
symptoms of fowl paralysis in poultry. This feature of the
disease in poultry had slipped my mind and was not recalled
until I recently found and re-read Dr. Durant's article.

It is possible that the cases of blindness just mentioned were
the result of that infection. They occurred in older birds and the
first cases to occur were in birds which had been exposed to this
disease during my experiments. They did not become blind until
after the conclusion of the experiments, however. During the
appearance of these cases, covering a period of about five years,
there were only two cases of neck paralysis among my birds, so
I failed to notice any connection between the two conditions. See
FOWL PARALYSIS.†

The second condition that sometimes results in blindness in
canaries is an inflammation of the conjunctiva. It is discussed in
some detail under the heading CONJUNCTIVITIS.

Blindness may result from infestation of the eyes with Manson's worm or from diphtheric lesions involving the eyes only
when the conditions are treated with gross neglect.

The only kind or sensible thing to do with blind birds is to
kill them.†

---

* **Note:** The cornea is the transparent covering of the front of the eye; the
iris is the colored area surrounding the pupil.

† **Note:** During the present season—1941—I have been able to cure this
condition by giving the bird, canary, a 1/10 grain dose of sulfanilamide
into the crop. See FOWL PARALYSIS.

BLISTERS. The spontaneous appearance of blisters around the eyes or vent is an indication of diphtheria. Such blisters should be opened and treated with potassium permanganate, sodium perborate or silver nitrate. The bird should be placed on the general treatment for AVIAN DIPHTHERIA—which see.

Blisters resulting from burns or contact with such substances as coal oil, turpentine, etc., will usually heal without special treatment, if they are not too extensive. Where the damage has been considerable it may be necessary to open the blisters and drain them. Raw burns should be treated with a tannic acid dusting powder.

BLOOD. That simple red fluid that comes out when you prick your finger and that seems to be so important to life consists of a straw-colored fluid called the **plasma,** a large number of red cells which float in the plasma, called **erythrocytes (erythro** means **red** and **cyte** means **cell**), and a few obscure bodies called leucocytes or white cells **(leuco** simply means white), so-called because they do not contain the iron pigment (hemoglobin) responsible for the red color of the blood.

Bird blood, according to the literature on the subject to come to my attention, is said to contain five kinds of leucocytes in addition to the red cells, and the description of each of these cells is usually appended to the account. That is the way I wrote this section in the original manuscript of this book. It all seemed so simple, but when I started searching microscopic slides for typical illustrations of the cells described, I ran into trouble. Since that time, I have spent more than three thousand hours over my microscope, studying bird blood; I have written and illustrated this section no less than five times; I have studied the most thorough work on human blood to appear (Osgood's Atlas of Hematology, Stacey, Inc., San Francisco, California, 1937); I have tested 65 different staining techniques, most of them original with me; and I have worried Dr. Zellermeyer—who has done research work in avian embryology—so much that I can no longer get him to talk to me. And after all this work, I am forced to warn you that, concerning what is to follow, I probably do not know what I am talking about and have grave doubts as to whether anyone else knows anything about the subject, either.

It appears to me that all the men who have worked with bird blood have simply applied what they have been taught concerning human blood, ignored what they did not understand, and let the subject go at that. So, in order to avoid that same error, and in

Figure 12.   BLOOD

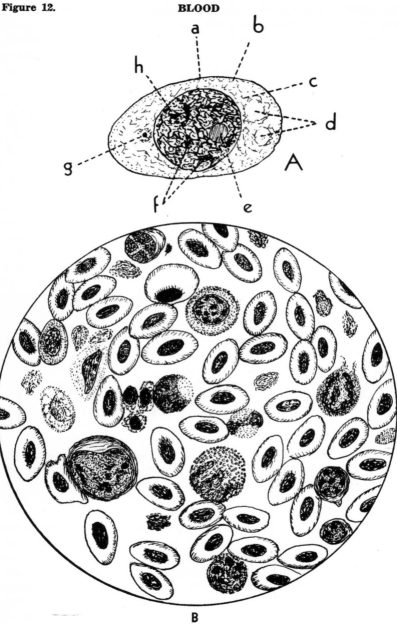

A

B

the hope of making this section of some value to those who may want to carry on from the point where I have left off, I am going to have to make it more technical than the general nature of this work would ordinarily call for. Those who are not interested in microscopic work can just admire my drawings and skip over the involved text.

Structure of a cell. Before going into the histology of bird blood, it is necessary for the reader to have some idea of the features that go to make up an ideal cell. And it should be understood that these features are common to all cells, from the lowest single cell animal to man. In fact, there is no quality or function found in the most differentiated cells of the most differentiated creatures that are not present in the lowest single-cell animals. Differentiation of the cells that make up the different tissues is obtained, not by something being added to the ideal cell, but by some one quality being expanded and developed, while other qualities are lost.

"A," Figure 12, gives a rough idea of the structure of an ideal cell, and shows the following structural features: "a," **cell wall** or **cell membrane;** "b," **ectoplasm** (from **ecto,** out; **plasm,** living matter); "c," the granular network of the cell body is called the **spongioplasm** (**spongio,** sponge; **plasm,** living matter); and the material filling the spaces between the meshes is called the **hyaloplasm** (**hyalo,** transparent). These two materials taken together are often called the **cytoplasm** (**kytos,** a cell), though this term is also applied to the entire cell body, as distinct from the nucleus. "d" shows two empty spaces called **vacuoles** (**vacuus,** empty). The large dark body in the center of the cell is called the **nucleus,** and the small round body shown within the nucleus, at "e," is called the **nucleolus** (little nucleus) and it plays an important part in cell division. The granular material inside of the nucleus, "f," is called **chromatin** (**chroma,** color) because it has an affinity for deep-colored basic stains. The small round body shown at "g" is called the **centrosome** (**centro,** center; **some,** body), while "h" indicated the nuclear membrane or wall.

It was mentioned above that many of these features are often lost in the process of differentiation by which special cells of the body become adapted to different structures and functions, but there are two essentials of a cell that can never be lost while the cell remains a cell—the **nucleus,** and some **cytoplasm,** though much of the latter may be lost without the cell losing its vitality, some small part always remains. And the material of which these two essential parts of the cell are made are always electro-chemical opposites, which makes of each living cell a small electro-chemical battery. It would lead us too far afield to go into that here, however. The only exception to this rule exists in the red corpuscles of mammalian blood, which have been reduced to a single function, that of carrying oxygen or carbon dioxide.

The cytology of bird blood. Bird blood consists of a straw-colored fluid that carries many different chemical substances in solution and a great number of cells in suspension. In addition it contains small bodies called **micrones,** because they are about one micron in diameter, which undoubtedly come from the food (they are more plentiful shortly after eating and scarce during fasts) and which probably consist of fat globules, since they take up fat-soluble dyes. There are also found in the blood small bodies called platelets, and many bits of protein material resulting from cell disintegration, which is going on at a very rapid rate all the time.

Of the cells found in bird blood the erythrocytes—red cells—are by far the most numerous. They make up about 99 per cent of all cells present. Moore has recorded red-cell counts on well chickens (Biannual Report of the Bureau of Animal Industry, 1895-6, pages 197-8) ranging from 3,500,000 to 4,500,000, with an average of about 3,800,000 red cells to each cubic millimeter of blood. He records white counts on well chickens as low as 14,500 to the cubic millimeter and as high as 26,500 to the cubic millimeter of blood. Ward and Gallagher, DISEASES OF DOMESTICATED BIRD, page 7, gives the average red count for healthy adult chickens as 3,250,000, and the average white cell count for healthy adult chickens as 26,000. These figures may be true for chickens, though I doubt it, since my own work on canary blood has in all cases given somewhat higher figures. I have found the average number of red cells in a cubic millimeter of blood from a healthy adult canary to be about 4,250,000, which may vary from a low of 3,800,000 to 5,000,000 in birds that show no evidence of illness. My white counts have varied from a low of 29,000 to a high of 50,000, with an average of 35,000 to 40,000. And, realizing the many sources of possible error resulting from attempts to apply the techniques of human cytology to bird blood, I cannot convince myself that men trained on mammalian blood, and who have not found it necessary to report special techniques for the study of bird blood, could possibly produce results that are wholly above question. So, while it is possible that canaries and chickens have different blood counts, I would have to do the counting myself before I would believe it.

The following tabulation of the bodies found in bird blood and their properties is compiled from the descriptions of bird blood I have been able to find in the literature:

Staining by Giemsa method.

Cell	Per Cent	Nucleus		Cytoplasm Staining	Granules	Size
		Shape	Staining			
Erythrocyte	99.25	oval	deep blue	pink	none	12x15u
Lymphocyte	40	round or oval	deep blue	pale blue	none	5 to 7u
Monocyte	18	round or oval	deep blue	pale blue	not mentioned	10 to 15u
Polymorpho-nuclears	35	broken, lobulated	blue	lighter blue	round or rod-shaped violet	10 to 15u
Mast cells	3	lobulated	deep blue	pale	small round violet	8 to 10u
Eosinophiles	4	lobulated	blue	pale blue	round bright red	12u
Plateletes		colorless bodies	granular centers		occur in clumps	3 to 4u
Shadow cells		oval	deep blue	colorless, irregular in outline		
		These are disintegrating red cells				
Microblasts		oval	deep blue	pink	These are red cells that are smaller than normal	

Macroblasts, red cells larger than normal. Microblasts and macroblasts are said to be absent from the blood of healthy adult birds but present in the blood of young birds.

Myelocytes (leucocytes from the bone marrow) are said to often occur in bird blood. They are described as being similar to Mast cells excepting that their cytoplasm is vacuolated.

The percentages of the erythrocytes are expressed in terms of total number of cells in blood; the percentages of leucocytes are expressed in terms of the remainder, or of the total number of leucocytes present.

"u" is the designation symbol for one micron, one one-thousandth of a millimeter; one twenty-five thousandth of an inch.

For a description of Giemsa's Blood Stain see Conn's BIOLOGICAL STAINS, or MERCK'S INDEX, 1940.

Normal bird blood. As I said before, I found myself unable to accept either the descriptions or the proportions of the cells described in the above chart, since the cells seen under my microscope failed to fall into the classes designated or conforming to the criteria given in the chart. This led me into a series of studies of bird blood to which I have devoted more than 3,000 hours during the last year; yet, the most important thing I have learned is that I still know practically nothing about my subject; but in plate 13, figures 1 to 26, I pass that nothing on to you.

These drawings were made with a magnification of 1350× and to a scale of $\frac{1}{16}$ of an inch to the micron, and they are reduced by one-third in reproduction. The sizes were not measured, but estimated from the size of the erythrocytes.

Figure 13.   **BLOOD**

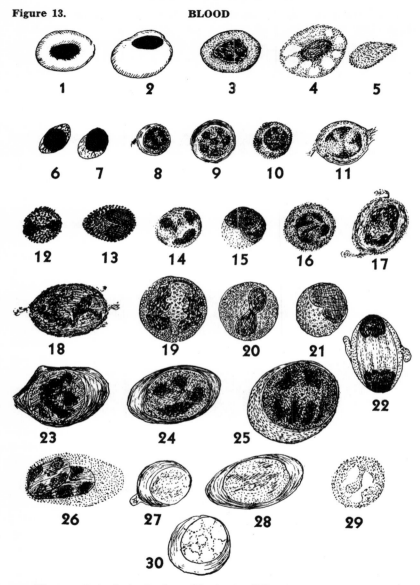

Figures 1 to 5, inclusive, illustrate different stages in the life and death of the erythrocyte as found in normal canary blood, staining with solutions "A" and "C" as described in supplement.

"1." Normal, healthy erythrocyte; 12 by 15 microns; nucleus, deep blue; cytoplasm, pale yellow, pale green, or pink, depending on reaction of solutions and staining time, and should in no case be deeply stained, which would indicate a too alkaline solution. Where the acidity of the solution is exactly right, the cytoplasm of the healthy erythrocyte stains a delicate pale green.

"2." Young erythrocyte that has just been released into the blood stream from the bone marrow.*

The odd shapes assumed by these cells result from the fact that their dense cell walls have not yet formed. The nucleus is concentrically located, deep staining, but usually take a more reddish stain than that taken by the mature cells, and some are seen in which the nuclei take a pink stain. The cytoplasm always stains slightly more yellowish or pinkish than that of the mature erythrocyte. In a count of 10,000 cells of the erythrocyte group I found 863 of these young cells.

"3." Old erythrocyte in which the cytoplasm has not yet started to break up. The cytoplasm takes a deep brownish or purplish color by my polychrome methylene blue stain and a dull, bluish-gray color by Wright's method. The nucleus is somewhat expanded and chromatin is gathered into dense-staining clumps, and the color is no longer a clear blue, but, rather, takes a brownish cast. Cells of this type would probably be greatly increased in pathologic blood, but I have not yet found the time necessary for investigating this. The color changes correspond to what Osgood (Osgood's Atlas of Hematology, San Francisco, 1937) calls **four-plus basophilia.**

"4." A **shadow** or disintegrating erythrocyte. This cell is slightly larger than a healthy red cell, while cell No. 3 is usually slightly smaller. The cytoplasm is vacuolated and stains a pale orange color, retaining very little of the dye. In unstained smears these cells are easily recognized by the fact that the cytoplasm has lost its hemoglobin. These cells were first observed by Moore (Biannual Report of the Bureau of Animal Industry, 1895-6, plate X; reproduced in part in figure 41), who made a careful study of the blood changes in **fowl typhoid** and who, in the course of this study, observed the leucocytes attacking the erythrocytes and converting them into shadow cells by extracting or setting free their hemoglobin. This process, as observed and illustrated by Moore, is shown

* **Note:** All blood cells are formed in the bone marrow, spleen, or lymph nodes. In a state of health, the lymphatic tissues—spleen and lymph nodes —produce only lymphocytes, while all other forms are produced in the bone marrow. In illness, however, the spleen may also take up the production of other leucocytes and erythrocytes.

in figure 40. The nucleus takes a dull purple or lavender stain and may or may not contain much granular chromatin.

No transition forms between cell "3" and cell "4" have been observed, though practically all stages between both of these forms and the next to be described are found, which convinces me that two distinct processes of erythrocyte destruction are going on in normal bird blood at all times. Both of these processes appear to be going on all the time, and both are increased by the administration of certain dyes and drugs, though my studies on this point are incomplete.

Moore's observations were too carefully made to leave any doubt about such cells resulting from the overactivity of the phagocytes in the course of severe bacteremic infections, but this does not account for the presence of these cells in normal blood.

"5." This is a small gob of free nuclear protein. On a fresh, unstained smear the nuclear wall, and, sometimes, the entire body can still be seen. But in stained smears it appears as a more or less structureless mass that takes a stain ranging in color from lavender to dull purple. These bodies never stain a bright color, regardless of the dye or process used. On smears stained by the Wright process, it is sometimes impossible to differentiate some of these bodies from certain of the leucocytes, and it is this fact that makes the Wright process worthless for bird blood. In a count of 10,000 cells these bodies were grouped with the shadow cells and together 1,462 were counted, which is about 1:6. They may vary from less than five per cent to more than 20 per cent in the blood of birds which appear to be in perfect health.

"6" and "7." These two drawings show two aspects of the same cell, but what this cell is I would not know. In fresh smears the cytoplasm of these cells contain lumps of highly refractile material which is probably of a lipoid nature, since in the blood of birds fed on fat soluble dyes these bodies are stained the same color as the micrones. And this brings up a question to which I have not yet been able to find the answer. Are these cells undergoing lipoid degeneration, or are they phagocytic for lipoid material? The nucleus of these cells is the deepest staining body found in bird blood and tends to take rather large amounts of acid dye. By Wright's stain, it stains a rich, velvety blue. It has a strong affinity for acid fuchsin, and with solutions containing this dye it takes a more or less reddish purple stain. By my stain it is stained purple, but its color is always richer and brighter than that of any other body present on the same slide. The cytoplasm takes a pale blue or pale orange stain, and the bodies observed in the fresh smears are always lost in the staining process, so that in stained smears the cytoplasm of these cells always contains numerous vacuoles. Counted with the leucocytes, these cells are found in normal bird blood in proportions ranging from 21 to 43 per cent. I have consulted a number of doctors and technicians concerning the identity of this cell, and most of them insist that it should be counted as a lymphocyte. Dr. Zellermeyer of the Public Health Service, who is probably the best qualified of the men consulted, says that it is possible that some of the lymphocytes of birds are phagocytic for lipoid material and that it has long been known that birds have two distinct types of lymphocytes which, unfortunately do not seem to have received much study, since this extra well-informed gentleman could not direct me to any literature on the subject.

"8." This cell fulfills the criteria laid down for the lymphocyte, both for human and bird blood, much better than the cell just described, and it resembles closely the lymphocytes observed in sections of fixed tissue. It is a small cell with a rather coarse granular chromatin in a nucleus that fills almost the entire cell. The chromatin has no definite arrangement, but in some of these cells a distinct nucleolus can be seen. The cytoplasm contains no granules. The majority of these cells have pseudopods. The chromatin takes a deep purple stain; the nucleolus a blue stain, which may be either lighter or darker than the chromatin; the nuclear protoplasm, **hyaloplasm,** usually stains some shade of purple or gray and is lighter than the chromatin. There is a distinct nuclear wall. The cytoplasm is rather deep staining and usually takes a blue or greenish color. It is rather opaque, but contains no granules.

Tissue section showing morbid processes indicates that the functions of this cell correspond closely to those of the human lymphocyte, which is a cell of repair and gives rise to the development of new connective tissue cells and the formation of scar tissue. This cell makes up from 11 to 16 per cent of the leucocytes found in normal bird blood.

"9." This cell differs from "8" in just one important feature, the wheel-shaped arrangement of the chromatin in the nucleus. It differs from "10" and "11" in that it has no granules in its cytoplasm. There is considerable variation in the size of these cells. In selecting examples for my drawings, I have tried to choose those that were as near typical as possible, but it should be understood that while the largest examples of cell "9" are always as much larger than the largest examples of cell "8" as the sizes of the drawings indicate, it is possible to find many examples of cell "9" that are much smaller than the largest examples of cell "8," but all of the cells from "6" to "15," inclusive, are always smaller than the erythrocytes, and, within that size range, each cell should be identified by its internal structure and staining reactions.

"10." This cell differs from "9" in that the cytoplasm is densely packed with medium sized granules that take a reddish-brown stain. This form can be differentiated from "16" only by observing the presence or absence of a continuous nuclear membrane, and this feature may be obscured by the density of the granules, making the differentiation impossible.

"11." In this cell the nucleus is larger and less dense than in cell "10," and the granules seem to be finer and not quite so plentiful, but I am convinced that they are merely two aspects of the same cell, but I am able to offer very little information concerning the true identity of any one of these cells. Dr. Zellermeyer tells me that the **star** or **wheel** arrangement of the chromatin is characteristic of plasmocytes, and that all cells displaying this feature should be so classified. But Osgood describes the human plasmocyte as a cell that may have a wheel-shaped arrangement of the chromatin, but is characterized by a dense, nongranular cytoplasm that takes a deep blue stain. GOULD'S MEDICAL DICTIONARY, 4th edition, 1937, defines the plasmocyte as any cell other than a leucocyte or erythrocyte found in the blood stream, and even includes such bodies as free-swimming malaria parasites in this classification. The answer to the question, it seems, is to be found only by more research, and in the meantime we had just as well accept Dr. Zellermeyer's suggestion and call them all plasmocytes, providing we keep in mind the fact that that is simply a name for something we know nothing about. These cells total about nine per cent of the leucocytes in normal bird blood.

"12" and "13." These are mast cells. They are very easy to identify by any good staining technique. With untreated methylene blue, the granules take a deep blue stain; the cytoplasm is colorless, and the nucleus a light gray; with my polychrome methylene blue, the granules take a deep red stain, and are the richest stained bodies on the slide, with the possible exception of the nuclei of cells of group "6"; the cytoplasm is pale blue or green, but is not easily seen, and the nucleus is deep blue or purple. In staining properties as well as structure, these cells closely resemble the basophiles of human blood. Concerning the function of the human basophile, little or nothing is known. They are increased in diseases associated with other abnormal cell formations, such as leukemias and anemias, but they are not increased as a direct result of either infection or poisoning.

The mast cells of bird blood have no pseudopods, but it is characteristic of them that the granules on one side at right angle to the nucleus usually appear to be located outside of the cell membrane, creating the suggestion that the cell is a phagocyte and that these external granules have a prehensile (adapted for grasping or holding) function similar to that of the diamond-shaped bodies in Moore's leucocyte, figure 41. They are increased in the blood in certain chronic infections and some conditions of abnormal metabolism, the exact nature of which I have not yet been able to determine.

Mast cells are said to make up three per cent of normal chicken blood, and I have found them in normal canary blood in proportions ranging from 0.5 to 2.8 per cent. In the case of one hen suffering from an obscure endocrin derangement, following overbreeding, I found them in proportions ranging from 20 to 24 per cent.

"14" and "15." These drawings represent two aspects of the same cell, which is undoubtedly a member of the granulocyte series. The granules stain a pale reddish-orange or pale lavender color; the cytoplasm is almost colorless, but may be pale yellow, pale blue, or pale green. The transparency of cytoplasm, the fineness of the granules and the tendency of the nuclear matter to appear to be located on the surface of the cell are characteristic of this cell. Pseudopods are not seen, but the granules have the same tendency of projecting themselves beyond the cell membrane as is observed in the mast cells, but, because of the fineness of the granules and their pale color, this feature is not easily demonstrated. These cells may make up from 0.5 to 2.5 per cent of the leucocytes in normal bird blood.

"16" and "17." These drawings are of typical polymorphonuclear leucocytes (neutrophile lobocytes). The color taken by the cytoplasm is probably pale blue, but it is very hard to see because of the dense granules taking reddish-brown stain. These cells vary greatly in size. They may be as large as "20" or as small as "8," though they occur most often in about the sizes indicated. The form shown in "16" is very common and very hard to differentiate, since it is necessary to convince oneself that there is not a nuclear membrane surrounding the circularly arranged masses of dense chromatin. The chromatin takes a deep purple stain and is broken up into angular clumps which seem to be embedded in a rather tenuous, stringy hyaloplasm. The granules appear round or rod shaped, but the round ones are probably rods presenting an end view. Pseudopods are usually observed. Cells of these types make up 11 to 14 per cent of the leucocytes found in normal canary blood.

These cells are the principal bacterial phagocytes of bird blood and they are increased in all of the acute bacterial septicemias. I have not, however, had the opportunity to work out the exact rate and extent of that increase.

"18." This is another form that I have not been able to identify. The cell varies considerably in size, though it is never smaller than "17," the long axis may attain a length double that of the long axis of the erythrocyte. The general color in stained smears is deep olive green. The cytoplasm seems to be a slightly lighter olive, but there are two kinds of granules which are very dense. One kind of granule takes a deep reddish-brown stain; the other type takes an olive stain. By partial staining, a distinct nuclear membrane can be demonstrated. There is a relatively small amount of dense chromatin which occurs in small, irregular clumps and takes a slightly lighter stain than that observed in the other cells that have been discussed up to this point. These cells make up about one to two per cent of the leucocytes in normal canary blood.

"19," "20," and "21." These are eosinophiles. The granules take a bright orange-red stain. The cytoplasm is pale green, and the nucleus stains a rather light, pale purple or gray and appears to contain less dense chromatin than any other cell. "19" is the most mature of the forms shown and "21" is the least mature. The function of eosinophiles has something to do with the destruction of poisons in the blood. They are increased by the administration of many toxic substances and in some chronic diseases, but usually disappear from the blood during the progress of acute, contagious septicemias. Eosinophiles make up from 3 to 4.5 per cent of the leucocytes in normal bird blood, but they may sometimes run as high as 6 per cent in the blood of birds that show no evidence of illness.

"22." This is a leucocyte undergoing mitosis. The nuclear material at each end of the cells seems to be made up of dissolving chromosomes. The granular material making up the threads connecting the two nuclei takes a lavender stain. The granules in the cytoplasm take an orange stain, and for general coloring this cell resembles "26" more closely than any other cell found, but that does not indicate anything concerning the type of cell it actually is. These forms can usually be found in the blood of a healthy canary, providing a large enough number of fields are examined, but I have never found more than five of them in a differential count of 1,000 cells.

"23" and "24." These are two aspects of the same cell. These cells undoubtedly are myelocytes (marrow cells), but that is about all I know about them. The cytoplasm takes a rather dense, dull olive stain; the nuclear protoplasm is gray and granular and more transparent than the cytoplasm, which contains no granules. The chromatin takes a deep purple stain, and one or more blue-staining nucleoli can often be seen. They may be either lighter or darker than the chromatin or so near the same density that the color difference is hard to distinguish. These cells may be present in normal bird blood in proportions ranging from 2 to 8 per cent. And they may vary in size from that of the erythrocyte to cells having twice the diameter of the erythrocyte.

"25." This cell has many points of resemblance to the one just described. Its distinguishing features are that the cytoplasm contains a great many rod-shaped reddish-brown granules; that the nuclear protoplasm is more densely granular and takes a deeper stain; that the chromatin, which may occur in round or irregular clumps, always has an orderly arrangement. There is a sharply defined nuclear wall and cell wall. Some of the clumps of chromatin, like the two larger ones shown in the drawing, seem to surround nucleoli, but I have not been able to wholly convince myself of this—that what appear to be nucleoli are not actually clumps of chromatin of slightly different density. These cells are present in normal canary blood in proportion averaging 4.33 per cent.

"26." This cell has more of the characteristics of the human monocyte than any other cell found in canary blood. No cell wall can be demonstrated, but its existence is indicated by the uniform distribution of the very fine, pale orange granules. The cytoplasm may be pale blue or colorless. The nuclear protoplasm stains a pale gray by my method, but is unstained by Wright's stain. By both methods the clumps of chromatin—which may be irregular, as shown, or cuboidal or pyramidal in shape are laced together by many pale lavender threads. There is a distinct nuclear wall, but it is very hard to see, and can only be seen good by placing the condenser in immersion contact with the slide and by lighting the microscope with a strong beam of parallel light rays, since any haze in the instrument will blot it out. These cells may occur in normal bird blood in proportions ranging from 7 to 17 per cent, the average being about 11.5 per cent.

Moore's leucocyte, figure 41. In connection with his work on FOWL TYPHOID, which has already been mentioned several times in this section, Moore described and illustrated a phagocytic leucocyte observed in the blood of chickens suffering from this condition. You will notice that in the diagramic illustrations of this cell attacking the red cells, it is shown as a cell having a round nucleus and numerous red-staining granules having the shape of double pyramids. In the drawings made from stained smears, however, this cell is shown as a blue-staining globule with the pyramidal-shaped granules lying on its surface, and no nucleus is shown, merely a slight deepening of the blue color over the center of the cell. Moore does not mention the fact that he was able to see no nuclei in these cells, and he probably assumed that there was a nucleus present that did not take the stain well. Moore makes no attempt to classify these cells, but other writers have classified them as polymorphonuclear leucocytes. They are, however, distinctly different cells from the ones illustrated at "16" and "17."

These cells are present in normal canary blood in the proportion of two or three per thousand leucocytes. The granules illustrated are composed of nuclear protoplasm, and they are connected with one another by very fine purple-staining threads. No other chromatic material is found in these cells. The granules are usually diamond-shaped (double pyramids) in cells seen in blood smears, but in cells seen in the spleen, liver and bone marrow, where these cells are much more plentiful than they are in normal blood, the nuclear protoplasm is often arranged in cuboidal-shaped clumps, which are always located on the surface of the cell. This characteristic sets this cell off from all others found in canary blood, spleen, liver, or bone marrow, with the exception of "15," which is much smaller.

"27," "28," "29," and "30" were drawn from incompletely stained cells without regard to scale, for the purpose of showing the reticula of the nuclei. "27" corresponds to "8"; "30" to "9"; "28" to "24"; and "29" to "16."

The appearance of a smear. In figure 12, "B," I have illustrated the general appearance of a blood smear, but this is an impossible smear in that it contains practically everything found in bird blood. No single field could possibly ever contain all of these different forms. What I have tried to do is to illustrate the general appearances of all of these different forms in relation to one another, and to do this in a single field, I have had to ignore proportional relationships. In actual practice, working with a smear as thin as this, which is just about as thin as can be obtained without breaking the film, not more than one or two leucocytes would be found in any single high-power field, and many would contain none at all. But while all of the cells illustrated could never be found in the same field, all were found on the same slide.

The leucocytes present are, directly at the bottom, "16"; to the right, "8" and "9"; to the left, "5" and "24"; directly above, "19"; to the right, "12" and "17"; to the left, "15," "7," "4," "5," "26," and "3"; in the center above these, "25," "2," and another aspect of "8."

BORIC ACID AND BORATES. Boric acid has been discussed under the heading ANTISEPTICS FOR THE EYES.

Sodium borate, "borax." This is valuable for cleaning paint work. As it is a mild antiseptic and an insecticide, a little added to the water in which cages are washed will help in keeping them bright and clean-looking and free from mites.

Sodium perborate. I have mentioned this drug before, and I will mention it again and again throughout these pages. I fully realize that there is not a medical man in the world who will agree with what I am about to say now, but it is my opinion that this is the least understood substance known to materia medica, and I venture to predict that fifty years from now it will be considered one of the most important. I have little hope of living to see my prediction fulfilled, but some day sodium perborate will be successfully employed in the treatment of developed rabies, tetanus, and streptococcus septicemia, and in probably a number of other highly fatal conditions affecting both man and animals. I claim priority in the discovery of these potentialities. My claims are based upon observations made over a period of more than ten years devoted to the study of bird diseases. I set them down here fully convinced they will be held more estimable by future generations than by my own. See ANTISEPTICS FOR THE EYES; AVIAN DIPHTHERIA; HEMORRHAGIC SEPTICEMIA; CANARY TYPHOID; PSITTACOSIS.

BOWELS. See DROPPINGS; INTESTINES; DIGESTIVE TRACT.

BRAIN. Birds have highly developed brains which differ from the brains of mammals in a few important particulars. The cerebrum is smooth, instead of being convoluted as is the case in mammals, and there are no nerve channels connecting it directly with the spinal cord. To my mind this second fact plays an important part in avian psychology. Birds, particularly the small flying birds, have reasoning powers that would often put an engineer to shame; still in many situations they appear to have no reasoning powers whatever. I believe this is because their actions are based upon coordinations entirely divorced from thought. In the wild state their lives constantly depend upon split-second actions. To carry out any line of reasoned actions, they must think those actions out slowly in advance. Once thought out, the action is executed at a speed which leaves no time for thought. I could fill pages with illustrations of these facts, but this is a book on bird diseases rather than avian psychology. The interested breeder may supply his own illustrations by watching baby birds and cripples solve their problems.

Figure 14 consists of two rather crude drawings of a canary's brain. "A" gives an idea of the appearance of the brain **in situ** when

Figure 14.   **BRAIN**

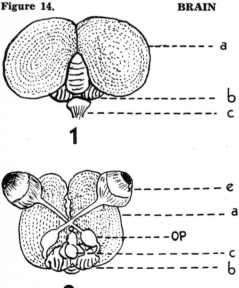

Fig. 1. Dorsal aspect

Fig. 2. Posterior aspect

a, Cerebrum

b, Cerebellum

c, Cord and medulla

e, Eyes

op, Optical plexuses

Sketched by the author from memory.

viewed posteriorly after the back of the skull has been removed and shows the relative size and location of the cerebrum and cerebellum, which, as can be seen, is located at back and base of the skull. The drawing "B" gives a rough idea of the size of the optic nerves, which are almost as large as the spinal cord, and the large optic thalamuses. This view is of the bottom of the brain, the part resting on the floor of the cranium.

Lesions are found in the brain in apoplectiform septicemia and B. paratyphosus B infection.

BREAD. Bread is of necessity a large item in the diet of caged birds, since there is nothing else so convenient for mixing egg food and other soft foods. It is easy to digest and very nourishing, but it is totally deficient in the vitamins necessary for the support of life, growth and reproduction. For that reason the breeder should be careful not to feed his birds too much bread, thus crowding out of their diet foods necessary to their well-being.

The bread that is fed to my birds is placed on top of my water heater and permitted to dry for one week. It is then crushed and sifted through wire cloth. About one tablespoonful of cod-liver oil is mixed into each seven pounds—a week's supply for my flock—of the resulting powder, which is then stored in a closed can until used. See EGG FOOD.

BREEDING BIRDS. Each fall breeders should be set aside for use during the following spring. About one-third more should be reserved than the breeder intends to use, since some are certain to suffer mishaps or be out of condition when the breeding season arrives. Breeders are best wintered in cold flight rooms, but enough heat should be supplied to keep their drinking water from freezing. It is essential that they get plenty of wing exercise and direct sunlight if they are to be good producers; so the flight room should have at least one window of southern exposure in which the birds can sun themselves. There should be several perches crossing this window-opening outside of the sashes, and the bottom sash should never be completely closed; then the birds can get almost the full force of whatever sun there happens to be, because the only thing it has to pass through is the window screen.

Seed of the best quality should be fed in creeps, and I find it advisable to use separate creeps for the different varieties of seed fed. My flight room contains six twenty-four-inch creeps—three for canary seed, three for rape seed. I also believe it advisable to supply a little soft food and tonic seed the year around, though, of course, the amount of egg material contained in the fall mixture should not be sufficient to bring the birds into breeding condition.

Where only one flight room in which to winter birds is available, it should be used for the females and the males wintered in cages.

BREEDING CONDITION. Birds are brought into breeding condition by increasing the amount of animal protein and reproductive vitamin in their diets, by added egg-yolk, tonic seed mixture, and either crushed hemp seed or wheat-germ oil to the soft food mixture, and, of course, by giving them all the green food they will eat. But this last should be done year around as a general health measure, regardless of whether or not it is desirable to bring the birds into breeding condition.

Male canary. Any male canary that is in loud ringing song and tight feathers is in breeding condition. Other indications of breeding conditions are carrying string or bits of paper in his beak; champing his beak as if he had worms; regurgitating his food and placing it between his toes or in cracks or trying to feed it to other

Figure 15.   **BREEDING CONDITION**

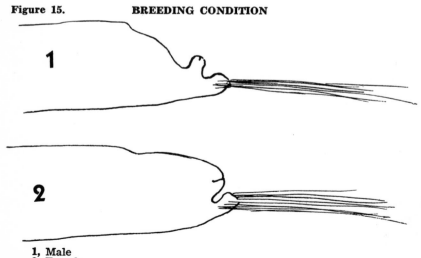

1, Male
2, Female
Notice the differences in the shape of the vents and abdomens.
Sketched by the author from memory.

males. If caged with other males he will try to make love to them, and fights follow the repulsing of his advances. He often masturbates, using any convenient object for his purpose, even the finger of his owner. Many male finches show breeding condition by a change in the color of the beak; the color becoming brighter and richer, in some varieties, becoming bright red. The vent protrudes and turns forward as shown at "1" Figure 15.

Females. Female canaries, and what is said of canaries usually applies to caged birds in general, indicate breeding condition by their loud, ringing calls, ceaseless activity and energetic efforts toward nest-building. When caged together, female canaries make use of each other in the gratification of their sexual desires, sometimes piling up four high. There is less serious fighting among the females than among the males, but usually more actual damage is done by them, since what they are interested in is nesting material, and they have no compunction about using the feathers of other birds. The physical evidence of breeding condition in females consists of the abdomen becoming enlarged and rounded in shape and the vent taking on the form of a lateral slit as shown at "2" Figure 15. See WHEAT GERM OIL; VITAMIN E.

BROKEN BONES. Fractures of the wings of small birds cannot be set for several reasons: first, human fingers are too large and clumsy to work with such small bones with any chance of success; second, the resentment of these little creatures against any form of restraint is so great that it is usually impossible to even make an examination of a broken wing without the struggles of the bird aggravating the injury; third, there is no way of affixing a splint or cast to the wing of a small bird without doing more harm than good. The best course to follow is to place the bird in a cage from which the high perches have been removed and observe the droop of the injured member. If the wing hangs in a graceful droop, as it would if the bird drooped it intentionally, place food and water within easy reach of the little cripple and go on about your business; feed and water at night for the next ten days, so that the bird will not at any time be disturbed or frightened into attempting to use the injured wing. At the end of that period the injury will be healed, and there is a good chance that the bird will not be crippled.

If the wing hangs at an awkward, abnormal angle, it must be folded against the bird's side in as natural a position as possible, and then held in place by passing a narrow strip of adhesive tape twice around the body in such a manner as to leave other wing free. Some breeders have reported good results from fastening the ends of the two wings together with string or a letter clip. This might work all right with larger, heavier birds, but I have found that the small flying birds will fight this form of restraint until the injured wing is damaged beyond repair. In practically all cases where restraint is necessary the bird will be crippled; often, however, they will be able to fly good enough to take care of themselves. I have known some of these broken-winged birds to make wonderful breeders.

Leg fractures located in the femur or tibia cannot be set, since the two upper divisions of the leg are enclosed by the skin of the side. Fractures of the metatarsus can be set and held in place by placing the shank in a tube made from metal foil or stiff paper. The tube must be left loose enough so that the swelling which occurs as part of the healing process will not stop the circulation in the foot, for, should that happen for only a very short time, the foot will be lost. I have found that regardless of the location of the break, a foot sling is one of the best ways of preventing the bird from being crippled. A tube can keep the metatarsus straight, but it cannot keep the foot from being twisted to the right or left,

Figure 16.   **BROKEN BONES**

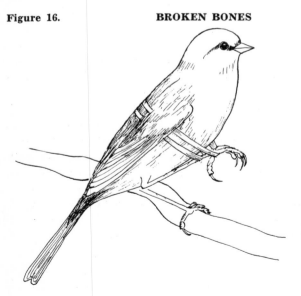

Freehand sketch by the author illustrating the correct method of putting a bird's foot in a sling in order to hold the bones of a broken leg in alignment during healing. Apologies to N. E. R. Carter, one of whose drawings was used as a rough model.

but by means of the foot sling, as illustrated in Figure 16, the foot can be held in the natural, normal position, and the bones will usually fall into their normal position and heal without difficulty. Sometimes it is necessary to make a loop around the bird's foot to keep him from taking it out of the sling. In affixing the sling the wings must be left free—otherwise the bird will be unable to get around and take care of himself. With the wings free, however, he will have little difficulty, even in a large flight.

Broken toes often result from permitting the claws to get too long or from keeping the birds in flights screened with fine-mesh wire cloth. The nails hang in the wire, and when the bird struggles to free himself, a toe is broken. Such injuries go undiscovered at the time and heal without treatment. Crippling of one of the front toes is not serious because it does not cause the bird to lose the use of the foot; injuries to one of the back toes, however, often causes the back claw to become stiff. When this happens to a female her usefulness in the breeding room is over. Her eggs will always be infertile because her foot is certain to slip at the critical moment. The situation is almost as bad when it is a male with a crippled back claw. He can no longer grasp the hen's wing with that foot, but the male does have some value as a singer.

I have only known one bird to overcome this handicap and make a good breeder. He was a hard-luck little fellow. His three nestmates had died of aspergillosis; his mother had been half sick herself and had hovered him too closely at first, causing the back claws on both feet to become **slipped** (see SLIPPED CLAW). Then, with only one baby to care for and him not able to stand in the nest, she made up her mind that it was time for a new start; so she quit him and let him get a couple of bad chillings. He grew to be about half the size of an ordinary canary of his type, which even normally was not large. The claws were set as soon as they were discovered, but one of them remained stiff. This little runt became accidentally mated with a large Yorkshire hen. I had other plans for her, but she was given a few days' exercise in a flight where this little fellow happened to be. She picked up with him and thereafter would try to kill any other male put in a cage with her. Because of the difference in their sizes, I would have expected nothing from this mating, even if both birds had good feet. The little runt solved his problem in a very unique and efficient manner, however. He would grasp the hen's wing with his one good foot, and instead of trying to balance himself, he would lean over on the other side, sometimes until his head was below the perch she was standing on, and then he would take good aim and go from there. Most of her eggs were good.

BRONCHITIS. See INFECTIOUS BRONCHITIS; AVIAN DIPH-THERIA.

BROODER PNEUMONIA. See ASPERGILLOSIS.

C

CAGES. I shall not go into a long-winded discussion of the various kinds of cages used for housing the different species of birds. That would take us far beyond the scope of this work, and beyond my qualifications, too, for that matter—for I am qualified to speak for but one group of birds on this subject, the small seed eaters. I do want to go on record, though, against that very popular and very stupid abomination, the round canary cage. That a bird is able to live in one of these contraptions says a great deal for his adaptability. It says nothing for the humanity or intelligence of his owner. Birds like corners for the same reasons that you like them; they give a sense of protection. This may be a throwback to the time when both of us crawled out of the sea and hid under a rock, but it is so very real that a large proportion of humanity would go mad if compelled to live in round rooms. Another thing, these cages offer no room for exercise, and what little room they do afford is taken up by the swing. I have watched birds bumping their heads on these swings until I felt that it would be a much better world if both cage and owner were dropped in the ash-can. If you are one of those faddists who must keep her bird in a nice round cage because that is the kind Mrs. Smith next door has for her bird, do have the sense and humanity to take the swing out and throw it away.

The best type of cage for the small varieties of singing birds is the box-type singing cage used by roller breeders. This cage is rectangular and has a solid top, back and ends. The bottom is a metal sand tray. Only the front is of wire. There are three perches—one at each end of the bottom rail and one in the middle, above the door. The least inside measurements should be 8"x12"x12". The seed and water cups should be on the outside, at the ends of the lower perches. At the end of the upper perch there should be a green-food hook. There should be two small dishes inside of the cage—one for mineral food; the other for tonic seed, soft food, etc.

Breeding cages should be constructed on the same general design. They should be at least 15"x18"x24" inside. There should be three perches: one at the lower left-hand corner; one about six inches from the first and resting on the second rail of the front; one about three or four inches from the other end and resting on the top rail of the front. This stair-step arrangement forces the bird to fly from perch to perch and leaves most of the upper part of the cages as unobstructed flying space.

The water cup is placed outside, at the end of the lower perch, a green-food hook is placed at the end of the second perch, and at the back end of the same perch there should be a round wire ring for holding the mineral-food cup. The fourth or fifth wire in the top panel at the right end of the cage—which is at the end of the top perch—is removable. The outside nest box is hung over this opening. The sand tray, which forms the bottom of the cage, rests on cleats. The ends are formed of wooden frames fitted with steel slides. Thus, when the tray and end slides are removed, three sides of the cage are wide open. You will have no trouble getting your hand inside with a big scrubbing brush. You will appreciate this feature the first time a really contagious disease gets into your plant. All cages should be finished with a hard zinc enamel that will stand boiling water for at least two minutes.

Another advantage of these cages is the fact that five or six of them can be hung in a row, the ends removed, and you have a ten or twelve foot flight cage ready for use. By having a couple of extra slides made of wire gratings you can use an extra breeding cage as a weaning cage when necessary. You can hang two of them side by side and you have a double breeder, if that is the method you prefer.

CALCIUM CARBONATE. Cuttlebone, egg shells, oyster shells, chalk, limestone, marble, and pearls are all largely composed of calcium carbonate. Birds do not get enough of this mineral in their ordinary diet; therefore, a supply must be kept constantly before them. This, true at all times, is doubly true during the breeding season, since the hen must have an extra large supply of this salt for making egg shells. For chickens, ground oyster shell is often used; for canaries, many breeders prefer cuttle bone. There are now on the market many mineral mixtures that are preferable to either of these substances, since they also contain many other mineral salts which the birds need in small quantities but do not obtain from the ordinary diet. See MINERAL FOOD.

CALCIUM GLYCERINOPHOSPHATE. This is a salt made from calcium carbonate and glycerinophosphoric acid. It is soluble in thirty parts of cold water but almost completely insoluble in boiling water. This is the substance into which the phosphates of food are converted before assimilation. Hence, it has been recommended as the most logical form in which to administer phosphates to run-down birds. It is used as a tonic for birds that are out of condition because of starvation, shipping about, acute illness, or from general neglect. It can be given in the drinking water in doses of from $\frac{1}{16}$ to $\frac{1}{8}$ grain to the ounce of water.

CALCIUM PERMANGANATE. I have never been able to learn why doctors pay so little attention to this salt. It is the calcium salt of permanganic acid. In chemical and physical properties it is very similar to the potassium salt, which is so widely used. Being less disagreeable in taste, no more poisonous to the body tissue and having antiseptic powers one hundred times greater than those of potassium permanganate, greater even than mercury bichloride (Merk's Index, 1907), it would seem that this salt is in every respect preferable to the potassium salt.

I have found no record of calcium permanganate having ever been used in the treatment of bird diseases, and I have not had the opportunity to test it for myself. But it appears to me that this substance might well replace potassium permanganate in the bird breeder's medicine cabinet, and that it might well be employed for both external and internal medication. It could be used in solutions of 1:10000 to 1:12000 and still have a greater germ-killing power than potassium permanganate solutions of the strengths usually employed, or it could be used in strengths having a greater germ-killing power but being no more toxicity than the strongest solution of potassium permanganate it is possible to make.

CALCIUM TRIBASIS PHOSPHATE. This salt is found in bone and is partly responsible for the white color of bird urine. The pure salt is not used in bird feeding or medicine, though most good mineral foods contain this salt in the form of steamed bone meal. See MINERAL FOOD.

CAMPHOR. This substance is a volatile gum derived from certain trees growing in subtropical, Asiatic countries. It has recently been synthesized by the duPont Laboratories from the gum of southern pine. Camphor has been extensively used in human medicine. It appears to be of little value in the treatment of bird diseases, however. In the past it was used in the bird room as an insecticide, for ridding cages of mites. It is now largely supplanted in this field by naphthalene and other substances which are both cheaper and more effective. See NAPHTHALENE.

CANARY NECROSIS; INFECTIOUS NECROSIS OF CANARIES. This disease has been studied by Binder, Miessner, Schern, and others. It is generally considered to be a form of hemorrhagic septicemia peculiar to canaries and other small seed-eating birds. This disease is not common in America, yet it does occur on rare occasions as an imported disease in shipments of German canaries. It is said to be quite prevalent in Europe, and in English bird literature it is often referred to by the name **Septic fever,** or simply as **septicemia.**

Etiology. The cause of infectious necrosis is a germ thought to belong to the hemorrhagic septicemia group, but differing from the germ of fowl cholera in that it does not cause disease in chickens. Pigeons, finches, mice, rabbits and guinea pigs are susceptible. The differentiation of this disease from fowl cholera by pathological lesions is much simpler than it is to differentiate the causative organisms by microscopic and cultural examinations.

Symptoms. There is nothing typical about the symptoms of this disease, unless the very fact that there is no outstanding set of symptoms which will set it off from other septicemic diseases is itself characteristic. The bird refuses food, gets very weak, and finally sits in the bottom of the cage and dies. There is fever but no one seems to have measured it. The sick bird lives from twenty-four to thirty-six hours. The period of incubation is from three to five days. All birds taken sick die. There are no spontaneous recoveries.

Morbid anatomy. The morbid changes in this disease are as unique as the symptoms are commonplace. The spleen is greatly enlarged and has a knotty or warty appearance arising from the presence of a great many yellow nodules (lumps) which vary in size from mere points to lumps of 1 mm to 1½ mm in diameter, and which make the organ so friable that it often breaks up while being removed. The liver, too, is plentifully studded with yellow nodules, which are irregular in shape and detachable from the surrounding tissue with difficulty. There may be yellow nodules in the throat and a yellow exudate in the pleural cavities.

The necrotic lesions closely resemble those of tuberculosis, and the two conditions might be confused if nothing of the history of the case were known. Tuberculosis is a chronic disease attacking the older members of the flock; canary necrosis is an acute disease affecting birds of all ages. The bird with well-developed tubercular lesions will be greatly emaciated and will have been sick for considerable time, but in canary necrosis well-developed lesions are found in birds in good flesh which have died after twenty-four hours of illness. "A" and "B" Figure 17 give a rough idea of the appearances of the spleen and liver in this disease.

Treatment. One writer recommends two grains of sodium sulphate (Glauber's salt) to each ounce of drinking water along with enough potassium permanganate to turn the water wine-red. Another breeder has recommended one teaspoonful of brandy, a few drops of paregoric, and a little red pepper be added to each one-ounce drink of water. The more authoritative writers suggest "kill and disinfect" as the only effective measure of control. Fortunately, this is one disease in which the "kill and disinfect" method, because of the short period of incubation and the short course of the illness, can be expected to be effective.

Figure 17. CANARY NECROSIS

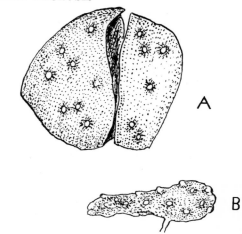

A, Liver

B, Spleen

These sketches, made from memory by the author illustrate the general appearance of the liver and spleen in Canary Necrosis. The nodules are very similar to those associated with tuberculosis.

Having never had this disease in my own flock, my experience with it is limited to the few occasions upon which I have been called upon to treat it in the flocks of others.

In all cases where I have treated diseases in the flocks of others, diagnosis has been based upon the examination of bodies sent to me, upon a description of the symptoms and lesions supplied by the breeder asking my help, or upon post mortems performed on the spot by some local veterinarian or at some laboratory in the neighborhood—this last has often been at my suggestion and the reports have usually reached me too late to be of any practical value in outlining methods of treatment. Sometimes I have had ample information of the most authoritative nature; at others I have been forced to base my diagnosis upon the sketchiest of material. In some cases I have received detailed reports of the results of my suggestions; in others I have learned of their effectiveness as much as a year or two later, when the breeder in question happened to refer someone else to me.

To all breeders writing to me who have described a disease having symptoms and lesions similar to those described above, I have given the following suggestions:

Give one teaspoonful of STROUD'S EFFERVESCENT BIRD SALTS in each quart of drinking water for the entire flock, sick and well alike, and one teaspoonful of STROUD'S SALTS NO. 1 in each quart of soft food used. If this does not bring the outbreak under control within three days discontinue the use of the effervescent mixture and add one teaspoonful of STROUD'S SALTS NO. 1 to each quart of drinking water, and please let me know the results.

In all cases to report back I have been told that the first line of treatment gave no noticeable results but that no birds died after application of the second line of treatment.

Sanitation. The sanitary measures suggested under the heading AVIAN DIPHTHERIA should be put into effect at once upon the appearance of any contagious disease in your flock. And when three or more birds die within a space of as many weeks with similar symptoms and lesions, you have a sound right for assuming that you are dealing with a serious disease which may be contagious. The sanitary measures should in all cases be maintained for a period of at least three weeks after the last sick bird has either died or recovered. I do not mean by this that your birds should be kept under unsanitary conditions at any time, although it is not necessary to be quite so strict when there is no disease on the premises.

CANARY SEED. Canary grass, probably a native grass of the Mediterranean basin, was cultivated for human food for centuries before the Canary Islands were discovered or the canary bird domesticated; but because this seed is one of the favorite foods of all small seed eating birds, and because canaries have long been the most popular of our pet birds, the two have become associated in name.

The seed is now cultivated almost exclusively for bird food. It is grown in practically all of the Western Mediterranean countries and in South America. Some varieties of canary grass are grown in the United States for hay and pasturage, and why the

American farmer has never thought of growing this seed for bird food is something I have never been able to figure out. There is no sound reason why some parts of the United States could not grow seed as good as any grown in Europe. The planting and harvesting could be handled by the same machinery that is used for wheat and the crop would be worth about four times as much.

Formerly the best grade of canary seed came from Sicily, but a few years ago much of the cultivated area was destroyed by volcanic eruption. In recent years Spain has been our chief source of high-grade seed. Now, however, Spain is disorganized by war and there is little of the very best variety of canary seed available. A fair second-grade seed comes from Morocco.

Canary seed is graded according to size, mammoth, super-mammoth, etc. These large seeds run from 52 to 72 seeds to the gram and are used almost exclusively for feeding the large English type canaries. Common singers, rollers and the other small varieties of canaries, can handle the smaller grades of canary seed better than they can these larger, more expensive grades. The seed for these small canaries, and other small birds, is first grade Moroccan seed, which runs about 108 seeds to the gram.

Good canary seed, regardless of where it was grown, must have a bright, shining, straw-colored husk, which must not have a greenish or brownish tinge. When your doubled-up fist is forced down into a bag of this seed it should sink into the seed with ease— (should it fail to do this the seed has been kiln dried)—and come out free from dust. Canary seed, when a mason jar is half filled with it, sealed and permitted to stand overnight, should not give off a musty odor.

Canary seed comprises one-half of the diet of roller canaries and three-fourths of the seed diet of the other varieties. Tame sparrows, some finches and parrakeets will eat little of any other seed while a supply of good canary seed is available.

CANARY TYPHOID. In 1929 I described a contagious disease of canaries that I then thought to be identical with fowl typhoid. The limited amount of study I have been able to give to this disease since that time has left grave doubts in my mind as to the correctness of my former opinion. In my book, "Diseases of Canaries," published in 1933, I discussed this condition under the heading, "An Unidentified Disease of Canaries."

Characterization. The disease is an acute, contagious septicemia attacking canaries, finches and sparrows. It is not known whether or not other species are susceptible. The disease is not very common, but I have had reports of its presence from points as widely separated as Massachusetts and California. Little could be learned about the source of the infection or its mode of transmission. It is noteworthy, however, that in five out of seven outbreaks occurring within a very short period and in widely separated sections of the United States, the owners informed me that they had been using a particular brand of bird food. One ingredient of this food was sun-dried egg yolk. Because I knew the manufacturer of this food, knew him to be a fine upright man, who by honest efforts had built up his business from a shoestring, I informed him of my findings. I am glad to be able to say that not a single case of this disease associated with the use of his food has since come to my attention.

Etiology. The cause of this disease is an organism that resembles more or less closely **B sanguinarium** and **B. pullorum** in its growth on gelatin and agar. It was also grown in milk, in which it produced no change other than increased acidity. Microscopic examinations were not made for the good and sufficient reasons that I had no microscope at the time and could not get anyone else to make them for me. I deeply regret that I have not been able to work out the identity of this disease, but maybe the information I am able to give will be considered of even more importance by practical breeders. In a moment I shall describe features of this infection by which it can be easily recognized in canaries and sparrows and outline an absolutely specific line of treatment. It may be, as first thought, that this disease is identical with fowl typhoid; it may be that it is caused by B. pullorum; and it is possible that it is an entirely distinct disease to which only the small seed eaters are susceptible. I am not able to accept the latter view, however, since the only evidence available indicates that a possible source of infection may have been improperly sterilized egg products.

Symptoms. While the causative agent of this infection is still shrouded in doubt, the symptoms are so characteristic and constant as to make positive identification very simple, so unique that descriptions sent to me from breeders in different parts of the country are almost word for word replicas of one another.

The birds usually take sick within forty-eight hours of exposure. The first day—or during the first phase of the illness, which may be of considerably less duration than a day—the bird fluffs out its feathers until it looks like a ball, sits hunched up, breathing a little faster than usual, and sleeping most of the time. During this first period of the illness the bird may stand on one foot. It eats little or nothing but drinks a great deal. The bowels are loose and the droppings watery, but their discharge excites little or no pain. During the second day, or second period of the illness, the bird eats nothing at all and drinks very little. Being very weak, the bird grasps the perch firmly with both feet, hardly ever leaving it. The droppings become thick, white and chalky in appearance and their passage painful. The bird either falls from the perch and dies, or having left the perch, is unable to return to it and sits in a corner of the cage until death comes, which is within from 12 to 48 hours after the onset of the first symptoms.

Morbid anatomy. I should have mentioned in the discussion of the symptoms that the abdomen is always greatly enlarged and dark in color. The most characteristic lesion of this disease is a characteristic enlargement of the liver to five or more times normal size. The pressure inside the abdominal cavity is so great that the liver will force its way out through a very small incision. In this case, unlike those enormously enlarged mulberry livers found in peracute diphtheria and psittacosis, the connective tissues of the capsule of the organ remain intact. The color of the organ is not greatly changed, though it may be of a slightly yellowish cast and be a little more opaque than normal. In some cases it may be a little darker than normal and contain small, point-like hemorrhages. One very noticeable characteristic of this disease is the presence of golden-yellow bands or lacings (ecchymosis) just below the capsule of the liver, running around the organ more or less parallel with its edges and separated from them by a space of from one to three millimeters. These lacings, examined with a hand lens, appear

Figure 18.   **CANARY TYPHOID**

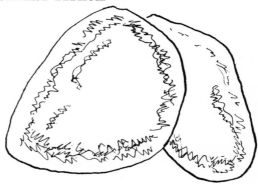

This sketch gives a general idea of distribution of ecchymosis in the liver of a canary affected with Canary Typhoid.

Sketched by the author from memory.

to be areas of fatty degeneration. The healthy, unclouded endothelium of the capsule is stretched over them like a covering of cellophane. Death is undoubtedly the result of pressure on the organs of respiration and circulation. Figure 18 is a sketch of the liver of a bird that died of canary typhoid.

The intestines are inflamed and there may be punctiform (point-like) hemorrhages in the deep-lying tissue of the duodenum.

The kidneys may be enlarged and a little lighter in color than normal. The spleen may be enlarged too, but there is nothing characteristic or of diagnostic value about these lesions.

The blood is clotted and very dark. There are no hemorrhages into any of the body cavities.

Control and treatment. As indicated above, this disease is highly contagious and may wipe out an entire flock within a very few days. The same sanitary measures as recommended for AVIAN DIPHTHERIA and other contagious diseases are required. They must be put into operation at once. There is a disadvantage in attempting to control this disease by sanitary measures, however, since we do not know how it is spread, excepting by contact. And it does spread throughout the plant very rapidly even though contacts are guarded against. On the other hand, the short period of incubation and the short course of the disease tend to operate to the breeder's advantage—for once the disease is stopped, it is stopped for good. I have never heard of it playing a return engagement.

Medical treatment for the sick can be effective only during the first phase of the illness, but it is then extremely effective. One teaspoonful of STROUD'S SALTS NO. 1, added to each quart of drinking water for the entire flock will stop this disease within 24 hours. There will be no new cases after the first dose of medicine is given, and those sick birds that are in the early stage of the illness will quickly recover. If my treatment is unavailable, one teaspoonful of sodium perborate or two ounces of commercial peroxide of hydrogen may be added to each quart of drinking water. There are reasons for believing that calcium permanganate or potassium chlorate added to all drinking water in the proportion of six drops of saturated solution to each ounce of drinking water would give the same results. All of these substances are powerful oxidizing agents that cause poisoning by oxidizing the hemoglobin of the blood to methemoglobin. I have not been able to figure out the relation between this poisonous reaction and the curative properties of these drugs, but I am certain that some such relation exists.

CANKER. See AVIAN DIPHTHERIA.

CANCER. Tumorous and cancerous growths occur in all species of birds. The structure of some of these growths closely resembles human cancer, and they are important for that reason alone, since they occur so rarely that most breeders would live out their lives without ever meeting a case of true bird cancer. Ward and Gallagher, "Diseases of Domesticated Birds," Macmillan Company, have made a digest of the literature on this subject to which the interested reader is referred.

Exudates occurring in air cavities and bone sinuses might be mistaken for cancer by the breeder unfamiliar with pathology, but a careful naked-eye examination is almost certain to detect the difference. Exudates are composed of dead material, not living, growing cell.

Tumor-like swelling of the joints, particularly those of the legs and feet are usually caused by chronic bacterial infections or gouty deposits of urate in the joints.* See GOUT; HEMORRHAGIC SEPTICEMIA; TUBERCULOSIS.

CARBOLIC ACID. This is a product of the distillation of coal-tar. It is used as an antiseptic, disinfectant, and insecticide. Because it is very poisonous to birds, it must be used carefully around the bird room. This warning applies to all of the coal-tar disinfectants. In one case to come to my attention, a breeder, wishing to rid his bird room of mites, took all of the birds out of the room and had it sprayed with a mixture of coal oil and coal-tar disinfectant. After permitting the room to air out for a few days he returned the birds to it. They all became ill, developed sores on their feet and abdomens and under their wings. Some had blisters around their eyes. A number died. Thinking that he was dealing with an outbreak of diphtheria, the gentleman wrote to me. I advised him to remove all birds from the room for at least a month and to return them to it a few at a time. He followed this advice and the birds that had not already died, recovered.

---

* **Note:** Recently, two birds were dissected that showed well-developed sarcomaform (like scarcoma, malignant tumors of the bone, muscles and connective tissues) tumors of the ilium, located directly below the posterior lobes of the kidneys. One bird had been killed because of blindness; the other had died of a hemorrhage from the liver. The growths were identical as to size, shape, and position, and, in both, that on the right side of the spine was slightly larger than that on the left side. It was later established that these birds had suffered from metallic poisoning resulting from the corrosion of a copper vessel that was soldered on the inside with a lead-tin solder. This suggests the possibility that myeloma (a highly fatal form of sarcoma involving the bone marrow in man) may result from chronic poisoning with minute quantities of heavy metals. See LEAD POISONING.

In another case a breeder who had read an article on hand washing had a bright idea for improving the process by adding a teaspoonful of Lysol to the water. He washed 75 birds. They all died.

CASCARA SAGRADA—U.S.P. This is the bark of a tree growing in the northwestern part of the United States. It is employed in human medicine in the form of an extract as a cathartic and tonic. There are many preparations of cascara, but the **Aromatic Fluid Extract** of **Cascara Sagrada,** which contains magnesia, compound spirits of orange, and 25 per cent glycerine, is the only one I have used on birds. It is a valuable constituent of a number of bird tonics. The following are useful:

(1) Aromatic cascara, one part; fluid extract of gentian, one part; licorice powder, one part; tincture of opium, one part; 50% ethyl alcohol, eight parts; glycerine, two parts.

Dissolve the licorice in the alcohol and then add the other ingredients; mix well; filter through paper; and bottle. Dose is three to ten drops to the ounce of drinking water. Also mixed with water in the proportion 1:5 and given into the beak in from one to three drop doses.

This preparation is fine for birds that have suffered an attack of food poisoning or apoplectiform septicemia and are so nervous they are about to jump out of their skins. With the opium omitted it makes a good general tonic for run-down birds.

(2) This is the same as (1) excepting that four minims of beachwood creosote are added to each ounce of the preparation. Doses the same as for (1).

This preparation is of value for the treatment of inflammation of the intestines and respiratory tract, but because of the creosote being irritating to the digestive mucosa it is not suitable for prolonged administration.

Cascara may also be combined with sarsaparilla, quassia and a number of other extracts with good results.

CASTOR OIL. Almost every poultry and bird book recommends castor oil as a cathartic for birds. The dose for chickens is usually placed at one teaspoonful, but some persons recommend twice that much. The dose recommended for a canary is usually two or three drops. Now, I do not know anything about the action of castor oil on chickens, but I do know that I have never seen a canary or sparrow survive a two drop dose of this nauseous substance; that is, of course, where the two drops were actually consumed. The way these little fellows fight against taking this substance usually assures that most of it goes on their feathers or on the giver—which only goes to show that the birds often have more sense than we who keep them. A single drop of castor oil is sufficient to make a small bird seriously ill. I know of no good results to be obtained from the employment of this substance, or any other drastic cathartic for that matter, in either human or bird medicine that could not be obtained by less drastic and more sensible means. I am not in favor of using oils as cathartics and laxatives for birds, but if you are one of those persons who just cannot resist the temptation to dose both your children and your birds with oils, I suggest that you use olive oil. It, at least, will do no harm.

CATHARTICS. Birds that are sanely treated never need cathartics. In fevers they may need saline laxatives; in some cases where they have become constipated as a result of being kept on too rich a diet, or on a diet of dry seed and no green food, they may be benefited by the use of syrup of buckthorn or cascara; but in most cases the bowels can be perfectly regulated by supplying the ailing birds with all the fresh green food they care to eat. It should always be remembered that indiscriminate dosing can always be depended upon to do more harm than good.

Of course, there are cases, particularly where the birds have been given a vermifuge (a substance for expelling worms), where a cathartic is necessary; but even in these cases a double dose of some good saline laxative will give better results than one of the more drastic cathartics.

CECA. These are the bind guts or appendages, two in number, that branch off from the main intestinal tract at a point just above the cloaca. They are present in robins, blackbirds, pigeons, chickens, turkeys, water fowls and a great many other species of birds; they are not present in canaries, sparrows, finches and some of the other species of small birds. In chickens and turkeys the ceca vary in length from four to seven inches. Their function is thought to be the absorption of nourishment that has escaped absorption in the main intestinal tract. They are the seat of lesions in coccidiosis and entro-hepatitis.

CEREBELLUM. This is the part of the brain to which the sensory nerves are connected. It is located at the base of the skull and partly overlapped by the cerebrum. See BRAIN. See "A," Figure 19.

CEREBRUM. This is the thinking brain. It fills the front and top

Figure 19.   CEREBELLUM AND CEREBRUM

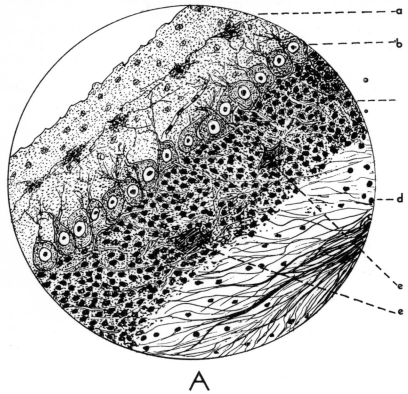

A

A, Cerebellum of a canary

a, Molecular layer, showing faintly the nuclei of the supporting cell; the "spider" or star cells, and a single capillary in which the blood cells are seen moving in single file.

b, The Purkinje (pronounced poor-kin'-gee) cells.

c, Granular layer, containing supporting cells and large star cells, two of which are shown.

d, Medullary or fibrous layer, containing nerve fibers and supporting cells.

of the cranial cavity and is divided longitudinally into two hemispheres. In birds there are no nerves connecting the cerebrum directly with the spinal cord. See BRAIN. See "B," Figure 19.

CHALK. This is a natural mineral composed largely of calcium carbonate and calcium sulphate. It is sometimes given to birds to peck at as a source of minerals. See MINERAL FOOD.

CHICKS, DEAD IN SHELL. Chicks may die in the shell from a number of different causes. If the hen that laid the egg received an insufficiency of minerals and vitamins while she was making it, the chick will be weak and very apt to die at hatching time. I once lost 85% of my chicks in the shell as a result of iodide defi-

Figure 19 (continued)

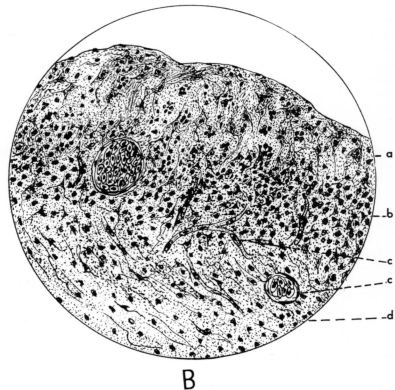

B

B, Cerebrum of a canary

a, Molecular layer of the cortex
b, Granular layer
c, A large and a small capillary
d, Fibrous layer

Notice that the order of the cellular arrangement is much less regular in the cerebrum than in the cerebellum. The large and small, generally triangular shaped cells, are the nerve cells, and they are scattered more or less indiscriminately throughout the area. The small, round bodies are the nuclei of the supporting cells.

Tissue fixed in ½ per cent silver nitrate and stained by a modification of Mallery's eosin-methylene blue process. The drawings were made free-hand by the author, using a magnification of 445×.

ciency. By adding a little potassium iodide to the drinking water (8 drops of saturated solution to each quart of water) the trouble was overcome and the same hens gave me full clutches of hatchable eggs. Since that time I have avoided trouble from this source by keeping before my birds a mineral food containing the correct amount of iodides.

Chilling is another cause of chicks dying in the shell. This is often caused by turning the lights entirely out at night. Sometimes hens will lay after they have been set. The shell of the egg is made during the night preceding laying. The canary hen lays a very large egg in proportion to her weight, and her blood does not usually contain enough lime to make a good shell and still take care of the other body functions. So, when she is making shell, the hen gets very hungry for lime during the night. Many hens will leave the nest to eat lime, and if the room is so dark that they cannot find their way back to the nest, the eggs in which development has started will be chilled and lost. Permitting the hen to bathe during the first ten days of incubation may result in the eggs getting chilled, and chilling during this period is pretty certain to kill the chick. After the tenth day the eggs can often be permitted to cool down to room temperature for twelve hours without killing the chick, but such chilling will delay hatching for several days.

Dryness is another common cause of chicks being found dead in the shell. When the air is too dry the chick sticks to the shell and cannot get his head around to open it. You know that at hatching time the chick opens the egg by turning round and round, dragging the tip of his beak against the shell until it is cut open. Naturally, when he is stuck, he cannot do this.

Dampness as well as dryness may prevent the chick from hatching. There is an air cell at the end of the egg. During incubation, evaporation of moisture from the egg causes the size of this air cell to increase. If the evaporation does not take place the chick will be so large that there will be no room for him to move his head, and he will be unable to open the shell. The solution for these two problems consists of withholding the bath from the hen during the first ten days of incubation and keeping it constantly before her during the last three days. By the tenth day the necessary evaporation has taken place; then the hen, returning to the nest after her bath and sitting on the eggs with her moist feathers, subjects them to a sort of a vapor bath which softens the membrane and guarantees against the chick sticking to the shell. The reader will notice that I have not mentioned loud noises as a cause of chicks being found dead in the shell. Toward the end of the first week of incubation, when the blood vessels are forming, it is said that any loud noise will cause the vessels to rupture and the embryo (developing creature before birth or hatching) to die. This is probably true in the case of larger birds. It is not true in the case of eggs from healthy canaries. I have had lightning strike the building in which my birds are kept a number of times during the middle of the breeding season without any chicks being killed—and if there is any noise louder than Kansas thunder at close range, I would like very much to know what it is.

Touching the egg may cause the chick to be killed. I have picked up canary eggs and held them to the light during all stages of incubation without killing the chicks but in other cases the chicks have been killed by touching the eggs. After the ninth day of incubation the danger is passed so far as canary eggs are concerned, but the eggs of some finches and those of canary hybrids will not stand touching before the eleventh day and are sometimes ruined by it then. I have found it a good policy to candle eggs without touching them. This can be done by holding the nest so that the light falls on the eggs obliquely. The infertile eggs will appear lighter in color and less opaque than the fertile eggs.

CHICKS, DEAD IN NEST. Baby birds may die in the nest from a number of causes. The nest may be too dark, and the hen, not being able to see, may be unable to feed the chicks, or she may bite their heads or feet off while she is cleaning the nest. Chicks are often killed by chasing the hen off the nest, for in her fright she may step on them or drive her claws into them. The feeding as well as the laying hen—and after the first nest the two are often the same— may leave the nest at night to eat; if she cannot see to return to it, the chicks are apt to be chilled and lost. Putting the lights out without first seeing to it that all the hens are on their nests is another fruitful cause of nest losses. I find it a good plan to turn the lights out one at a time; thus darkening the room gradually and giving the birds plenty of time to get settled for the night. A single light is shaded with a piece of paper and left burning. This is sufficient to permit the hens to return to their nests, should they leave them during the night, but it does not interfere with the sleep of the other birds. Chicks may be lost by chilling at feathering time. Many hens do not hover their chicks after the tenth day. If there are three or four chicks in the nest they will be able to keep each other warm, but if there are only one or two birds in the nest and the weather is chilly, they are apt to be found dead in the morning.

During the first two or three days of life, chicks are often dragged out of the nest in the hen's feathers. They are found on the floor of the cage, stiff and cold. Chilling at this age is not fatal, however. If these apparently dead babies are returned to the nest and thawed out they will be as good as new in a few hours.

There are a very few cases where the hen is so anxious about her new babies that she is afraid to leave the nest to get food for them. This is more often the case with young hens rearing their first nest than with more experienced birds. If she is mated with an older cock, he will bring her the food and see that she attends to the babies, but if she is alone or mated to a young cock, the babies may be lost. Such losses need not occur in the large bird room, however, since the young babies may be given to some good feeding hen and her older babies given to the young mother. Chicks four or five days old will tell that young hen what she is supposed to do in language she cannot misunderstand.

Mites may kill chicks in the nest by sucking all the blood out of their bodies. It is easy to tell chicks killed by mites, for their bodies are white and bloodless.

For every chick that is lost from all of these causes combined, a hundred are lost because the old birds are not given food that is fit for a baby bird to eat. Those breeders who are forever cursing their hens for not feeding should spend a little time looking into their feeding methods. It is natural for a hen to feed her babies. If she does not do so, it is 100 to 1 that the fault is that she has no food fit to give them or that she, herself, is half sick from eating stale food and is unable to feed them for that reason. This is certain to be true where a number of hens in the same flock refuse to feed. See ASPERGILLOSIS; RED MITES.

CHINOSOL. This is a complex organic dyestuff with powerful antiseptic properties. It is used in human medicine as an antiseptic for the mucous membranes and as a contraceptive.

In 1931 William C. Dustin recommended the use of chinosol for the treatment of aspergillosis. I have not experimented with this drug in the treatment of contagious diseases. I have tested its toxicity for canaries and found that it can be given in the drinking water in solutions of from 1:5000 to 1:15000 for two or three months at a time without causing serious poisoning. A two per cent solution introduced into the nostrils gives good results in some cases of nasal infection.

CHLORIDE OF LIME, CALCIUM HYPOCHLORITE, BLEACH-ING POWDER. This preparation is produced by passing chlorine gas over freshly slaked lime. It comes on the market as a creamy-white powder with a strong, suffocating odor of chlorine, and which draws moisture from the air (deliquescence). Fresh chloride of lime contains about 35 per cent chlorine gas, but, if exposed to the air, it loses this chlorine very rapidly. It is this property of giving off free chlorine which makes this substance one of the most powerful disinfectants known; its cheapness makes it one of the most prac-tical for use where large areas or large masses of material, like city drinking water and chicken yards, must be treated. It has been found that the most resistant bacterial spores are killed within a few hours in water containing chloride of lime in the proportion of 1:300000. There is no quicker or surer way of disinfecting the poultry yard than sprinkling it liberally with chloride of lime, turn-ing the surface under, and then either sprinkling it with water or waiting for a rain. The gas will work its way through the soil, destroying all forms of life. The fact that the gas is soon evaporated (**lost** or **dispersed** would probably be better words), prevents this substance from permanently poisoning the soil.

Chloride of lime may be used for cleaning floors, walls, etc., but because of the unsightly lime deposits it leaves behind, most persons prefer to convert it into the sodium salt. This is done by adding three pounds of carbonate of soda to each gallon of water used, bringing the water to a boil, and then adding one pound of chloride of lime for each gallon of solution. The solution is then permitted to cool, filtered through cloth or paper, and stored in tightly corked jugs. One teacupful—six ounces—of this solution added to three gallons of water will give a solution which will kill all forms of microscopic life very rapidly.

Caution. Any of these solutions of chloride of lime will take the skin off the hands so fast you won't know what it is all about. A drop of the strong stock solution spattered into an eye might cause blindness. Chlorine attacks iron, causing it to rust badly. Birds or chickens should never be permitted to come in contact with fresh chloride of lime. Where it is used for cleaning up yards, the chickens should be kept out of those yards for at least three weeks, and certainly until there has been at least one good rain.

CHOLERA. See FOWL CHOLERA; HEMORRHAGIC SEPTI-CEMIA; HOG CHOLERA; B. PARATYPHOSUS B INFECTION.

CHRYSANTHEMUM FLOWERS, PYRETHRUM. This is a brown-ish-yellow powder made from the petals of a flower native to

Western Asia and Asia Minor. Its constituents are: volatile oil; chrysanthemic acid; pyrethrotoxic acid; chrysanthemic; and possibly a crystaline glucoside. It is very poisonous to all insects but

Figure 20.   **CIRCULATORY SYSTEM**

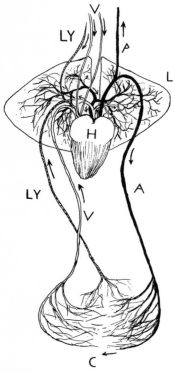

A diagrammatic sketch of the circulatory system of a bird.

H, Heart

A, Arteries

L, Lungs

V, Veins

LY, Lymphatics

C, Capillaries

Drawn by the author.

harmless .to animals and birds, and for that reason it is the best and safest powder that can be used in nests.* I never use this pow-

---

* **Note:** Many of the makers of insect powder have abandoned the use of pyrethrum flowers and substituted a mixture of the active principles extracted from the flowers and roots of this plant and sold under the name PYRETHINS. I believe that these substances have recently been synthetized. Powders containing 0.60 per cent of pyrethins are many times stronger than those formerly on the market containing 85 per cent pyrethrum flowers. They may be used in the nest lining and the nest may be liberally powdered at the time the bird is set. They should not be used after the eggs are set or on babies under ten days old, and my limited experience to date indicates that it is not necessary. No mites have been found in nesting material of nests that were powdered at the time they were made but not powdered thereafter. Examinations were made at the time the babies left the nests. The nests were slowly heated to a temperature that would have caused any mites present to crawl out onto a white paper, where they could have been easily seen.

der on birds big enough to fly, excepting hens with babies, but
for powdering nests, it is invaluable. I make it a practice to powder
each nest with pyrethrum when I give it to the hen, when I set
her, two days before the babies are due to hatch and when the
babies are ten days old. See SODIUM FLUORIDE.

CIRCULATORY SYSTEM. The circulatory system of birds consists of the heart, arteries, veins, capillaries, and lymphatics. Figure
20 gives in diagrammatic form a rough idea of the arrangement and
functions of these parts.

Heart. The heart, the central organ of the circulatory system,
is a powerful muscular pump, the function of which is to force
blood through the arteries. Avian hearts vary considerably in
shape. The heart of an ostrich is short and thick, that of a chicken
is somewhat elongated, and that of a canary is broad across the
auricles with the ventricular portion long and tapering. It is from
$\frac{3}{16}$ to $\frac{1}{4}$ of an inch wide at the top of the ventricles and quite a
bit wider above that point. The upper part of the organ, i. e., the
auricles, are a dull, silvery-gray in color; the lower part, the ventricular portion, is of the reddish-brown color common to muscular
tissue.

There are four cavities in the heart. The two upper cavities
are called **auricles**—as you may have guessed—while the two lower
cavities are called **ventricles.** It is the function of the auricles to
receive blood from the veins and deliver it to the ventricles; it
is the function of the ventricles to deliver the blood to the arteries.
From this it is seen that the ventricles have by far the most difficult part of the task and, to perform it, they are constructed of
thick, heavy walls formed from innumerable bands and layers of
interwoven muscular fibers. These heart muscles and those of the
gizzard are designated **smooth** to distinguish them from the **striated**
muscles of locomotion. They differ from the latter in that the
fibers lie directly against each other, while each fiber of a striated
muscle is enclosed in a sheath of serous membrane. The avian heart
differs from the mammalian heart in that there is no tricuspid
(three leaf) valve. The right auricular-ventricular opening is closed
by a strong muscular fold or flap.

When the auricles are relaxed, blood from the veins flows into
the right auricle and blood from the lungs flows into the left auricle
through the pulmonary vein. At the same time the ventricles are
contracting and blood from the right ventricle is being forced into
the pulmonary artery for aeration in the lungs, while blood from
the left ventricle is being forced into the aorta for distribution

throughout the body. At this instant the heart is said to be in **systole.** Then the ventricles relax while the auricles contract, and blood flows from the right auricle into the right ventricle and from the left auricle into the left ventricle. At this instant the heart is said to be in **diastole.** One systole and one diastole make up one complete heart beat.

The reader may have noticed that in all of my descriptions of diseases I have made no mention of the rate of the pulse—the first thing the doctor determines when he calls on you. The truth of the matter is that it is not easy to take a bird's pulse. According to Loer, who opened the birds and held their hearts in his fingers in order to count the beats, a chicken's heart beats about 135 times per minute; a pigeon's heart about 145. Ducks have a heart beat—determined by listening to the heart through the chest wall—by **ausculation,** that is, of from 150 to 180 times per minute. I have never been able to determine the rate of a canary's heart beat. I have read statements that fixed its rate at anywhere from 300 to 1,000 per minute. When a canary's breast is held against the ear, the heart sounds can be plainly heard; they cannot be counted, though, for they sound like the roar of an aeroplane motor. This subject should be studied by means of a microphone and an electrical recording device, but I have read of no such studies being made.

The lower part of the heart is enclosed in a serous sac called the **pericardium.** In some diseases this sac fills with serous, fibrinous, or gelatinous exudate. This condition is called **pericarditis,** which simply means inflammation of the pericardium. There are other conditions in which bacteria sometimes lodge and grow on the inner surface of the heart, setting up an inflammation there. This causes a change in the shape of the heart valves and prevents them from closing tightly; thus permitting some of the blood to be forced back in the wrong direction, **regurgitated.** This is called **endocarditis.** See AVIAN DIPHTHERIA; PSITTACOSIS; FOWL CHOLERA; FOWL TYPHOID.

The arteries. On leaving the heart the aorta (the largest of the arteries) gives off a large branch which passes up the neck and may be plainly seen where it passes over the crop. The aorta itself makes a "U" turn and extends down the length of the body, close to the spine, as far as the coccygeal (tail bone), giving off numerous branches along the way.

Veins. The veins parallel the arteries throughout the body and are considerably larger, which is necessary because the blood in the veins moves much slower than that in the arteries. As the blood in the veins is also under much less pressure than that in the arteries, the walls of the veins are much thinner than are those of the arteries. Figure 21 gives some idea of the appearance of a cross section of a small artery and its accompanying vein and of their relative size and structure.

Figure 21.

The general construction of a vein and artery.

A, Artery

V, Vein

a, v, n, the small artery, vein and nerve that supply the walls of the larger vessels. Notice that the artery is empty and the vein is filled with blood. This is usually the case after death. Sometimes the lymphatic will also be contained in the same stroma (muscular coating) with the vein and artery. In structure it is identical with the vein, but can be distinguished from it by the fact that the lymphatics do not contain blood cells. In health they are usually found empty or containing a few lymphocytes. In morbid conditions they may be packed with lymphocytes, which are easily distinguished from the red blood cells.

Freehand sketch by the author, using a magnification of about $445\times$.

CIRCULATORY SYSTEM

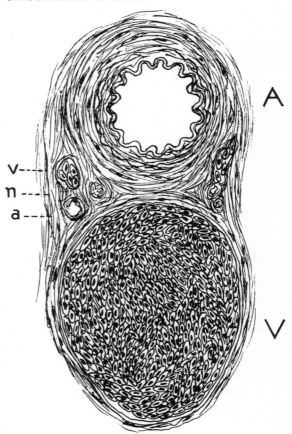

The blood from the body is returned to the heart by a single large vein called the **ascending aorta.** Blood from the head and neck is returned by means of two veins, which are connected by a cross-branch at the base of the skull. I cannot escape the opinion that it is this provision which permits birds to sleep with their heads turned back **over their shoulders** without getting cricks in their necks.

Capillaries. These are small vessels which weave their way through all of the soft tissues of the body and carry blood from the arteries to the veins. They are so small that the blood cells have to pass through them in single file in some places. Their walls are so thin that they cannot be seen under the microscope. The capillary is seen as a string of blood cells. It is here that the chemical transfer of oxygen for carbon dioxide takes place. Much of the fluid (plasma) of the blood escapes through the walls of the capillaries and flows between and around the tissue cells, bathing them at all times.

Lymphatics. It is the function of the lymphatics to return tissue fluids to the blood stream. The main lymphatic duct enters the ascending aorta just above the right auricle. Unlike mammals, birds have no superficial lymphatics and their **deep seated** lymphatic system contains very few glands. The two largest are located in the neck, at the point where it passes between the clavicles, one on each side; there are several small ones located at the base of the jaw, near the quadrate; but for the most part they are replaced by plexuses (complex knots of tubes or nerves are called plexuses) of small lymph ducts.

The function of mammalian lymph glands appears to be that of guarding the blood stream from harmful substances or organisms picked up by the lymph from the tissue. When a foci of infection develops the lymph gland through which that area drains becomes enlarged and inflamed and very sore, as you very well know from the many times those in your neck, armpits, or groins have become much sorer than the pimple that started the trouble, but they stop the infection from reaching the blood stream. The few lymph glands that birds do have seem to be located in such a manner as to guard the principal avenues by which infection is most likely to gain entrance to the blood stream.

In canaries the two lymph glands in the neck are about the size of maw seed; those at the base of the jaw are normally invisible to the naked eye, though I have seen them as large as number eight shot in a case of mastoiditis. In tuberculosis the lymph glands at the base of the neck are often involved and may contain gritty deposits.

CITRIC ACID. This is the acid of citrus fruit—oranges, lemons, limes, grapefruit. Because it is non-poisonous, it is a valuable constituent of many medical preparations for both human and avian use; and, because it can be converted into solid citrocarbonates, it is very useful in the preparation of effervescent mixtures. Effervescent mixtures containing citric acid are much more valuable in the treatment of fevers than are those which contain only tartaric acid. The action of tartaric acid is principally on the bowels; that of citric acid is principally on the kidneys.

CITROCARBONATE. There is no chemical compound by this name, but when one part of dry powdered citric acid is mixed with two parts of bicarbonate of soda, the mixture becomes moist, doughy, very cold, and gives off carbon dioxide, causing the paste to swell. Now, if this mixture is dried in a warming oven, crushed to a powder, and placed in tightly stoppered jars, where it will keep indefinitely, you have the preparation we are now discussing. One teaspoonful of citrocarbonate added to a glass of water makes a delightful effervescent drink of sharp, pleasing taste and slightly alkaline reaction. It acts as an anti-acid in the stomach and blood and as a mild antiseptic and diuretic in the kidneys. It is wonderful for restoring the alkaline balance to the blood stream and for gently promoting the removal of waste products through the kidneys. It is the best known pick-me-up for the morning after. In human medicine it is administered in doses of one to two teaspoonfuls in a glass of water three or four times per day. Thousands of persons take this preparation night and morning with considerable benefit to their general health, for it is, or is a constituent of, most of the effervescent mixtures on the market.

Effervescent mixtures can be made in three ways: by using tartaric acid and bicarbonate of soda (Seidlitz powder); by using acid sodium phosphate and bicarbonate of soda (effervescent sodium phosphate); and by using citric acid and bicarbonate of soda (Citrocarbonate). Each of these preparations has its own particular virtue; they have the common virtue, however, of rapid solubility. Salines, like sodium sulphate and normal sodium phosphate, and drugs, like the salicylates, which are not readily soluble in cold water, can be gotten into solution quickly and conveniently by incorporating them in effervescent mixtures, which makes them easy and pleasant to take and combines their virtues with those of the drugs added to them. Some of these preparations are extremely valuable.

Citrocarbonate can be used in the treatment of fevers; for the reduction of fat; for bringing over-fat birds into breeding condition; for restoring the alkaline balance of birds suffering from septicemic diseases, for tightening the feathers of birds in soft moult, and for reducing the enlarged livers and swollen feet resulting from too close confinement and overfeeding on rich, protein foods—this is a gouty condition.

I believe that I am the first to suggest or use citrocarbonate and the effervescent mixtures containing it in the treatment of bird diseases. It is one of the foundation stones upon which rests STROUD'S SPECIFIC, which has saved more birds from fatal septicemias than any and all other preparations combined.

CLEAR EGGS.   Clear eggs may result from a number of causes. The male may be infertile; the male and female may not have mated; coition may not have been complete (see BROKEN BONES); the hen may have been in a weakened, run-down condition and unable to produce hatchable eggs; the bird's diet may have been deficient in some material essential to reproduction; or the eggs may have been chilled before they were set or shortly afterwards. Whenever the breeder is confronted with this condition he should consider all the possibilities before he starts to blame the persons from whom he purchased his stock—the chances are always better than even that the fault lies in their owner or environment rather than in the birds themselves.

During the winter of 1939 and 1940 I had a chance to examine microscopically the testicles of more than 100 sparrows that had been killed in traps. Between the months of November and February, not one testicle containing spermatozoa was found. The cells of the germinal layers of the testicular epithelia were largely exfoliated and filled the lumins of the tubes. See GENERATIVE SYSTEM.

It is reasonable to assume that a similar seasonal sterility occurs in caged birds, which should be a forceful argument against off-season breeding.

Birds that have become sterile because they have been fed on mustard seed, or have received an insufficiency of the necessary vitamins will usually recover their breeding powers as soon as the dietetic errors have been corrected. The best foods for overcoming sterility are natural foods. For chickens this means live insects, raw meat, wild greens, permission to run on a piece of new, clean ground that has been recently spaded or plowed; for canaries it means fresh egg food, good hemp seed (see HEMP SEED), dandelions, chickweed, and other flowering or seeding weeds and grasses; for sparrows and finches it means, in addition to the above, plenty of live meal worms or other insects. See VITAMIN E; STERILITY.

CLOACA. This is the terminal pouch at the lower end of the intestinal tract into which the bowels, ureters, and **vasa deferentiae** of the male, or oviduct of the female, empty.   See DIGESTIVE TRACT.

COCCIDIOSIS. This is a disease in which the mucous cells, usually those of the intestinal tract, are invaded by a protozoan parasite (**protozoa** are single-cell, microscopic animals) known as **Eimeria (Coccidium) avian,** and to which all species of birds are susceptible. It causes enormous losses among birds held in crowded, unsanitary quarters or on long-used, worm-contaminated ground; particularly

Figure 22.   **COCCIDIOSIS**

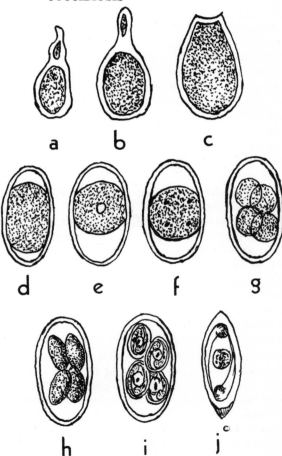

Coccidium Avian

The figures "a" to "j" show progressively the stages of development of the organism during the oocyst (egg) stage of its existence as worked out by Fantham — After Fantham, London Zoological S o c i e t y, 1910.

Note:. These are only a few of the forms taken by this organism, but they are the ones most easily recognized under the microscope.

among chickens, pigeons, turkeys and closely confined and crowded birds of zoological gardens.

Etiology. The life history of the coccidium avian has been admirably worked out by Fantham, Proceedings of the Zoological Society, London, 1910, page 708.

In Figure 22 the illustrations (a) to (j) show some of the stages in the development of the parasite that are easily recognized under the microscope. These forms can usually be found in the intestinal contents.

Briefly, the parasite, taken in with the food, invades an epithalial cell of the duodenum, where it grows and multiplies at the expense of the host-cell. When the original host-cell has been destroyed the parasites desert it and invade new cells. This continues until large areas of the intestinal mucosa, so necessary for the absorption of nourishment, have been destroyed. Since the organisms multiply very rapidly, both by sexual and asexual reproduction, large numbers of them are passed out in the droppings, to pass the infection along to other birds by contaminating food and water. The coccidium assumes many forms, but the ones most easily recognized under the microscope are those of the **oocyst** (egg) stage which are illustrated in Figure 22. In this stage the cell is oval in shape, with the granular mass in the center surrounded by a highly refractive zone with double-contured borders.

Diagnosis. Diagnosis is established by examination of the dropping and recognition of the parasites which are usually abundant. The material is placed in a watch glass and broken up with a little salt solution. A loopful (a **loop** as used here refers to a piece of platinum or nichrome wire with a small loop on one end and provided with a handle on the other. It is used for transferring cultures, etc., and is sterilized by passing it through the flame of the lamp) or two of the resulting emulsion is placed on a slide, covered with a cover glass, and examined under the microscope. The oocysts vary in length from 25 to 35 microns and in width from 15 to 20 microns. Once seen they are fairly easily recognized.

Symptoms. The symptoms and course of coccidiosis depend to a large extent upon the age of the bird attacked. In young chickens the disease develops rapidly and is highly fatal. The birds display the usual symptoms of illness: listlessness, unkempt feathers, loss of appetite, and a tendency to sleep in the daytime. There is diarrhea—usually of a light or whitish color, though sometimes it is bloody before death. Very few affected birds survive. In older birds the disease runs a more chronic course. The appetite may

appear to be good, even ravenous at feeding time, but the sick bird
makes little effort to find food during the intervals between regular
feedings. There is a persistent diarrhea and great emaciation. The
bird becomes very weak and eventually dies.

   Morbid anatomy. The lesions of coccidiosis are usually confined
to the intestinal tract, though in young chickens the liver may be
involved. In geese the kidneys are apt to be affected. Figure 23
is a microscopic drawing from a section of a rabbit's liver showing
the presence of coccidia. The duodenum, which is the primary seat
of the infection, practically always shows morbid changes, and in
chickens and turkeys one or both ceca are usually plugged with a

Figure 23.

COCCIDIOSIS

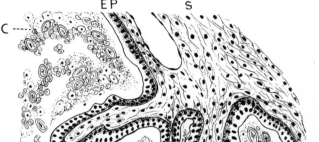

SECTION OF
A RABBIT'S
LIVER SHOW-
ING COCCIDIA.

Ep, Epithelium

S, Stroma of
connective tissue

C,C, Coccidium
oviforme sur-
rounded by pus
cells and degen-
erated liver cells.
After Thomas
and Kitt.

bloody or cream-color mass consisting of feces, degenerated mucous
cells, and parasites. When the liver is involved, its surface will be
studded with small, whitish, necrotic spots.

   Treatment.* Fantham has recommended the use of crude

---

* Note: In the July, 1941, issue of the American Canary Magazine, Ralf H.
Masure, bacteriologist, who had just completed a study of the cause of
death in 41 bodies of birds brought to the Institute Biologicico of Sao Paulo,
Brazil, pointed out that most wild tropical birds carried a few coccidium
in their intestines, but so long as the bird is able to pass these out, with no
chance of self reinfection or cross infection, no illness results. But where
the caged bird is permitted to pick among its own droppings and reinfect
itself over and over again, a fatal illness is very apt to develop. He points
out that keeping such birds for a period in boxes or cages the bottoms of
which are made from half inch mesh wire cloth will prevent reinfection,
and the birds soon become free of the parasite. What this means to the bird
breeder is very simple: Quarantine and cleanliness. Recently the new
drugs, succinylsulfaguanodine and succinylsulfathiazol have been used effectively against this condition. Dose: canary, 1/10 grain daily for three
days, while watching for symptoms of poisoning; chicken, 5 grains daily;
turkey, 10 to 15 grains daily. The drugs are used in tablet form and administered into the crop.

catechu in the drinking water in the proportion of one-third tea-spoonful to the gallon of water. Mercury bichloride in the drinking water in the proportion of 1:6000 and potassium permanganate 1:500 have also been recommended. Mr. L. A. May, Reseda, California, carrying out some experiments with STROUD'S SPECIFIC under my direction, reported the treatment of 250 six-week-old pullets with a mixture of three parts STROUD'S SALTS NO. 1 and one part of STROUD'S EFFERVESCENT BIRD SALTS given in all drinking water in the proportion of one teaspoonful to each quart of water for a period of three weeks. He wrote:

"When I gave these birds the treatment three weeks ago, I would not have given a dollar for the bunch. I never saw a worse lot. I was over to look at them this morning. Could hardly believe my eyes or that they were the same chickens. They had all come out of it and are progressing nicely. Nothing else done. I wanted a good test. The same dirt and litter is still on the floor. I am convinced that you have something."

Because canaries during a large part of their lives are caged alone or in small groups, coccidiosis is not a serious disease among them. Only in neglected flight rooms, where the droppings are allowed to accumulate month after month, and into which new birds are being constantly introduced, would there be danger of this disease ever assuming serious proportions. The few cases to come to my attention have all run very chronic courses. The birds lived for months, becoming progressively weaker. Because of the lack of microscopic equipment at the time, diagnoses were not established during life.

COLDS. Birds are subject to colds just the same as we are, and their symptoms are identical with ours. The infected bird sneezes, coughs, and has a nasal discharge. The cause of the condition is as much a mystery as is the cause of human colds. Epidemics (**Epizootics,** rather) of colds arrive from no known source and sweep through the bird room with great rapidity and without rela-tion to weather or season. They are rarely fatal, however.

Treatment. One of the best internal treatments for colds is a mixture of STROUD'S SALTS NO. 1 and STROUD'S EFFER-VESCENT BIRD SALTS in equal parts added to the drinking water in the proportion of one teaspoonful of the mixture to each quart of water. AMMONIAC, AMMONIUM CHLORIDE and I.Q.S. (which see) are all valuable in treating this condition. Potassium iodide, one drop to each ounce of drinking water, sometimes gives good results in those cases that turn chronic. The real object in treating a cold, however, is not to effect a cure—though that, of course, is desirable—but to get the jump on what may be the first symptoms of a serious disease. Many of the most serious bird infections start with symptoms which cannot be distinguished from those of a common cold. For that reason all birds showing these symptoms must be kept under close observation. See DIPH-THERIA; ASTHMA; ASPERGILLOSIS; INFECTIOUS BRON-CHITIS, etc.

Figure 24.   **CONJUNCTIVITIS**

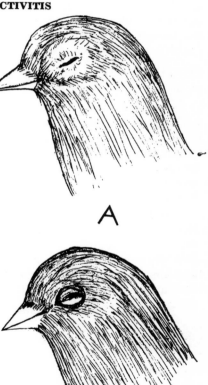

Freehand sketches by the author showing two types of conjunctivitis.

- **A,** All of the tissues around the eye are involved and the eye is swollen shut.

- **B,** Only the conjunctiva is swollen, and the swelling forces the lids apart.

A

B

There are some cases in which the suborbital sinuses become involved and the nostrils plugged. This may cause a large swelling above the beak. The best way I have found of clearing up these cases is to put the bird on the ammonium chloride treatment and also clean out the nostrils once or twice daily with a little NASAL OIL (which see). This is done by digging as much as possible of the deposited material from the nostrils with the point of a clean inoculating wire (a piece of number 22 platinum or nichrome wire fixed in a handle), and then introducing the oil into the nostrils by dipping the wire into the oil and holding it upright with its point in the nostril. The small droplets of oil run down the wire and into the nostril without it coming in contact with the feathers. This is very desirable, since this, and most oils, will blister a canary's skin and cause the loss of feathers.

CONJUNCTIVITIS. This, as the name indicates, is an inflammation of the mucous tissues of the eye, of the conjunctiva.

Symptoms. Usually the first symptom noticed will be large swelling of the eye. Often the eye will be entirely closed and the feathers matted over it—stuck together by the dried discharge. In other cases the swelling may be confined to the inner surfaces of the lids, and then, instead of being closed, the eye will be held open by the interference of the inflamed tissue. Then, again, the only symptom may be a watery or viscid discharge. See Figure 24.

Etiology. I have been able to gather little or no information concerning the cause or causes of this condition. In some cases resulting in blindness I have reasons to suspect the presence of some protozoan parasite, probably a coccidium; but so far I have been unable to demonstrate it to my own satisfaction. In many cases a diplococcus resembling the pneumococcus is found.

Treatment. The most effective treatment I have found for all eye infections consists of anointing the affected eye twice daily with a two per cent yellow oxide of mercury ointment. See ANTISEPTICS FOR THE EYES. The affected bird should be kept away from his fellows, since there are reasons for believing that this condition may be slightly contagious. The majority of the birds associated with an infected bird do not develop this condition, but a few of them are pretty certain to do so. If treatment is begun at once and continued until the eye returns to normal, that is until the inflammation has disappeared, the sight may not be lost. About half of the cases I have treated resulted in blindness. There are some cases where the birds go blind without showing symptoms of conjunctivitis. One or both eyes may be affected. Every bird to develop this condition had a history of exposure to some bird suffering either with conjunctivitis or nasal infection. See note under FOWL PARALYSIS; BLINDNESS.

COLOR FOOD and COLOR FEEDING. If certain vegetable coloring matters are fed to canaries during their moulting season the color will be taken up by the blood stream and deposited in the growing feathers.

The red coloring matter of flower petals, particularly of red nasturtiums, and the coloring matter of red pepper and of saffron are used for this purpose—the latter are preferable, since the flower petals must be fed fresh and are not always procurable. Formerly, cayenne pepper was used. Experiments have shown us, however, that paprika produces just as good coloring in the feathers and is far less harmful to the birds, although they do not like the taste of it as well as they do that of the cayenne pepper. There are now many mixtures on the market for color-feeding birds. The one that has the most standing with experienced fanciers of the English type birds, who are the men who developed color feeding, consists of from four to nine parts of paprika to one part cayenne pepper with three ounces of olive oil added for each pound of the mixture.

The pepper mixture is added to the egg food or other soft food for about three weeks before the birds are expected to begin moulting. At first, only a trace of the mixture is added, but the proportion is gradually increased until at the height of the moult one part of pepper is mixed with three parts of food. By taking all other food away for several hours each morning, each bird is forced to eat one-half teaspoonful of this pepper food daily. Birds that are being color-fed must not be exposed to direct sunlight during the process, for strong light will fade the color as fast as it is deposited. To overcome the resulting deficiency in vitamin D, many breeders now replace a part of the olive oil with cod-liver oil. It is a good plan to mix a little crushed hemp seed into the mixture.* Several times each week and for three weeks after the last of the pinfeathers have disappeared from the head, the colored birds are given an iron tonic. This fixes the color in the feathers, and it will then be retained until the next moult. For this purpose I have found one drop of I.Q.S. added to each ounce of drinking water

---

* **Note:** Because of a stupid piece of legislation requiring the sterilization of all hemp seed, instead of effectively punishing those guilty of smoking hemp, there is now no hemp seed on the American market that is fit for a bird to eat.

to be satisfactory. A good iron tonic can be prepared, if one desires, as follows:

Pour into a beaker one ounce of Ammonium Chloride cough
mixture, add twenty drops of diluted hydrochloric acid, one
teaspoonful of a saturated solution of copperas (iron sulphate) .
and enough water to make up to four ounces. Filter through
paper and store in a tightly stoppered brown bottle. Dose is
one to three drops to the ounce of water.

Recent experiments on the color-feeding of white canaries. In
the last few years the American people have become color conscious. They have come to demand beautiful colors in everything,
and there has been considerable interest in the development of
brightly colored birds. Canary breeders have attacked this problem
along two distinct lines of experimentation. The first has been
directed towards the breeding of fancy colored birds by developing
the mutations which have naturally occurred in canaries and has
led to the development of whites, silver-grays, blues, fauns,
browns (cinnamons) and combinations of these colors. The second
has been directed toward the introduction of new and unusual
colors into the canary strain by hybridizing. This, too, has been
largely successful, since it has been found that males produced by
crossing canaries with the Black-Headed South American Siskin
are partly fertile. (See RED CANARIES.) This line of breeding
has given birds containing varying amounts of red pigmentation
in their feathers and ranging in color from bright lemon yellow
to deep copper red. These birds are very beautiful, and their colors
are natural, but they lack the size and lines of the perfected canary
strains which can be produced in yellow and white with considerable ease. To every breeder who has ever looked at one of these
white birds the thought has come: "If these fellows could just be
color-fed."

In 1937 I made up my mind to do something about it. Using
for my purpose some of the more common water-soluble dyes, I
carried out a long series of feeding experiments. Tests were made
with indigo carmine, neutral red, congo red, eosin, methylene blue,
and gential violet. The dyes were given in the drinking water in
proportions ranging from 1:12000 to 1:800 for periods of from two
to five weeks. Indigo carmine was the only one of these dyes to
produce symptoms of poisoning. Congo red was largely destroyed
in the body. Methylene blue, neutral red, and eosin were eliminated
by the kidneys. Neutral red was the only one of these dyes to be
carried into the feathers in detectable quantities—and even in this

case the amount of dye reaching the feathers was too small to have any noticeable influence upon their color.

Dr. C. H. McLaughlin, Dade City, Florida, writing in the August, 1938, issue of "All-Pets," says that he has heard of chickens being produced in bright-red and sky-blue plumage by feeding the birds on methyl blue and methyl eosin during the moulting season. I have not tested these dyes. I hope to do so during the coming season (1939).

After considering the reactions of the water-soluble dyes and of the coloring matter from pepper—which, by the way, is oil soluble, I obtained from the duPont Laboratories a series of fat soluble dyes consisting of the following:

duPont Oil Red
duPont Oil Orange
duPont Oil Brown
duPont "Anthroquinone" Violet Base
duPont "Anthroquinone" Iris Base
duPont "Anthroquinone" Blue AB Base
duPont "Anthroquinone" Blue Sky Base
duPont "Anthroquinone" Green G Base

After the solubility and color tests, the brown was discarded as being unsuitable for my purpose; the orange, since this color is easily produced both by breeding and color-feeding-with-pepper, was set aside as being of little importance. Feeding tests were made with the "Anthroquinone" Iris Base; "Anthroquinone" Blue Sky Base; "Anthroquinone" Violet Base; and Oil Red, with the following results:

"Anthroquinone" Iris mixed with dry food in the proportion of 1:1000 to 1:300 and fed to feathering nestling canaries was unabsorbed. When two per cent of cod-liver oil was added to the mixture the dye was absorbed, was partially eliminated through the kidneys and partially deposited in the body fat. There was some evidence of toxemia, an increase in the number of leucocytes in the blood and a decrease in the number of red cells. The birds maintained their rate of growth and did not seem seriously ill though they were constantly short of breath. The dye was not carried to the feathers, and when its administration was stopped that part of it that had been deposited in the fat was eliminated through the kidneys in about one week.

"Anthroquinone" Sky Base was fed to nestling canaries in the proportion of 1:300 to the dye weight of the food used. Two per cent of cod-liver oil was added to the dye food. The dye was absorbed at once and the fat, feet and beak became a deep, dirty, bluish-green in color. Part of the dye was eliminated through the kidneys. Dye once deposited in the body was not eliminated through any of the organs of excretion, however. It gradually disappeared after a period of about four months. There were no toxic symptoms. The dye was carried into the feathers in amounts just sufficient to give the feathers a dirty appearance.

"Anthroquinone" Violet Base was used under the same conditions. It caused the beak and feet to become a deep blue, the fat and flesh to take on a very deep violet color. When the daily dose of dye per bird was less than four milligrams per gram of body weight, it had no influence upon the coloring of the feathers, but when the consumption of dye was greater than that the feathers came out a rich lavender. This substance was fed to some birds for periods exceeding four months without noticeably injuring their health. The deposited color does not fade easily, but with time it appears to lose its blue factor, taking on a pinkish cast. As this is written it is impossible for me to tell just how long the color will last, how long it will take to eliminate the color from the tissue, or whether or not the process as I have worked it out will be of any practical value.

Oil Red was used on another group of white babies. Thirteen were used altogether in my tests with this dye. The dye was absorbed more rapidly than any of the others tested. No effect was noticed upon the baby feathers up until the time the birds had left the nest, so the dye was discontinued. All the tissues of the body, with the exception of the nervous tissue, had been permeated by the dye, which gave them a fiery red color. Sections from muscular tissue stained with methylene blue were perfectly differentiated without counter staining, having retained enough of the red for that purpose.

Sometime after these birds had left the nests and been taken off of the red dye it was noticed that the bases of the large flight feathers had come out a nice pink. They were put back on the dye and fed through the baby moult. Those birds receiving better than two milligrams of dye per day for each gram of body weight moulted out a beautiful pastel pink. Their livers became enlarged, however, and there was some evidence of toxemia. There were no fatalities; the effects of the dye wore off gradually after its administration was discontinued. The color in the feathers faded very rapidly when the birds were exposed to direct sunlight. It was more permanent when they were kept indoors, however.

During the feeding process some of the dye is eliminated through the kidneys, but that part of the dye that has once been incorporated in the tissue is retained in the body for some months.

CONGESTION OF THE LUNGS. In making post-mortem examinations it is often desirable to be able to distinguish between simple congestion and pneumonia. This is done by cutting out the inflamed area and dropping it in water. Congested lung tissue will float in water; pneumonic tissue will sink.

CONSTIPATION. Constipation is usually brought about by feeding a bird on a straight seed diet. The bird will have trouble forcing a passage and the dropping will be firm and dry. A difficult passage alone does not indicate constipation, however, since most birds suffering from diarrhea also have trouble forcing a passage. The diarrhea sets up an inflammation of the vent, causing its walls to adhere and the passage to become difficult and painful. The correct treatment for constipation is always the addition of a liberal supply of fresh green food to the diet. The breeders should realize that in the wild state most birds live in an environment affording green food in unlimited quantities.

CONTAGIOUS DISEASES. Strictly speaking, a contagious disease is a disease that can be transmitted by contact; an infectious disease is one that can be transmitted by any means whatsoever. Thus, you can contract a cold or scarlet fever or diphtheria, either directly or indirectly; but you are infected with malaria through the bite of the malaria-carrying mosquito; you are infected with typhoid by taking into your body food or drink contaminated with the germ of that disease. You could sleep with a typhoid or malaria patient with perfect safety; you could not do that with a diphtheria or scarlet fever patient. All contagious diseases are of necessity infectious, but there are many infectious diseases which are in no sense contagious. Fowl cholera, avian diphtheria, canary necrosis, and canary typhoid are good examples of contagious diseases of birds. On the other hand, fowl paralysis, apoplectiform septicemia, and aspergillosis are strictly infectious. An infectious disease, once its mode of transmission is known, can be controlled by breaking the chain of events necessary for its passage from one individual to another. Destroy the mosquito and there can be no malaria; use no sour egg food and see that food and water have no chance to become stale in the cages and you will lose no birds from fits; keep your birds from contaminated ground and see that none of their green food comes from contaminated ground and there will be no fowl paralysis in your flock.

The above distinction should be kept in mind. When you are reading the description of any particular disease you want to know just what measures are necessary to keep it from spreading through your flock. If the disease is described as highly contagious, you know at once that your birds must be separated into groups of as few as possible and strictly quarantined, one from another; but if it is described as infectious, you know that some one line of action will break the chain of infection. Some diseases that were once thought to be contagious are now thought to be infectious. It is claimed by some poultrymen, probably with good reason, that forcing the brooder chicks to stand on one-inch wire mesh which prevents them from ever coming in contact with each other's droppings, will stop the spread of bacillary white diarrhea through the brood, which would place bacillary white diarrhea in the strictly infectious class of diseases. Such a precaution would be of no value towards controlling cholera or diphtheria.

CREOSOTE. This is the produce of the destructive distillation of organic matter. Beachwood creosote, which, because it is the least toxic, is the only kind used for internal medication, is often employed in the treatment of intestinal and respiratory infection. See CASCARA. Coal-tar creosotes are the basis of coal-tar disinfectants and are all highly poisonous. See CARBOLIC ACID.

CRESTS. Many birds in the wild state have their heads adorned by crests of feathers. This is not true of canaries, chickens and pigeons, however. Crests in these birds have resulted from mutations. A **mutation** is some change in the germ plasm of the reproductive cells which causes a corresponding change in the development of the individuals produced from those cells, called **sports,** which have occurred since domestication. In most cases, certainly in all cases with which I am familiar, the factor responsible is what is known as a **lethal dominant.** Such birds can never be bred true. When bred crest to crest at least one-fourth of the young, those receiving the crest factor from both parents, die at feathering time or before. See BALDNESS.

CROP. This is an expansion of the esophagus located on the right side of the neck. See DIGESTIVE TRACT.

DIAGNOSIS. "My bird is dead. Why did he die? I treated him well, but he just puffed up and died. Please tell me why?" Every breeder who has ever written anything on the care and treatment of birds has received hundreds of requests like the above. And it is not only the novice breeder who offends in this respect, either; in fact, he is far from the worst offender, for he is usually so wrapped up in his birds that he can describe their every move and action in the most minute detail, while breeders with years of experience often seek advice without giving any more information upon which to base a diagnosis than is contained in the above quoted sentences. There might be some excuse for the novice breeder; there can be none for the old hand. He should be so trained in the observation of his birds and so familiar with every detail of their anatomy that the most minute change in the bird's conduct or the smallest abnormality in the condition or appearance of its organs would stand out before him like a headlight in a fog. When this is not the case, it simply illustrates that he is too lazy to use his eyes.

Observe the symptoms. Any abnormal conduct on the part of a bird may be the first symptom of illness. If a bird that has been out of condition starts singing his little head off two or three weeks after being placed with some newly acquired stock or, if a hen, starts the most energetic spell of nest-building, it may mean that the bird has come into condition and is just feeling fine, but it may mean diphtheria. If a bird that is in fine song stops every once in a while in his singing to pant for a few moments, it may mean that he is too warm, but it may mean fever, probably of diphtheric origin. If a bird that has always been steady and friendly jumps in fright as you approach his cage, it is pretty sure to mean that he is in a highly nervous condition as the result of poisoning or disease.

In some diseases a bird eats more than normal; in others he eats less than normal, or not at all. In some, a bird puffs out his feathers; in others, he carries them more closely. I shall not attempt to list in this section all abnormal conducts possible to a bird; that is the function of this entire work, and even then I shall probably fall far short of my goal. What I want to do and am trying to do here is to impress upon you the importance of noticing little things. As this is written, among the stack of books scattered about within easy reach, is one very thick, very old volume containing 1100 pages of fine print. The title is—"Loonis's Practical Medicine." This work is long since out of date, but for many years it was a standard medical textbook, and some of the best doctors who have ever lived have used it as the foundation of their medical training. It devotes pages to describing the symptoms and morbid changes in the most minute detail, telling how the patient's face looks, how his lips look, how his tongue looks, how his breath smells, how his urine looks, how it smells, how it tastes (don't laugh, that is true), and how the feces looks and smells and then devotes two or three lines to treatment.

I once knew one of the old doctors who got his training from this book. Many times have I seen him take a patient's temperature, break the thermometer in two and call to his assistant, "Bring me two thermometers. This damn thing was wrong." And he was so well trained in observing the little things that indicate fever in a human being that it took two new thermometers to convince him he was wrong—usually they just demonstrated that he was right. Modern doctors depend on and trust instruments, but these old fellows depended upon and trusted their eyes, their ability to see and notice little things. It is this same ability that the bird breeder must develop in order to be able to treat the ailments of his birds intelligently.

Notice the little things.

The color and consistency of a bird's droppings may only indicate that he has been eating some particular food, but they may be important indications as to the state of his health. Considered in connection with other facts, they may be the deciding factor between a correct and incorrect diagnosis, the thread upon which hangs the life of every bird in your flock. Normally the droppings are white and black. The white part is urine; the black part is feces. The feces can and will be affected by the nature of the food, but there are few foods that have any influence upon the color of the urine; so any change in its color is pretty certain to indicate some pathological condition. Learn to notice these things, to remember them. Usually they will indicate nothing, but when a disease does get into your flock, they will indicate plenty. Your habit of noticing and remembering will then come in very handy.

Morbid changes. After studying a sick bird's actions, examining his abdomen, studying his dropping, taking his temperature, noting his respiratory rate, and considering all facts in connection with his history and environment, you have a picture of the external symptoms of that particular disease. Those symptoms have a meaning, however, only in relation to the changes taking place within the body and of which they are simply indications. It is these morbid changes which form the subject matter of the science of pathology. Many pathological changes can be observed only by the employment of equipment and technique of such refinement as to tax the resources of the world's finest laboratories, the resourcefulness and skill of its foremost scientists; but the great bulk of pathological data can be observed by anyone with two eyes and the patience and will to see. See POST-MORTEM EXAMINATIONS. To illustrate how simple such examinations often are, a woman wrote to me concerning a disease in her flock. She was totally ignorant of bird anatomy—so much so that she mistook the oil gland for a diphtheric sore. At my direction she performed a post-mortem examination and reported it as follows: "I opened the bird as you suggested. The liver was as big as a hickory nut; the heart was as big as a kidney bean; the lungs were kind of blue and spotted looking. These are the only organs I know the names of. I do not know if they should look as they do or not." She had never examined a bird before, but the best laboratory in the world could not have given me more valuable information. For what she had given me was sufficient to enable me to identify the disease and save the balance of her flock.

It is one of the main purposes of this book to supply the reader with as true a picture as possible of every disease with which I am at all familiar, of every symptom, of every lesion, to the end that he may learn to make his own diagnoses. I can tell him what he should find in each case, but I cannot make his observations for him. If he will not make them for himself there is nothing in this book that can do him or his birds any good. I have outlined treatments which have saved the lives of thousands of birds, but they cannot save his birds until he learns to apply them to the conditions for which they are intended. That is the whole purpose and object of diagnosis.

DIARRHEA. Any inflammation of the intestines or cloaca is apt to cause the secretion of an abnormal amount of fluid. The droppings become soft, viscid, pasty or watery, and the bird is said to be suffering from diarrhea. Because the inflammatory liquids are usually strongly acid in reaction, they are apt to irritate the delicate tissues of the vent. This makes the passage painful and causes the bird to whip its tail after each passage. During the time between passages the inflamed walls of the vent tend to become stuck together, which causes the bird to strain in order to force the next passage.

Diarrhea is a symptom of many diseases of minor and major importance. The real seat of the trouble may be in the digestive tract, in the urinary system, or in the blood stream. Persistent diarrhea may sometimes continue over a long period of time without having any deleterious effects upon the general health—this is often the result of parasitic infectation of the intestinal tract or improper diet.

Etiology. To enumerate all of the various reasons that may cause a bird to have diarrhea would be to repeat much of what has been written elsewhere in these pages. Often, as has been so often mentioned, the cause may be some septicemic disease; in other cases digestive disorders set up by the use of stale, mouldy, or rancid food may be at the root of the trouble. Some of these conditions are discussed under the heading DIGESTIVE DISORDERS. I will risk the charge of boorishness by repeating one thing, however: **Fresh green food never is and never can be the cause of diarrhea.**

Treatment. The treatment of diarrhea should always be directed towards removing its cause. Inflammation of the bowels which results from the use of stale, mouldy or otherwise unsuitable foods can only be corrected by correcting the diet. Such cases may be helped by giving the birds plenty of fresh green food and black loam—see AVIAN DIPHTHERIA; FOWL CHOLERA—but the improvement can only be temporary, if the cause is not removed. Bismuth subnitrate mixed with sugar and dusted on bread may help—see BISMUTH. In other cases STROUD'S SPECIAL PRESCRIPTION is of value.* It, too, may be dusted on bread, but it is better given in the drinking water.

DIET. It is not the purpose or object of this book to discuss the diets of all the different species of birds. That would take a whole book in itself. The interested reader should consult some work dealing with the species of birds in which he is interested. I am qualified to discuss the diets of just one small group of birds, the small seed eaters—canaries, finches, sparrows. The general principles of dietetics, however, are about the same for all living

---

* **Note:** STROUD'S SPECIAL PRESCRIPTION is a 50:50 mixture of STROUD'S SALTS NO. 1 and STROUD'S EFFERVESCENT BIRD SALTS. Where these products are unavailable, fair results can be obtained by mixing sodium perborate, citrocarbonate, and "Sal Hepatica" in equal parts and administering it in the drinking water in doses of from one to four grains to the ounce of water.

creatures. Our bodies are made up of just about the same elements, and we must get those elements from our food. I shall discuss these principles in their application to the diet of a canary; the breeder with an active imagination will be able to apply them to the needs of his own particular species. The canary eats seed; the chicken eats grain; the parrot eats nuts. The canary eats chickweed; the chicken eats alfalfa or cabbage; the parrot eats bananas and other fruit. Each has a body made of bone and flesh, and clothed in feathers. Each requires protein, carbohydrates, fats, mineral and vitamins. The cow can get these things from grass because she has machinery adapted to digesting grass; we get them from the cow because our machinery is best suited to digesting beefsteak.

The general diet of the canary is a mixture of canary and rape seeds. For the roller canary the mixture is at least one-half and sometimes two-thirds or three-fourths rape seed. For the large type canaries the proportions are reversed. The type canaries, with large bodies and thick feathers, need the energizing carbohydrates and feather-building materials found in canary seed. The roller with his smaller body and thinner feathers needs the heat-producing oils and proteins from the rape seed. If the type canary were fed on the roller's diet he would not be able to maintain his body and grow his fine coat of feathers. If the roller were fed on the type bird's diet, his song would become loud and faulty.

In addition to the regular diet of rape and canary seed, all canaries require small amounts of the elements contained in hemp, flax seed, niger seed, dandelion seed, and all will enjoy and thrive on all manner of fresh seeding plants and grasses, from the hair-like wire grass to broomcorn. For animal protein the canary requires a little good egg food. The following feeding schedule is one that for years I supplied to the purchasers of my birds. It is out of date now, since there is no good hemp seed, but it still illustrates the principle involved.

FEEDING SCHEDULE

Keep in front of the bird at all times clean sand; canary and rape seed, mixed half and half; mineral foods or cuttle bone; wild greens, such as dandelions, chickweed, or seeding grasses in summer. In winter, when there are no wild greens available, use cabbage, apple or spinach. Also give him the following extras:

Sunday ....Crushed hemp seed
Monday ....Egg food
Tuesday ....Tonic seed

Wednesday ....Egg food
Thursday ....Crushed hemp seed
Friday ....Tonic seed
Saturday ....Egg food

These extras are fed in little dishes, known as **egg** drawers, holding about one-fourth as much as a teaspoon.

During the moulting season the extras are mixed together and the bird is permitted to eat as much of them as he wishes.

Sparrows do best on a basic diet of straight canary seed, but they require small amounts of a good tonic seed mixture and plenty of green food and animal protein. They will eat egg food, but they prefer bugs and insects. They will not eat rape seed.

Most finches require a diet containing canary seed, red millet, niger, maw, flax and hemp, but most of them can be gradually broken in to live on the canary's diet. Most finches prefer insects to egg food. Of course they need green food, and all of these birds love seeding plants and grasses.

Practically all of our domesticated birds, excepting pigeons and birds of the parrot family, require some form of animal protein.

All birds, excepting those that are strictly carnivorous (living exclusively on animal food) need a supply of minerals. Those that eat seed and grain must have a supply of gravel of suitable size for their gizzards. The best bird gravel is riverbed silica, since it is insoluble in gastric juice and has rounded edges. Crushed quartz, because of its razor-sharp edges, may cause inflammation of the gizzard; crushed limestone and mica are too soft and soluble to be of any value for grinding food. Canaries, sparrows and small finches use grit that will pass a sixteen-mesh screen; pigeons use grit that will pass an eight-mesh screen; and chickens use grits that will pass a six-mesh screen.

DIGESTIVE DISORDERS. The most common causes of indigestion in caged birds are: the feeding of stale, mouldy or rancid food; the lack of sufficient minerals, vitamins or gravel of suitable size; the failure to feed green food; a diet that is unnatural to the particular species being fed; lack of sufficient exercise; and the failure of the owner to vary the diet to take care of the bird's seasonal needs— the most common example of this last is the failure of canary owners to supply their birds with additional animal protein during the breeding and moulting seasons. See BALDNESS. The symptoms of indigestion resulting from a number of other causes will be mentioned as this discussion continues.

Symptoms. The abdomen becomes enlarged; the intestines are usually visible through the abdominal wall; the appetite may appear to be normal, but in many cases the bird only goes through the motions of eating, shelling seed and then spitting them out, while it is actually starving; in some cases the appetite is actually abnormal. The bird consumes very large quantities of food, which passes through the body undigested. There is usually an abnormal thirst. Most birds suffering from indigestion scatter their seed badly. When your bird does that do not be fool enough to try to starve him into eating the discarded seed. It will be better to supply him with some food which he can eat. This habit of scattering seed results from one of three causes: it is a habit acquired by the bird from being fed on mixed seeds, some of which he likes better than others; the bird has a natural craving for something that he cannot find in his seed cup; or the seed is unfit for a bird to eat. In these last two contingencies digestive disorders are certain to make their appearance sooner or later. There are cases where the thirst becomes so great that the bird will drink the drinker dry within a couple of hours and the bottom of the cage is always moist from the thin, watery droppings, the feces of which is soft and yellow but unmixed with the copious watery discharge. If this condition is permitted to continue for any great length of time the bird becomes very weak and greatly emaciated. During attacks of indigestion the droppings are usually grayish-white, or yellow in color; they may be of watery, viscid, pasty or gummy consistency.

Digestive symptoms are present in the following diseases: AVIAN DIPHTHERIA, yellow droppings, abnormal appetite; FOWL CHOLERA, yellow droppings, abnormal appetite; APOPLECTIFORM SEPTICEMIA, gastro-enteritic form, green droppings, the bird is constantly hungry but swallows little food; COCCIDIOSIS, droppings grayish-white, appetite ravenous at feeding time, the bird makes little effort to eat between regular feedings; NEPHRITIS, droppings yellow and of gummy consistency, appetite is good but there is a preference for soft food; B. PARATYPHOSUS B INFECTION, appetite good, droppings green or bloody; AVITAMINOSIS B, droppings bright yellow, there is no appetite; TAPEWORM INFESTATION, droppings frothy, some contain fresh blood, appetite ravenous. This is not a complete list, for digestive symptoms of one kind or another are associated with most diseases. Many of the conditions mentioned occur in acute and chronic forms; it is only in the chronic forms of these diseases that they could be confused with purely digestive disorders.

Diagnosis and treatment. Because digestive symptoms are associated with many diseases, it is often impossible to make a diagnosis of indigestion without first considering the history and environment of the ailing bird. If the bird has an abnormal thirst but little or no fever; if the paper under his perch is always moist from droppings; if he refuses to eat seeds but is always begging for soft food and eats great quantities of it; if he eats canary seed in preference to rape seed; if the rape seed he does eat can sometimes be found in the droppings, partly digested; if he has been exposed to no contagious disease; and if the symptoms did not make their appearance directly following a sudden change in the weather, a possible chilling, there is sound reason for believing the bird is suffering from an aggravated case of indigestion and that the seed, or some particular seed in his diet, is at fault. Such a bird requires a complete change of diet. New seed of the very best quality must be obtained. If the season is spring or summer, he must have all the seeding pepper-grass and other seeding grasses and plants that he cares for—in winter a good tonic seed mixture should be kept before him at all times—and plenty of black loam. Either winter or summer it is no trouble to cut a large piece of sod from clean ground, place a piece of it upside down in a glass bath dish, add enough water to keep it moist and keep it before the ailing bird. You will be surprised how much of the dirt he will eat. Enough of STROUD'S SPECIAL PRESCRIPTION—see note under heading DIARRHEA—must be added to the drinking water to control the abnormal thirst. Start with a small pinch of the powder and increase it until the bird is drinking normally; then continue with that dosage for a week or more as required.

Where the offending agent is mouldy seed—canary or millet seed is most apt to be at fault—the droppings will be gray and of a gummy or viscid consistency. The offending item must be located and removed from the diet. If aspergillus infection has not taken place, the bird will respond quickly to treatment with STROUD'S SPECIAL PRESCRIPTION. In fact, this type of indigestion will often clear up in a single day, while the type of described in the preceding paragraph often requires weeks of treatment. Birds so far gone with both these types of indigestion that they had fallen into coma, have been saved by introducing into the crop a large dose of STROUD'S SPECIAL PRESCRIPTION in strong solution, and then following the regimen outlined above.

Why a big dose of this preparation introduced into the crop will snap a bird out of coma is something else about it that I do not know. The condition discussed in this paragraph is identical with NESTLING DIARRHEA, which is usually caused by the hen picking up bits of food that have become mouldy on the floor of the cage.

Stale hemp seed causes fatal attacks of acute indigestion. The affected bird refuses all food, drinks lots of water, puffs out his feathers and sleeps a little bit in the daytime, and usually dies within twenty-four hours or less. The offending seed can be found in the proventriculus or the gizzard.

Deaths from acute indigestion are often the result of indigestible matter finding its way into the gizzard. Birds of all ages may be affected, though the condition is much more common in baby birds than in adults. Almost any kind of seed hull is apt to stop a baby bird's gizzard, but in the only cases of this kind in adult canaries to come to my attention, the hulls of canary or niger seed were found. There was only one case of the former. The hull of an extra large canary seed had been swallowed, and the hard point of the hull had stuck into the soft tissue at the lower end of the gizzard.

The bird is hungry but cannot eat. It will take food into its mouth and then spit it out again. It stands stiff-legged and makes frequent efforts to force a passage, but is able to pass nothing more substantial than a little viscid fluid. Gas forms in the crop. These symptoms are the result of a spasmodic contraction of the pyloric valve (the valve between the gizzard and the duodenum), which always follows the introduction of any indigestible substance into the gizzard.

There is no treatment for this condition in adult birds. Their gizzards are full of rocks. Anything that those rocks will not grind up is too resistant to be handled by any treatment one might administer. The gizzards of baby birds are often stopped with rape seed hulls, however, and these birds can often be saved by hand-feeding them on apple pulp and olive oil. The bird is first given all the oil it will take, and when it will take no more, it is given all the apple pulp it will take. The feeding is done with a match stick. The bird is induced to open its mouth and the oil is dropped in from the end of the match stick a drop at a time. The apple pulp is prepared by taking a bite of fresh apple and chewing it until it is reduced to a semifluid state—this is fed in the same manner as the oil. This treatment is continued until the obstructing object is passed or the bird dies. Once the obstruction is removed the bird's appetite returns and he is quickly restored to normal.

DIGESTIVE TRACT, its construction and functions. Beginning at the mouth and extending through the body to the vent, the digestive tract is a continuous tube lined throughout its length by a continuous mucous membrane which is actually an extension and modification of the skin. In various sections of the canal the membrane is modified and elaborated for the performance of different functions. See Figure 25.

Figure 25.   **DIGESTIVE TRACT**
Diagram of the Digestive Tract of a Bird.

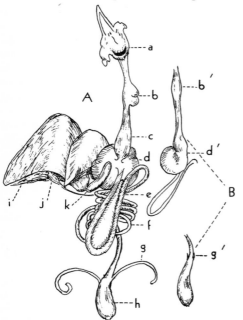

A, The digestive organs of a chicken.
B, Parts from the digestive tract of a canary showing the differences in structure in small birds.
a, Mouth, tongue, and gullet.
b, Crop; b^1 crop of a canary or sparrow.
c, Glandular stomach or Proventriculus.
d, Gizzard; d^1 gizzard of canary or sparrow.
e, Duodenum, the first section of the intestines, which encloses between its horns the pancreas.
f, Small intestines.
g, Ceca, the blind guts; g^1 rudimentary ceca of a small seed eater.
h, Cloaca, the common pouch into which empties the intestines, the ureters, and the generative ducts.
i, Liver.
j, Gallbladder and duct.
k, Spleen.

Note: There are minor differences in other species of birds. In pigeons the pancreas is lobulated; in water fowls the gizzard is small and compact and the crop highly developed; in soft-billed birds the gizzard is thin-walled and pouch-like.

Mouth. This is a cavity enclosed by two mandibles which form the beak. In psittacine birds (birds of the parrot family) and a few other species, both mandibles are movable. This is also true of most baby birds, but in the majority of species the bony support of the upper bill becomes firmly fused to the bones of the head as the bird develops. The upper bills of canaries become immovable between the fourteenth and eighteenth days of life. In all of the small seed eating birds the mandibles are triangular in shape, the lower fitting snugly into the upper. For the last third of its length the edges of the lower mandible turn inward to form a chewing surface which the bird uses to shell seeds and to chew food for its young. The tongue, fitted snugly into the cavity of the lower mandible, is long and pointed and near its base, is pierced by the opening of the larynx. Just back of this opening there is a step-like projection for forcing food back into the pharynx.

Esophagus. This is an elastic tube running down the right side of the neck and entering the body cavity through an opening between the clavicles. It carries the food from the mouth to the crop and from the crop to the proventriculus. It consists of an elastic muscular tube lined with a thick mucous membrane composed of many layers of squamous epithelial cells. (**Squamous** means **scaly** and is applied to the flat pavement cells of which the surface of the skin is composed. In both man and birds they cover, in addition to the surface of the body, the exterior divisions of all openings and tubes communicating with the surface of the body: The digestive tract above the stomach and below the ceca in birds and the sigmoid flexture in man; the urogenital tract below the ureters.)

Crop. In canaries and the other small seed-eating birds the crop is merely an expansion of the esophagus located in the right side of the neck, but in some species—pigeons for one, it is a well developed organ. The crop is provided with a large circular muscle which keeps up a slow peristaltic movement that feeds the food down through the esophagus to the proventriculus at a slow, uniform rate.

Proventriculus. In the left side of the thoracic cavity and extending into the upper part of the abdominal cavity there is an expansion of the esophagus called the **proventriculus.** This is the glandular stomach. It differs from the mammalian stomach in several important particulars. Its sole function is the secretion of gastric juices for the digestion of proteins. There is no provision for the storage or mixing of the food. It simply pours the gastric juices into its lumen as the food passes through on its way to the gizzard.

The proventriculus is provided with two kinds of glands: simple, tubular glands which are identical with the stomach glands found in man—"i," figure 26—and large, pear-shaped glands—"g," figure 26—which are different from any glands found in the human digestive tract, being much more elaborate in structure. To give you an idea of how small these elaborate structures really are, the entire structure illustrated represents from $\frac{1}{12}$ to $\frac{1}{24}$ of the circumference of this small organ, yet to show both the cells and the

Figure 26.   **DIGESTIVE TRACT**

A GASTRIC GLAND FROM THE PROVENTRICULUS (STOMACH) OF A FEMALE CANARY, RECONSTRUCTED AND CONVENTIONALIZED.

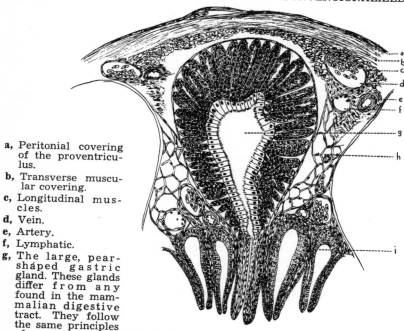

a, Peritonial covering of the proventriculus.

b, Transverse muscular covering.

c, Longitudinal muscles.

d, Vein.

e, Artery.

f, Lymphatic.

g, The large, pear-shaped gastric gland. These glands differ from any found in the mammalian digestive tract. They follow the same principles of construction in all birds, but in larger birds, where the wall of the organ is thicker, the gland is correspondingly more elaborate.

h, Fatty and elastic connective tissue contain small veins and arteries.

i, Tubular glands. These line the entire length of the digestive tract of both birds and mammals, from the back of the esophagus to head of the rectum, their functions differing according to their location. They are the only type of gland found in the human stomach. Their reaction to histological stains indicates that their secretion is highly acid in character, and their function is probably the secretion of hydrochloric acid.

The staining of the pear-shaped gland indicates that the secretion is almost neutral in reaction—neither acid nor alkaline.

It was necessary to reconstruct and conventionalize this drawing, since in not one section in ten thousand would all of these features be found lying in a single plane; also, using a magnification that would show the entire thickness of the wall, it would be impossible to see the details of the cellular construction.

structure, I have had to draw the cells much larger than they actually are.

Gizzard. The gizzard is a large, bulbous, muscular organ located in the upper left-hand side of the abdominal cavity. Its inner cavity has two almost-flat faces which are covered with heavy, horn-like linings with thick corrugated surfaces. These are the grinding surfaces, and they move against each other with a slow circular motion, driven by the most powerful muscles nature has created. They are "smooth," unstriated muscles, the same as those of the heart. It is function of the gizzard, with its powerful muscles, its horny surfaces, the gravel it contains, and by the aid of the strong gastric juices secreted by the proventriculus, to reduce the hardest seeds to a semifluid state. It is during this grinding that the digestion of proteins takes place.

Duodenum. From the gizzard the ground food passes into the duodenum through the pyloric valve. This, the first section of the intestines, is in birds something more than a mere gut. It is in reality a highly developed organ consisting of two long horns which are almost parallel, the second of which returns almost to the spot where the first leaves the gizzard. Between the two horns of the duodenum, closely attached to them, and binding them together, is the pancreas. The function of the duodenum is the completion of the digestion and absorption of proteins. Near the upper end of its ascending loop are located the openings of the pancreatic ducts, two, sometimes three, in number, and a little above these openings are the openings of the gall ducts—the first of which supplies secretion from left lobe of the liver; the second of which supplies secretion, through the gall bladder, from the right lobe of the liver. The function of pancreatic fluid is the digestion of starch; the function of bile is the digestion of fat. The former is slightly alkaline in reaction; the latter is strongly alkaline. I have not illustrated the general structure of the duodenum at this point, since most of its features are shown in other drawings made from morbid lesions. See FOWL CHOLERA, LEUKEMIA, etc.

Figure 27 gives two beautiful illustrations made from sections of the lower intestines. The lower drawing, with the low villi is from the lower part of the intestines. The two drawings are hardly necessary, but the sections came out so beautifully that I could not resist drawing them. The cuts are made at rather acute angles, as is shown by the directions of the muscular fibers.

Small intestines. This is a long coiled and convoluted tube filling the lower part of the abdominal cavity and emptying into the cloaca. It is here that absorption is normally completed.

Ceca. These are two blind guts attached to the main intestine just above the beginning of the cloaca. Their function is probably the absorption of any nourishment from the food that has escaped absorption in the intestines proper. Canaries have no ceca.

Cloaca. This is a common pouch for the reception of the discharges from the bowels, the ureters, and the sexual ducts.

Figure 27. DIGESTIVE TRACT

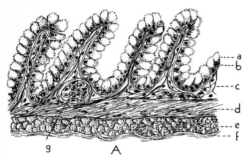

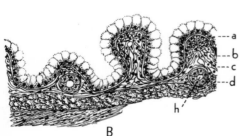

A, A section from the upper part of the small intestines.

B, A section from the lower part of the small intestines. This is indicated by the shape of the villi, the large humps, whose function it is to absorb nourishment.

a a, Goblet cells which seem to perform the double function of absorbing nourishment and secreting mucus.

b b, Basal membrane upon which the cells rest.

c c, Elastic connective tissue.

d d, Inner muscular layer.

e, Outer muscular layer.

f, Peritoneum.

g, A small blood vessel.

h, A mucous gland.

Magnification about 250×.

Sections and drawings by the Author.

DIUROL. This is an arbitrary name applied to certain prescriptions used in the treatment of diseases of the kidneys. The prescription that I have found most serviceable in the treatment of uremic conditions is discussed under the heading UREMIA.

DROPPINGS. See DIGESTIVE DISORDERS. The following tabulations of the colors and consistencies of bird droppings is for the most part based upon my observations of canaries; but, from the reports of diseases in other species, they appear to be of almost universal application:

White, thick, dry and chalky..............Canary typhoid
    canaries, sparrows, finches

White, thin and watery or viscid.........Nestling diarrhea
    probably all species

All species	Aspergillosis
Baby chicks	Bacillary White Diarrhea
probably all species	Nephritis

Gray, gummy and stringy......................Nephritis
    Aspergillosis   Nestling Diarrhea

Bright yellow, thin.......................Avitaminosis B
    probably all species

Dull ochre yellow, soft or gummy..............Diphtheria
    all species

all species	Cholera
canaries and sparrows	Indigestion
turkeys	Entro-hepatitis
parrots	Psittacosis

Dull yellow with colorless, gray or white fluid....Nephritis
    probably all species

| probably all species | Gout |

Green, bright, transparent, viscid...............Diphtheria

| Chickens, canaries | Apoplectiform Septicemia |
| probably all species | B. paratyphosus B inf. |

Brown, dry, scanty.................Sporadic pneumonia
    canaries and sparrows

Bloody ....Diphtheria
                              B. paratyphosus B inf.

Frothy white with gas bubbles and fresh blood..Tapeworms
    chickens, canaries and probably other species

This list is admittedly incomplete, but it may be of some service by suggesting headings under which the breeder may search for the other symptoms displayed by his ailing birds.

EGG BOUND. When a hen ready to lay is unable to pass the egg she is said to be **egg bound.** This is of probably more or less common occurrence in all species of birds, but it is particularly common in birds bred in close confinement. Young canary hens and pullets are often affected. Old hens that have been in high production and all over-bred pet birds are also very susceptible to this condition. In the case of young birds the trouble is ascribable to immaturity, to the underdevelopment of the oviduct and cloaca; in old birds, however, an inflammation of the oviduct is usually at the root of the trouble. There are many cases, too, where spasmodic contraction of the os-uteri **(os** means mouth; **uteri** pertains to the uterus. The **os-uteri** is the sphincter protected opening between the oviduct and the cloaca) follows a sudden change in the weather, and birds that would normally have been able to pass their eggs without difficulty are unable to do so. This condition may also result from a malformation of the egg or an obstruction of the os-uteri by concretions of egg material or by tumors. The most common cause of egg-binding in canaries is a spasmodic constriction of the os-uteri brought on by sudden changes in the weather.

Symptoms. The symptoms of egg-binding, of course, vary with the size and habits of the affected bird but are otherwise substantially the same in all species. In fact, any person who has ever seen labor in a woman, a dog or a cat could not fail to recognize the same condition in a bird, and egg-binding is simply a case of prolonged and ineffective labor. The chicken hen will be observed to be restless, to leave the flock frequently and go to the nest. Soon the cloaca will become inflamed as a result of the constant straining, and prolapse or eversion of the oviduct may occur, or the bird may continue her efforts to lay until she is exhausted. She may be seen standing in a corner of the yard, stiff-legged and straining, her whole appearance indicative of labor. If not relieved, the hen will probably die within twenty-four hours.

Should prolapse result, the other birds will be attracted by the sight of the protruding tissue, peck at it, tear chunks of it away, and so injure the affected hen that she must be destroyed. See PROLAPSE OF THE UTERUS.

The canary hen may be found dead on the nest. Often, however, she will leave the nest and seek a corner of the cage, where she will stand stiff-legged, straining until she dies. Death will not be long in coming, either. I have saved canary hens with eggs broken inside of them as late as four o'clock in the afternoon, but I have never known an egg-bound hen to live until noon. See EGG BROKEN; EGG RUPTURE. They are often dead before ten o'clock in the morning.*

Diagnosis. The presence of the egg may be determined by feeling the abdomen. In the case of a chicken, the well-oiled finger may be introduced into the cloaca; in a canary the great size of the egg in proportion to the size of the abdomen makes the determination of its presence very simple.

Treatment. The bird must be caught at once—this is usually easy, since she hates to move. There are a number of lines of treatment. The most popular is the steam bath. The bird is held over the open mouth of a large-mouthed bottle or jar that has been filled two-thirds full with hot water. The abdomen is steeped in the rising vapor. This method will sometimes cause the tissues to relax and the egg to pass. The best method, in my opinion, at least the best for me or any person who can manage it without slips or blunders, is to deliver the hen of the egg at once.

A chicken hen must be placed on her back and held by an assistant. A well-oiled finger is introduced into the cloaca, worked gently but firmly through the os-uteri—which, by the way, is always on the left side—and up into the oviduct until it comes in contact with the egg. Then with the thumb and forefinger of the other hand a gentle pressure is exerted on the egg through the abdominal wall, forcing it downward as the inserted finger is being slowly withdrawn. The egg will usually follow the finger. The hen, if she has been attended promptly, will be no worse off because of her harrowing experience.

Canary obstetrics are sometimes more complex. The bird is taken into the hand and turned on her back. She is then shifted to the other hand and held in such a manner that the thumb and forefinger grasp the abdomen at a point behind the egg. See Figure 28-A. By the application of a firm and gentle pressure the egg is gradually forced down towards the vent. It is at this point that the element of danger enters the operation. To move the egg, a

---

* **Note:** A canary hen always lays early in the morning, about one hour after getting up, which is usually between five and seven-thirty, though on rare occasions one will lay as late as nine-thirty or ten o'clock. They never lay later than ten o'clock, and any bird seen straining much after eight or eight-thirty should be given prompt attention.

considerable force is required,.but a canary's structure is not strong. If you are one of those persons who have a constant fear of crushing the bird every time you hold one in your hands and have to hold yourself back to keep from doing that, you had better get some steady-nerved friend to perform this operation for you. The pressure must be applied gently and smoothly and sufficient force must be used to move the egg. There need be no fear of breaking it, for under the even pressure of the body it will stand a great deal

Figure 28.   **EGG BOUND**

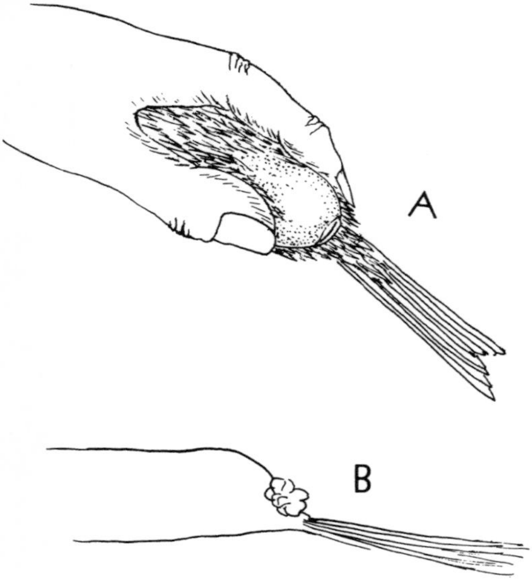

A, This sketch illustrates the manual method of delivering the egg.

B, This sketch shows the way in which the pro-lapsed uterus extrudes from the vent.

Freehand sketches by the author, made from memory.

more pressure than the hen can survive. Should the egg become visible when the vent is forced open, all will be well. A small drop of olive oil is applied to the end of the egg, some of the pressure is relaxed to let the egg slip back a little; then, when the pressure is again applied, the egg will slip out without difficulty. In performing this operation the operator must keep his mind free from any morbid fear about applying the needed pressure, and his hand steady. I have performed it hundreds of times without killing a bird. In the case of sickness or injury of a bird due to lay the next day, I have frequently delivered the egg at once in order to keep it from interfering with and complicating the main problem.

There are cases, however, where spasmodic contraction of the sphincter is so great that the egg cannot be forced past it. The egg can be forced down and will be forced down and out of the vent, still enclosed in the uterus, which, of course, will then be in a state of complete prolapse. To deliver the egg in such cases the spasmodically contracted muscles of the sphincter must be caused to relax. This can be done by dipping a small brush into a little tincture of belladonna, dragging it over the lip of the bottle to remove most of the drug, and applying it to the os-uteri. The most minute quantity of belladonna will usually cause the muscles to relax. It is not necessary or desirable to force the uterus into prolapse. As the vent is forced open it will be easy to see whether or not the sphincter is going to open, and in those cases where it refuses to do so, the belladonna can be applied to the os-uteri as soon as it becomes visible, the pressure relaxed for a moment, and a new effort, which may this time be successful, made to deliver the egg.

In those cases where prolapse has occurred, as soon as the egg is delivered the prolapsed tissue must be forced back into place and induced to remain there by injecting into the vent, with a blunt-nosed eye dropper, a little cold solution of common salt, STROUD'S SALTS NO. 1, or sodium perborate. See Figure 28-B.

EGG, BROKEN. This is not a very common condition with canaries. My first experience with an accident of this kind was with a sparrow hen during my early days as a bird keeper. What I did not know about birds at that time would have filled several books the size of this one—frankly, I often feel that the condition has not improved much, either. No treatment was attempted. The bird died of peritonitis forty-eight hours after the accident. In a number of cases occurring since, I have been able to deliver the broken eggs in much the same manner as described for delivering the egg from an egg-bound hen. In several cases occurring in a large flight room, it was late in the afternoon before the birds were discovered straining. They were caught at once by throwing a large, soft towel over them. In the first case the jagged, broken shell could be easily seen and felt through the abdominal wall. There was a little fresh blood around the vent. It was evident that any attempt to manipulate the egg would result in fatal injury to the hen. As a stop-gap measure, in the hope of guarding the hen against the development of peritonitis, a strong, warm solution of STROUD'S SALTS NO. 1, was injected into the cloaca, and the bird was placed in a small cage until I could think of something else to do for her. A few minutes later the broken egg was found on the floor of the cage; an hour later the hen was returned to the flight; the next morning she laid as usual. She incubated her eggs and raised her chicks. There have been several other such cases since and the results in each have been the same. None of these hens suffered any apparent injury from the experience.

EGG EATING. Many breeders complain of their birds eating their own eggs. This vicious habit, as well as the habit of plucking feathers from their fellows and chewing the butt ends, which some birds acquire, are the birds' only defenses against the stupidity of their owners who lack sense enough to supply them with the animal protein necessary to their physiological well-being. They satisfy this natural craving in the only ways open to them. Under the same circumstances you might do the same thing. A healthy, well-cared-for bird will never develop these habits.

EGG FOOD. To keep birds in health, to enable them to rear their young, to prevent them from developing the habits mentioned in the last paragraph, it is necessary to supply them with some form of animal protein. Naturally, the best form of animal protein for small singing birds is the same kind they would supply for themselves if they were living in the wild state—bugs and insects. It is not always possible to have a source of such food at hand, however. Long experience has shown us that food mixtures containing egg materials offer a practical, if not wholly satisfactory substitute for insect food.

Preparation. There are many ways of preparing egg food. The basis formula is to take one fresh fowl's egg, boil it for one hour, permit it to cool in the water in which it was boiled, remove the shell,* press the yolk and white through a piece of wire cloth, add enough dry, ground bread to the mixture to absorb the excessive moisture, mix well by rubbing between the palms of the hands. The resulting mixture should be moist enough that a handful of it grasped in the hand will retain its shape as the hand is opened, but fall apart as it is dropped back to the table or mixing board. If the egg food is too dry the birds will not eat it so readily; if it is too moist it will sour quickly. Many things may be added to this basis mixture; a little sugar and salt; tonic seed; crushed hemp seed; red pepper; cod-liver oil; wheat germ oil, etc. For many years I used to add salt, tonic seed, and hemp to my egg food mix-

---

* **Note:** The shells of these eggs are saved and used later for mineral food.

ture; but experience taught me that for feeding babies every item added to the mixture is also another source of trouble which must be watched. Were I now to go back to the use of fresh egg food, I would add nothing to it but ground bread and a little salt. Only one of the seeds in the tonic mixture has to be stale for the mixture to kill every baby bird to which it is fed.

There are two great objections to the use of fresh egg food. First, since the food sours quickly, it must be prepared twice daily; second, the great danger from spoilage. The birds in picking over the food always scatter a lot of it on the floor of the cage. These crumbs become mouldy and sour very quickly; then apoplectiform septicemia, nestling diarrhea, food poisoning, and aspergillosis may make their appearance. This objection holds true to a greater or less extent for practically all soft foods, but there are many foods which are far safer than fresh egg food. The breeder who thinks that any mixture can be entirely safe is just sticking his chin out, however. The price of freedom from disease, like the price of liberty, is eternal vigilance.

The market is glutted with prepared foods that have been developed for the express purpose of overcoming the objectionable features of fresh egg food. Some of these preparations are good; some are indifferent. I do not presume to pass judgment on them, however. I have never made it a practice to feed my flock exclusively on any of these preparations. There are a couple, however, that are of considerable value for special purposes.

SPRATT'S PATENT LIMITED, Newark, N. J., puts out a mixture under the name SPRATT'S COD-LIVER OIL CANARY FOOD. This food has one objection: the birds do not naturally like its taste; they have to be educated to eating it. It is invaluable for the hand-feeding of baby birds, however.

I have tested almost every possible system of feeding breeding canaries, and I have raised good birds by most of the systems tried. The method I am using now, which has given me better results than any other, is as follows:

Take 12 ounces of cracked hard wheat; place it in a can having a tight top; add enough water to cover the wheat; place can in the water bath and boil for one or two hours; permit to cool overnight; remove from the can and add one-half ounce of KRAFT'S Domestic-Spray egg-yolk pow-

der,* five ounces of SCARLETT'S COD-LIVER OIL NES-
TLING FOOD, and enough dry, ground bread to bring the
mixture to the desired consistency.

I used to add crushed hemp seed to this food when it was to
be fed to the hens making eggs in order to supply them with the
reproductive vitamin; but, since there is now no good hemp available, I mix into each ten pounds of ground bread used, two table-
spoonfuls of cod-liver oil and one-half teaspoonful of wheat germ
oil. For conditioning birds for the breeding season these oils should
be added to the food about six weeks before it is desired to start
breeding. The wheat germ oil must be discontinued in May, otherwise you will never be able to get your hens into moult in August.
If too much of this oil is used the hens will never moult; they will
breed themselves to death.

The great value of this mixture is that it does not sour easily,
contains all the elements necessary to life, growth and reproduction, and is very cheap.

EGG RUPTURE. Sometimes a chicken hen will rupture her oviduct in her efforts to pass an abnormally large or malformed egg,
and the egg will escape into the abdominal cavity. Other eggs
will pass through the opening. If this condition continues the ab-

---

* **Note:** for the last three years, 1939, 1940, 1941, I have replaced the egg
powder with meat and bone scraps. My present formula is as follows:
  Sunflower seed flour—made by running fresh sunflower seed
  through a fine grinder and sifting the resulting mass through a fine
  screen, which will remove most of the hulls—resulting from the
  use of five pounds of seed is mixed with five pounds of dry ground
  bread; two pounds of ground rape seed; two pounds of ground flax
  seed; two pounds of ground sesame seed; one-half pound each of
  hulled oats and maw seed; one ounce of salt; eight ounces of meat
  and bone scraps; two ounces of cod-liver oil and one-half ounce of
  wheat germ oil. This is thoroughly mixed and stored. It is mixed
  with cooked wheat as described above for feeding. The food is
  mixed only once per day, and if not mixed too moist or placed in
  dirty dishes, it will not spoil in 24 hours in the hottest weather, so
  needs to be mixed and fed but once each day. As a supplementary
  soft food the birds are given moistened dry bread twice each day.
Since I have been using this mixture there have been no babies lost in
the nest and there has been no feather plucking and no cases of food
poisoning.
* **Note:** The KRAFT'S Domestic Spray egg-yolk powder mentioned above
is put out by the Kraft-Phoenix Corporation, Chicago, and is worthy of
special mention. This product is not manufactured primarily for bird
food. It is very concentrated and only a small amount need be used to
add sufficient animal protein to take care of the bird's needs. The one-
half ounce per day mentioned in the above mixture makes enough food to
feed one hundred canaries. Foods containing the Kraft powder do not
sour easily. Some breeders use it mixed with SPRATT'S COD-LIVER OIL
CANARY FOOD in the proportion of one teaspoonful of the powder to a
teacupful of the SPRATT'S food, moisten the mixture with a little boiling
water and feed it at once. It is contended by many that this food never
spoils. They go so far as to mix the surplus from one day in with the
fresh food for the next, but I think that is forcing one's luck a little too far.

domen will become greatly enlarged, sag behind and eventually peritonitis will develop and the bird will die. The only possible treatment for this condition would be surgical, and in most cases its employment would be impractical.

Ruptures of the nature just described cannot occur in a canary. The egg is so large in proportion to the size of the abdomen and the bird that there would be no place for it to go. A rupture, or laceration, of the os-uteri does occur, however. It is then possible for waste materials from the cloaca to enter the uterus and set up an inflammation which may spread to the peritoneum and cause death.

Case history. The hen, two years old, laying on her second nest of the season, passed an extra large egg on the second day of her clutch. On the third day she did not lay; on the fourth day and fifth day she laid very small eggs with roughened shells. She was set on the fifth day. On the morning of the third day of incubation I noticed her standing high on the nest. The weather was warm and I thought she was just airing the eggs as they sometimes do. That evening I saw her leave the nest, stagger over toward the seed cup, stumble over it, and make her way to a corner of the cage, where she fell forward, bracing herself with her wings to keep her abdomen from touching anything. I noticed that her breathing was very rapid, close to three hundred per minute. She appeared to be in great pain.

I transferred the eggs to another nest, and while doing so I noticed that the large egg was stained with blood. I then caught the hen.

Her abdomen was swollen to three times normal size; the blood vessels, normally invisible to the naked eye, were in some cases almost 1 mm. in diameter. The whole abdomen was very much inflamed, and the lower part of it, surrounding the vent for a distance of 10 to 12 mm., was a dirty blue-black in color. The internal pressure forced the vent open, and the lining of the cloaca had the dull yellow appearance associated with suppuration (pus formation). It was evident that the bird was almost at the point of death from peritonitis.

"Well, Little Lady," I said as my thumb slipped to the back of her neck to break it, to put her out of her misery, "you have been a good little bird, and I am very sorry for you but this is the best thing I can do about it." But was it? She was not the first bird I had seen at the point of death, and some of the others had been snatched back to life and health.

I mixed a strong solution of STROUD'S SALTS NO. 1, three or four grains to half an ounce of warm water—and fed it to her from a match stick, drop by drop. She was so near death that I was afraid to attempt to inject the solution into her crop with a medicine dropper. After some difficulty she was induced to swallow about ten drops of the solution. I arranged some nestling material for her in the corner of the cage, making her as comfortable as possible. I would not have given one cent for her chances of living for an hour. I was so certain that she would be dead in the morning, that when I got up I put some culture tubes in the water bath, to melt the agar, before I looked into her cage. When I went to the cage to get the body, however, I found a very lively little lady awaiting me. She began cursing me at once because her nest was empty. Her eggs were returned to her, she hatched them and raised the babies, and she raised two more nests of babies that same season. When she was examined that next morning the abdomen had returned to normal size and color, excepting the area that had been blue-black the night before. The color was normal but the tissue below the skin had fallen away as if it had been gouged out with a spoon, leaving deep depressions into which the skin had sunken. See PERITONITIS.

EGGS, CLEAR, INFERTILE. See CLEAR EGGS.

EGG STRUCTURE AND FORMATION. The yolk, which is formed in an ovarian capsule, consists of a light-colored, club-shaped core around which deep yellow material is deposited in concentric layers. By feeding the hen on alternating days on cotton-seed oil or on fat soluble dyes, the alternate layers may be made to stand out, which makes it possible to determine just when each was deposited. The approximate composition of the yolk is: 33 per cent fat; 18 per cent protein; 48 per cent water; 1 per cent ash. The yolk of a hen's egg is about one inch in diameter; that of a canary's egg is about ¼ inch in diameter. When the yolk has attained its full size the capsule ruptures and permits it to escape into the abdominal cavity, from where it is carried to the first division of the oviduct. See Figure 30.

At the point where the surface of the yolk forms the base of the club-shaped core there is a milk-white spot called the **blastoderm,** or germinal disc. It is at this point that fertilization takes place and cell division begins.

In the first division of the oviduct the yolk is enclosed in a thin layer of dense albumen from the poles of which numerous strings of this dense material protrude. As the egg passes down the oviduct, layer after layer of albumen of decreasing densities are deposited. When it reaches the narrowest part of the oviduct two thin, tough membranes are formed. These later separate at one end, giving raise to the air cavity. In the meantime the strings of dense albumen attached to the dense covering of the yolk have become twisted into heavy ropes and attached to the inner shell

Figure 29.   **EGG STRUCTURE AND FORMATION**
STRUCTURE OF THE EGG.

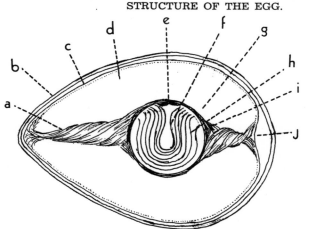

a, One of the chalaza — twisted, rope-like strands of dense albumen by which the yolk is suspended in the center of the egg.

b, Shell.

c, Shell membrane.

d, Fluid albumen.

e, Blastoderm or germinal disc.

f, Club - shaped body of white yolk.

g, Dense albumen.

h, Yellow yolk, deposited in layers.

i, Vitaline membrane, which surrounds the yolk and is very thin and chalaziferous (pronounced kal-a-zif'-er-ous and meaning hard, like a hailstone) membrane which is much thicker and is composed of dense albumen.

j, Air cell. It is in this end of the egg that the bird's head develops, and the air space permits it to turn in the shell at hatching time.

Drawn from memory by the author.

membrane at opposite ends of the egg. These ropes of dense albumen serve to suspend the yolk, which is lighter than the albumen, in the center of the egg. Without this provision the yolk would rise to the top, come in contact with the shell membrane, stick to it and thus make the formation of a normal chick impossible; which is exactly what happens when an egg is permitted to lie in one position for too long a period. As the egg becomes stale the strength of these ropes is lost. See Figure 29.

In the last division of the oviduct, the uterus, lime is deposited in the outer of the two shell membranes, which then becomes the

shell. The secretion of lime for the shell takes place during the
night preceding laying. For this reason canary hens are always
hungry for lime during the night the shell is being made. As their
eggs are so large in proportion to the size of their bodies, they
cannot form the shell from the lime in their bodies without causing

Figure 30.   EGG STRUCTURE AND FORMATION
Diagram Giving the General Appearance of the Sex Organs
of a Female Bird.

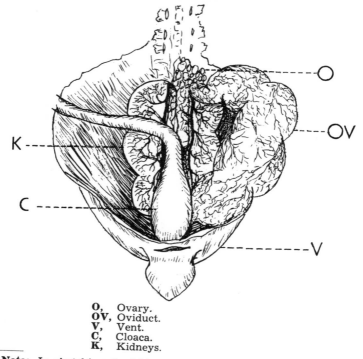

O,	Ovary.
OV,	Oviduct.
V,	Vent.
C,	Cloaca.
K,	Kidneys.

Note: In sketching the kidneys I have indicated the general location
and distribution of the blood supply, but have made only a feeble attempt
to indicate the ureters. In the drawing of the male's sex organs, under the
heading GENERATIVE SYSTEM, the ureters have been indicated in detail
while the circulation has been neglected. These two sets of vessels follow
parallel courses throughout most of their length, are often enclosed in the
same stroma, but they run in opposite directions. The renal arteries and
veins originate in the aortas at a point just above the upper margin of the
kidneys. The ureters, of course, originate in the kidney tubules and proceed
to the cloaca. The normal blood vessels appear red; the normal ureters
and uriniferous tubes appear white. Many of the interesting details of
these structures can be studied in fresh specimens with the aid of a
hand lens.

Sketched from memory by the author.

Figure 31.   **EGG STRUCTURE AND FORMATION**

A SECTION FROM THE OVIDUCT OF A CANARY.

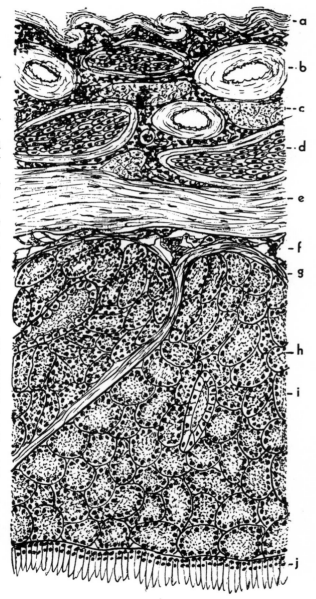

a, peritoneum

b, artery

c, t r a nsversely cut muscle

d, vein

e, l o ngitudinally cut muscle

f, i n t e r stitial connective tissue

g, stroma of the glandular element

h, gland, made up of many t u b u l a r secreting vessicles

i, i, s e c r e t ion ducts

j, t r a n sitional epithelium

Tissue fixed in mercury a n d iron solution; demetalized in acid iodine; stained in toto in a slightly acid solution of hematoxylin and phloxine; embedded in paraffin and mounted in balsam.

P r e p aration and drawing by the author. Magnification about 400x.

serious depletion. Too, there is a point of depletion below which no lime will be given up by the body for the formation of shell; so, if the bird has no chance to eat lime while the shell is being made, the shell is apt to be thin, and the chick hatched from that egg will be weak.*

Figure 31 shows a reconstructed section of the oviduct of a laying canary hen.

EGG YOLK. See EGG STRUCTURE; EGG FOOD.

EGG YOLK POWDER. See EGG FOOD.

---

* **Note:** A canary's egg weighs from 2 to 2.6 grams, and the hen weighs from 24 to 30 grams. If their eggs were in the same proportion to body weight, a chicken hen weighing 5 pounds would lay an egg weighing about 6.5 ounces.

FAVUS. See FUNGOID SKIN.

FEATHERS. Feathers are a modification of the skin and arise from the epidermal cells in much the same manner as does our own hair and nails and the scales of reptiles; in fact, like our own hair they originally arose from the scales of the birds' reptilian progenitors.

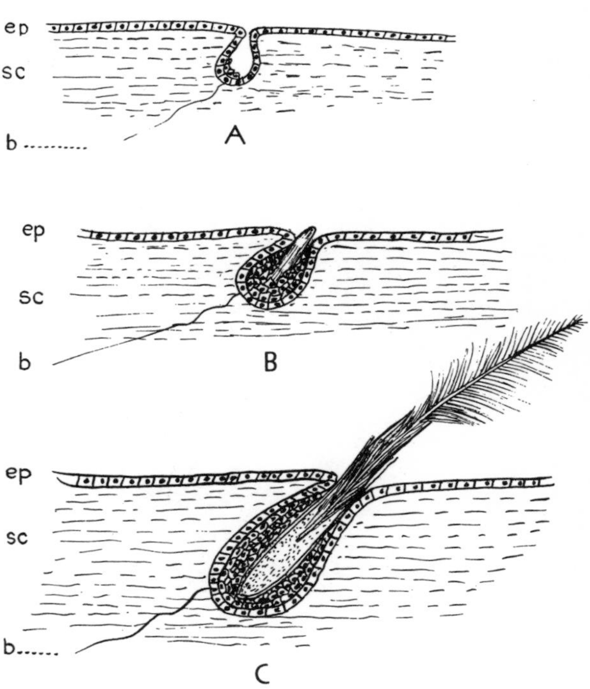

Figure 32.

FEATHERS

Diagrammatic illustration of the development of a feather, after Tom Hare, Cage Birds, London, October 31, 1931, as modified by the author.

A, A small dent appears in the skin and some of the epidermal cells sink below the surface, forming the beginning of the feather follicle.

B, The epidermal cells lining the feather follicle divide rapidly until the follicle is filled and the feather starts to form in the center of the bunch of cells.

C, This sketch shows the feather well on the road to complete growth.

ep, Epidermus.

sc, Subcutaneous tissue.

b, Blood and nerve supply.

Figure 32 shows, diagrammatically, three stages in the development of the feather. First, a small group of skin cells grows downward into the soft tissue below the skin and establishes contact with a blood and nerve supply, as shown in drawing "A." This is the beginning of the **feather follicle,** as it is called. Second, the cells continue to divide, and a hornly tube is formed and pushes

its nose up through the opening of the follicle. This tube is filled
with blood. This stage is shown in drawing "B." Third, the feather,
shaft and web, forms inside of this tube, which continues to rise
above the surface of the skin until it loses contact with its nourishment supply and becomes dry and brittle. The bird combs this
dry tube away, and the web of the feather spreads out and assumes
its normal position. Figure 33 is a drawing of a developing feather
in a canary embryo.

Figure 33.   **FEATHERS**

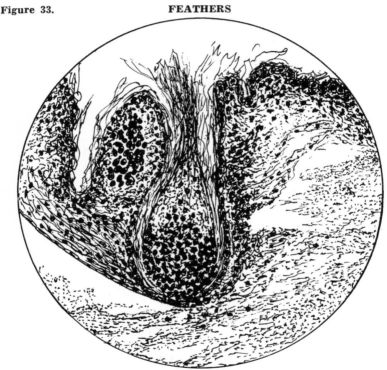

A freehand drawing of a developing feather from a section of a 12-day
canary embryo.
    Author's section and drawing. Tissue fixed in mercury-iron solution
and stained in toto with hematoxylin and phloxine; embedded in paraffin;
cut on hand **mike;** and mounted in balsam. Notice that below the skin there
is still a large mass of only slightly organized albumen. Magnification about
400 ×.

FEATHER LICE. About forty different species of feather lice are
known to infest the feathers of various species of birds. No less
than fourteen varieties have been found on chickens, seven on

pigeons, and six on pheasants. The species I have found on canaries is also common on chickens, sparrows, finches and pigeons.

These lice are not bloodsuckers. They live on the scruff of the feathers and skin, and they never willingly leave their host. They consume feather oil and cause the feathers to become dry and brittle; they lay their eggs on the shafts of the flight feathers, attaching them to the sides of the shaft on the under sides of the feathers by means of a gummy substance secreted for that purpose. The larvae, as soon as they hatch, start to eat their way across the web of the feather at right angle to the shaft. Sometimes a single louse larva will eat its way across three or four feathers of a young canary before the bird combs it off. Of course, a mature bird in vigorous health will comb the larva off before it gets across the first web. See Figure 34.

Figure 34.   **FEATHER LICE**

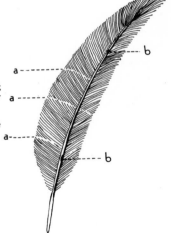

A LOUSE-EATEN FEATHER.

a,a,a, Lines eaten in the feather web at right angle to the shaft. These are eaten by the louse larva.

b,b, Nits attached to the shaft of the feather.

Sketched by the author from memory.

These straight lines eaten out of the webs of the flight feathers by the lice larvae are not only the best indication as to the presence of lice, but an infallible index to the extent of the infestation. In testing various methods of ridding birds of lice, I have found no better way of comparing results than by catching all the birds once each week, inspecting the flight feathers, and pulling out all feathers showing evidence of being worked on by the larvae. The number of feathers removed divided by the number of birds in the flock gives a numerical index of infestation.

Some species of lice are partial to certain parts of the body, as the head, neck, fluff of the rump, etc.

Injuries caused by lice. While, as stated, lice do not suck their host's blood, they injure it in other ways; they irritate the skin and interfere with the bird's rest; they suck the oil from the feathers and cause them to become dry and brittle; they will often bother the canary hen so much that she will leave her nest; and they will damage the flight feathers of young or ailing birds so badly that it becomes impossible for them to fly or take care of themselves. Such birds are often left exposed to dangers having fatal results. And what is worst of all, the presence of lice on your birds always means the presence of red mites in your room or cages.

Treatment. There are literally hundreds of good ways to rid a flock of birds, any kind of birds, of lice and keep it so, but they all boil down to just one thing—keeping eternally and everlastingly at it. The attack must always be made from two angles at once. First, the lice and nits on the birds must be destroyed; second, those lice that have been combed off by the birds must be given no chance to crawl back—if none of the lice combed off by the birds could ever crawl back on them, the birds would need no aid from men in solving this problem. In the wild state, where they sleep in trees, it is unusual to find louse marks on their feathers. When the breeder sees to it that his chicken houses, bird rooms and cages are kept clean by weekly cleanups and frequent sprayings, half of the battle against lice has been won. For years I have kept canaries in a large flight room. These birds are caught and powdered not more than once or twice each year. The room, however, is kept clean; all equipment is either washed or sprayed once each week; no litter is permitted to accumulate; and the birds have a bath constantly before them; during the breeding season the nests are powdered with pyrathrum. Lice have given these birds no trouble, though there is a constant source of infestation in the sparrows that visit the windows. There are other birds kept in cages in a part of this same room, but to keep them free from lice it is necessary to powder them once each week. Under these same conditions, it is necessary to powder young weanlings and ailing birds once every two or three days. In the large flight it takes the combed-off lice longer to find their way back to the birds, since they must travel greater distances. In the case of the caged birds the short distances are in the louse's favor. Of course, the sick birds and babies neglect their combing. Some breeders recommend the use of quassia and other chemicals in the bath water as a means of ridding the birds of lice, but in the clean room such measures are unnecessary for the birds in flight and ineffective for those in the cages. So long as water-bathing birds have the bath constantly before them and dust-bathing birds are supplied with well-filled dust boxes—more of this presently—those members of the flock which are in good health will keep their feathers pretty clean.

Dust-bathing birds: chickens; turkeys; guinea-fowls; sparrows, etc., can be aided in their fight against lice by adding one pound of sodium fluoride to each five pounds of dust used in the boxes. Sparrows are both water and dust bathers as are a number of the small finches. Canaries, as a rule, do not bathe in dust, but they will sometimes pick up this habit when they are associated with dust-bathing birds.

Closely confined poultry and birds kept in cages cannot keep themselves clean without the aid of their owner or attendant. There must be frequent and regular delousings. The simplest way of delousing pigeons and poultry is to dip the birds in a solution containing one ounce of sodium fluoride to each gallon of water. This should be done on a warm day or in a warm room, so that the birds will be able to dry themselves without chilling.

The bird is grasped firmly by the folded-back wings and plunged into the solution until all but the head is submerged. With the free hand the body feathers are ruffled to permit the solution to reach the skin. The head is ducked under for an instant, or a little of the solution is soused over it with the hand. The bird is then permitted to drain for a moment or two and released. The cost of dipping chickens, including the cost of labor, is less than one cent per bird. The advantage of dipping birds over dusting them is that dipping destroys both lice and nits.

For small caged birds, canaries, sparrows, finches, parrakeets, etc., dipping is inadvisable. These birds are very sensitive to chilling and are apt to develop acute or chronic inflammations of the kidneys—see UREMIA; NEPHRITIS. Then, too, the dipping is apt to detract from their value by injuring their feathers. The best method I have found for delousing small birds—this method is original with me and was mentioned in my book, "Diseases of Canaries," published in 1933—is to powder them once each week with a mixture of three parts white flour and one part sodium fluoride.

The mixture is kept in a pepper shaker or sifter-topped can. The bird is placed in the hand on its back, and the powder is dusted over the breast and abdomen, and the feathers are given ruffle with the finger to cause the powder to sink into them. Under the wing, over the back, under the other wing are all powdered in succession as the bird is turned in the hand. The powdered bird is then placed in a clean cage from which food and water have been removed. Sodium fluoride is poisonous, not highly poisonous as some substances are, but poisonous enough to cause trouble should any great amount of it get into food or water, and for that same reason it must never be used on setting or brooding hens or in the nests. In the strength suggested it is not harmful to the skin. It will kill all lice on the bird, but has no affect on the nits. Therefore the powdering should be repeated at regular intervals. See CHRYSANTHEMUM FLOWERS.

FEATHER MITES. The depluming mite, **Cnemiodocoptes levis** (don't try to pronounce that unless you want to choke), sometimes causes chickens to lose feathers. Pigeons and pheasants, too, may be infected by this parasite, and there is one report of a similar mite being found on a canary.

The mite infests the feather quills at a point just below the surface of the skin. Only the body feathers are involved. At first the infestation appears as a small spot on the back or neck, and from there it gradually spreads over the body.

Treatment. Several methods of treatment have been recommended for the control of depluming mites. Sulphur ointment and carbolic ointment have been used effectively by some poultrymen. A solution of one part creolin; eight parts glycerin; and four parts each of water and alcohol is also said to be effective. I have had no chance to experiment with these mites, but I doubt that anything will kill any mites more effectively than a 0.75 per cent solution of sodium fluoride—one ounce to the gallon of water. The affected part should be repeatedly washed with the solution.

Feather mites on canaries. Some years ago a department writer for "Cage Birds," London—who wrote under the pseudonym "Sub Rose," probably because the department was conducted by a woman, while canary breeding in England is strictly a man's sport—published a letter from a correspondent describing a depluming mite that the correspondent had found on one of his canaries. The mite in question was probably closely related to the depluming mite of poultry, if not identical with it—in any case, their modes of operation were identical. Disregarding the two long hair or hair-like processes radiation posteriorly from the mite, its body was about 1/200 of an inch long and 1/250 of an inch wide. It infests the lower part of the quills of the body feathers and eventually cuts them off. The writer had discovered the mite by examining the quill of one of the dropped feathers under his microscope, but the size of the mite is such as to make it easily visible under a good lens.

The writer of the letter reported that hand-washing the bird with "Life Buoy" soap had cured the condition.

This article was quoted, copied, or reprinted by most of the American bird journals—and right then and there the American bird breeders went stark, raving, feather-mite mad. With utter disregard for the treatment recommended by the writer, hundreds of "goos," salves, and what-nots appeared upon the American market for the treatment of feather mites. Every poor bird that had lost a few feathers from any cause whatsoever was smeared with from one to a dozen of these dopes and "goos"—most of which blistered the skin; none of which did any good. And in all the years I have been associated with birds not one case of genuine feather-mite infestation of a pet bird has ever come to my attention, though I have been called upon hundreds of times to treat the injuries stupid persons had inflicted upon their birds by smearing them with feather-mited concoctions.

FEATHERS, FLUFFED. A bird fluffs out his feathers when he is cold, when he is tired, when he is angry, when his feelings have been hurt, when he is sleepy, or when he feels bad for any reason whatsoever. Most sick birds fluff out their feathers, but in the early stages of two of their most serious diseases — the acute hemorrhagic form of apoplectiform septicemia and diphtheria—the feathers are carried close to the body. The way a bird carries his feathers may be an indication that he is not well; it is not a positive indication of any particular disease, however.

FEATHERS, INGROWN. See LUMPS.

FEET, CARE OF. Every time a caged bird is caught for any purpose his feet and beak should be inspected—for his claws and bill, like your own claws, grow at a rate that was fixed by nature during the millions of years he lived in the wild state, a rate sufficient to take care of the wear of a rather strenuous life. Cage life does not provide that wear; so, naturally, the beak and claws become overgrown and must be trimmed at frequent intervals.

To do this take the bird in your hand; hold him on the level with the edge of a table, with one of his feet resting on the table; and then, with a sharp knife, snip off the over-grown claws. The cut should be made at a point just beyond the end of the blood vessel which runs down the center of each claw for about half of its normal length and which is easily visible.

The beak can be trimmed in the same manner. It is the sides and point of the upper mandible which become over-grown. The point of the bill is snipped off in the same manner as the claws, though it is best to cut on an angle and from both sides, so as not to leave the bill blunt. The sides are cut by resting the point of the bill on the table, slipping a thin, sharp knife inside of the mouth and cutting downward, towards the point of the bill. To cut back towards the corner of the mouth would be to invite a serious accident. And this is not such a safe operation in any case. The edges of a bird's bill are very hard, but only the edges. Just below them the tissue is very soft. If the knife is not held under firm control at all times, the force necessary to cut through the edge of the bill may cause it to slip and cut half of the bird's bill off instead of just the over-grown edge. See BLEEDING.

Figure 35.   **FEET, CARE OF—**

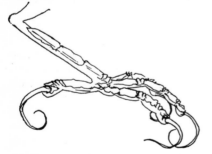

This sketch illustrates a condition of the feet all too common in caged birds.

Sketched from memory by the author.

The scales of the feet, too, as illustrated in Figure 35, are replaced at a uniform rate of growth compatible with existence in the wild state and are apt to become over-grown in captivity. The wild bird is out in all kinds of weather. His feet are in water dozens of times every day. During damp weather they are moist from the time he leaves his roost in the morning until his return to it at night. As the new scales grow, he has no trouble shedding the old ones. In captivity, however, many birds have trouble shedding the old scales, and as the new scales grow, under the old ones, the accumulation becomes thick and unsightly—see Figure

35—the feet become enlarged, misshapen and sometimes crippled. This may be avoided by scraping off with your fingernail **any** accumulation of scales you find on your bird's feet. In most cases the scales will come off easily. If they do not, rub the bird's feet with a little olive oil. This will loosen the scales so that they can be taken off the next time the bird is caught. See SCALY LEG, but do not have a scaly-legged fit. If your bird is infested with this mite, there is nothing to get excited about. Just clean his perches by washing them in hot soap and water and anoint his feet with olive oil.

An outsider should always be called in to tend to a parrot's feet and beak. Parrots have good memories for persons, and should the owner hurt the parrot, Mr. Parrot is apt to collect a chunk of finger the first chance he gets—and you can take my word for it, he really can collect.

FEET, DIRTY. Birds kept in dirty cages cannot avoid having dirty feet. There are some cases of indigestion in which the droppings are very soft and gummy, and such a bird confined in a small cage will always have its feet **gummed-up** with droppings. Birds kept on a diet too rich in proteins, particularly a diet containing milk or too much egg food, develop a condition closely related to gout in man. See GOUT. The feet become swollen, tender, and give off a viscous discharge which keeps them constantly moist, and makes any dirt they come in contact with stick to them.

Such birds should be put on a correct diet and given plenty of flying exercise. The feet may be washed in a little boric acid or sodium perborate solution. See DIGESTIVE DISORDERS; GOUT.

FEET, SWOLLEN. Swollen feet may indicate gout, as has just been mentioned, mosquito bites, bedbug bites, diphtheric lesions, chronic bacterial infections, or they may be the result of injuries.

Diphtheric lesions on the feet are usually confined to a single toe or a single joint. The swelling is not pronounced, but judging from the fuss the birds make over it, the sore is extremely painful— they throw about nine fits every time the foot touches anything. The discharge, if any, will be clear and viscous.

The sore caused by a mosquito bite is always extremely painful, but less so than a diphtheric sore on the feet. The swelling is much greater than that associated with the diphtheric lesion, and it is often surmounted by a blood clot. Sometimes the bite causes the whole foot to swell and the condition to be mistaken for gout. Frequently a claw or one or more joints of the toe is lost. See MOSQUITOES.

The swellings resulting from chronic bacterial infection of the joints frequently rupture and give off a purulent discharge. They are usually an aftermath of AVIAN DIPHTHERIA or FOWL CHOLERA—which see.

Bumblefoot. This is an abscessed condition of the ball of the foot affecting the larger breeds of poultry. It is thought to result from bruises received in jumping from high perches. It is necessary to open the swelling and clean it out. To stop the bleeding the incision is packed with gauze moistened with a ten per cent solution of chloride of iron, which is covered with a dry dressing to keep out the dirt. The next day the chloride or iron dressing may be replaced by a dry dressing.

FITS. See APOPLECTIFORM SEPTICEMIA; STRYCHNINE POISONING; B. PARATYPHOSUS B INFECTION; AVITAMIN-OSIS B.

FOOD. See DIET; EGG FOOD; GREEN FOOD; MINERAL FOOD; VITAMINS; etc. Birds may be divided into two general classes: those which subsist on a diet of grain and seeds are called **hard-billed** birds; those that live largely on fruit and insects are called **soft-billed** birds. At one extreme, we have the pigeons and psittacine birds, which eat no animal food; at the other, we have the **wing-feeders,** swallows, swifts, etc., which live exclusively on insect food. Most birds, however, fall between these two extremes. Some birds live on insects during one season and grain during another. Most of the seed-eating birds feed their young on insects. But regardless of their general dietetic habits, their elementary requirements are practically identical.

The food elements are: carbohydrates; proteins; fats; fiber; minerals and vitamins.

Carbohydrates are compounds of carbon, oxygen, and hydrogen in which the last two elements are present in the same proportion in which they are found in water. Starches, sugars and celluloses are the most important of the carbohydrates. Starches are found in larger or smaller quantities in practically all vegetable foods, but carbohydrates are also present in small quantities in such animal foods as milk, blood, muscular tissue, liver and egg yolk.

Proteins, strictly speaking, are compounds containing nitrogen in addition to carbon, hydrogen, and oxygen. A closely related group of compounds usually included under this same designation, though chemically distinct, contain sulphur and are known as caseins and albumens. The three—protein, casein and albumen—occur closely associated in the germs of seeds and in practically all animal products. Generally, though, one group will predominate: as casein in milk; albumen in blood and egg white; protein in muscular tissue. The bodies of some seed—hemp, rape, maw and niger, for instance—are rich in fats and proteins and contain little starch. The bodies of other seeds are rich in starches and contain little protein and fat. Canary seed and millet belong to this latter class. The bodies of peas and beans contain little oil but are rich in starches and proteins.

Fats, like the carbohydrates, are compounds of carbon, hydrogen and oxygen, but they contain a much smaller proportion of the latter element. They are found in the fat of animals and in the oils of seeds and grains. Egg yolk is rich in fat. Fats as they occur in nature are made up of two distinct chemical compounds in close chemical combination—glycerin and a fatty acid. This combination has a tendency to break up under the influence of heat, atmospheric oxygen, bacterial contamination. The substance takes on a disagreeable odor—the odor of the free fatty acid and becomes unfit for food. We refer to substances in which this change has occurred as being **rancid**.

Minerals (ash) are present in small quantities in practically all foodstuffs, particularly in bonemeal, fishmeal, seeds, grains and green foods. They differ from the other food elements in that they are also found free in nature. One of the most important sources of minerals is the drinking water. The mineral elements entering into avian economy are: potassium, sodium, calcium, magnesium, iron, copper, sulphur, phosphorus, chlorine, iodine, bromine, fluorine. There may be other minerals that are required in minute quantities, too. We still have plenty to learn about this subject.

Most of the minerals necessary to the maintenance of life, growth and reproduction are present in the diet and drinking water, but there are some cases where this is not true. Some localities may be deficient in some of the essential elements. See IODIDES. Most birds require certain mineral in excess of the quantities in which they are normally found in food and water. In the wild state these elements are probably often obtained by the digestion of gravel in the gizzard. Many wild birds deliberately search out calcium deposits. This subject will be discussed in more detail under the heading MINERAL FOOD.

Fiber is composed cellulose, a carbohydrate, which makes up

the connective tissue and cell membranes of all plants. Most warm-blooded creatures are unable to digest cellulose, but it plays an important part in maintaining normal digestive processes. Fruit and green food are the principal sources of fiber.

Vitamins are complex chemical compounds necessary in minute quantities for the maintenance of specific physiological processes. Until recently, they were little understood and the part they play in the processes they affect is still shrouded in mystery. In the last few years, however, great advances have been made in our knowledge of vitamins, and a number of them are now manufactured synthetically. This subject will be discussed in more detail under the heading VITAMINS.

Carbohydrates are the structural elements of plants and the fuel elements of animals. They are converted into sugars for use as fuel and into fats for storage. Animal structures are built up of protein and mineral elements. And while the animal body can in cases of necessity break down proteins and use them as fuel, doing so produces excessive quantities of poisonous, nitrogenous waste products, disposal of which places an added burden on the kidneys.

FOWL CHOLERA.* **Synonyms:** Bird fever; chicken cholera; avian pasteurellosis; cholera gallinarum; fowl septicemia; and hemorrhagic septicemia of birds. This is an acute, highly contagious, septicemic disease of chickens and a great many other species of animals and birds. It is the form of hemorrhagic septicemia to which chickens are particularly susceptible. The disease takes three forms: peracute, acute and chronic.

Symptoms. In the peracute form there are no symptoms. The bird drops dead, suddenly; often from the perch at night. Sometimes it puffs out its feathers and sleeps for a few hours before dying.

In the acute form the most noticeable and characteristic symptom is the ochre-yellow color of the droppings. These droppings are identical with those described in detail in the discussion of avian diphtheria—thick, pasty-yellow in the early stages of the disease; often green, brownish or bloody just before death. The bird eats and drinks almost up to the time of death but chooses soft food rather than seed or grain. The caged bird will often be found continually picking at the sand in the bottom of the cage as if looking for something that it cannot find. If opportunity per-

---

* Note: The relationship of fowl cholera to hemorrhagic septicemia in other species will be discussed under the heading HEMORRHAGIC SEPTICEMIA.

mits, these birds will consume large quantities of black loam and derive benefit from it.* In the early stages of the attack, the temperature may go as high as 113 degrees F., or higher, but in the more chronic cases the temperature is usually subnormal before death—sometimes sinking as low as 96 degrees F.

The chronic form of the disease is marked by persistent or intermittent diarrhea, drowsiness, depression, emaciation and death. The abdomen is usually enlarged and inflamed. During the latter stages of the illness there may be swellings of the joints.

The early cases of an outbreak of fowl cholera are usually of the peracute form, since the birds of least resistance will be the first attacked, or, at least, the first to die. Later the disease runs an acute course. Chronic cases appear toward the end of the outbreak.

Morbid anatomy. In the peracute form few changes will be found at post-mortem examination. There are almost always punctiform hemorrhages in the heart walls and in the walls of the duodenum, however, and the latter can usually be seen through the outer wall of the intestine. Hemorrhages in other parts of the intestines, in the skeletal muscles, and in organs other than the heart and duodenum occur only very infrequently. The intestines are filled with a cream-colored, pasty mass, which may be stained with blood. The liver may contain a number of small, white, necrotic spots scattered throughout its mass. There may be a bloody, fibrinous, or gelatinous exudate into the pericardium. Often this exudate is sero-fibrinous and contains numerous specks of jelly-like material. And though it is not found in all cases, when it is present, this gelatinous material is always evidence of hemorrhagic septicemia. If the disease runs a rapid course, fowl cholera is indicated, but when the development of the symptoms is more gradual, a careful search should be made for diphtheric lesions.

In some cases of fowl cholera there may be congestion of the lungs or pneumonic consolidations. In all cases stained smears from

---

* **Note:** This was the first fact of therapeutic value to crown my early experiences with birds. It was told to me by a very sick little sparrow. He got down on the floor and began searching for something, and the burnt ends of matches would take his eye. When he would taste them, however, his disappointment was plainly evident. "What, I asked myself, would this little fellow find on the ground, if he were living in the wild state, that would satisfy his craving? What is there that is black and possessed of possible therapeutic properties?" Loam appeared to me to be the only possible answer. I sent for some at once, and though it came too late to be of any value to the little fellow who had told me about it, it enabled his mate to recover. She had taken sick a day after the male and was still able to eat soft food when the loam arrived. The first day she must have eaten twice her weight of it. Three days later she was well.

the blood or organs, examined microscopically, will reveal the presence of numerous plump, bipolar-staining rods. See Figures 36 and 37.

Figure 36.

FOWL CHOLERA

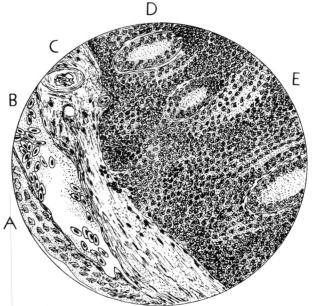

Section through a duodenal ulcer in the intestine of a sparrow that died of FOWL CHOLERA. A great many chickens, several cows and a few pigeons died in this same outbreak. The sparrows and pigeons were infected by going into the chicken yard and cow lot to eat. This particular bird fell out of the air and I picked him up before he was dead.

A, Muscles of the outer wall of the duodenum cut transversely.

B, Intramuscular space filled with blood.

C, Inner muscles are cut longitudinally and show two small arteries and a lymph capillary.

D, One of three glandular structures shown in this field which were not entirely destroyed. The location of several other tubes and their direction can be inferred from the configurations of the pus cell, although the structures have been destroyed.

E, Dense masses of infiltering pus cells.

Freehand drawing by the author made from tissue fixed in mercury-iron solution and stained in toto with hematoxylin and phloxine, imbedded in paraffin and cut on a hand microtome of the author's own construction.

It may interest some of my readers to know that when this drawing was made I was suffering from lobar pneumonia and meningitis and was almost as dead as the sparrow was when he fell into my hands. Temperature 105°.

Treatment. Fowl Cholera, as has been mentioned, is very closely related to avian diphtheria and, in fact, is often the real cause of death in diphtheric outbreaks. The treatment should be the same as the general treatment recommended for diphtheria.

The same sanitary measures as are recommended for diphtheria should be employed. And in cholera, because of the shorter period of incubation, more sudden and violent onset, and shorter course, sanitary measures give much better results than can be expected from them in the control of diphtheria. Then, too, bacteria are far more easily destroyed than is pox virus. See AVIAN DIPHTHERIA.

FOWL PARALYSIS. This is a comparatively new disease in America. I have found no mention of it in books on birds or poultry published as late as 1927. For my knowledge of this disease in poultry, I am indebted to an article which appeared in the

Figure 37.   **FOWL CHOLERA**

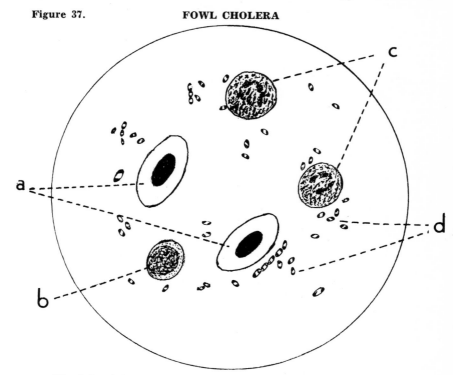

Blood from the same sparrow mentioned under figure **36.**
a, Red blood cell.
b, Lymphocyte.
c, Polymorphonuclear leucocytes, pus cells.
d, The cholera organisms.
Free-hand drawing by the author using a magnification of $1350\times$. Smear stained with eosin and methylene blue.

"Poultry Craftsman," Los Angeles, California, 1931.* See note, page 172. I regret, however, that the article has been misplaced, the date of the issue and the name of the author forgotten. The condition first came to my attention as a disease of canaries in 1929, and I had been studying it for two years before I became aware that in certain localities it had become a formidable disease of poultry.

Characterization. Fowl paralysis is an infectious disease of young birds in which one of the nerves of the neck is always affected in a characteristic manner, causing the head to twist to the right in such a manner that in some cases the bird is unable to pick up food or take a drink of water. A mild attack causes the

Figure 38.   **FOWL PARALYSIS**

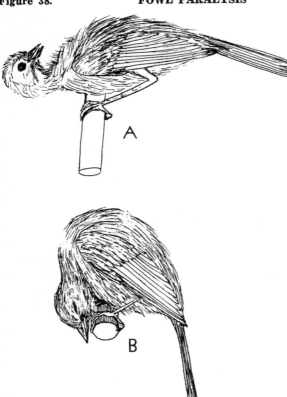

A, An acute case. This bird being unable to pick up food cannot live.

B, This sketch illustrates the position assumed by the chronically infected bird during sleep.

Sketched from memory by the author.

bird to carry its head at an awkward angle during the day and sleep with it hanging between the feet at night. See Figures 38 and 39.

The disease is reported to have first made its appearance in the eastern part of the United States, and at the time the article mentioned above was written, it was said to have become very common in certain localities in Missouri and Iowa. It has come to my attention, as a disease of canaries, as far west as New Mexico. Young chicks are attacked shortly after being put on the ground. Losses in some outbreaks run as high as sixty per cent. Chickens six months old or older are immune, and the disease has not been

Figure 39.   **FOWL PARALYSIS**

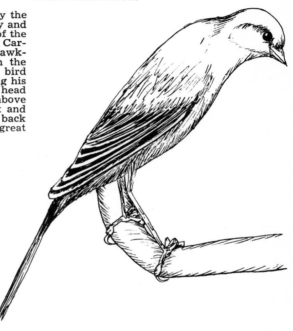

This sketch, made by the author from memory and with the aid of one of the drawings of N. E. R. Carter, illustrated the awkward way in which the chronically affected bird holds his neck during his waking hours. The head cannot be lifted above the line of the back and the feathers on the back are combed with great difficulty.

Note: I have recently discovered that a single one-tenth grain dose of sulphanilamide given into the crop of a canary in this condition will destroy the causative agent of the disease. The bird will completely recover in the course of from five to six months in a large flight.

observed in chicks under fifteen days old. Canaries over four months old take the disease rarely and in a mild form. Fatalities in canaries occur between the fifteenth day and eighth week.

Etiology. So far as I have been able to learn, the cause of fowl paralysis is still undetermined, but there are some reasons for believing that it may be caused by a protozoan parasite that either attacks the nerve of the neck directly or, multiplying in the digestive tract, elaborates a poison which has a selective action on the nerve of the neck analogous to the action of lead on the radius and ulna nerves and wood alcohol on the optic nerves. This latter view is supported somewhat by some experiments to be·recounted presently.

Symptoms. In the acute form the first symptom noticed is a peculiar twisting of the neck to the right. If it is a young bird in the nest or not yet weaned, it will be constantly crying for food but unable to take the food offered by the old birds. I have seen an old cock climb up on the wires of the nest box and get over one of these babies in his efforts to get in a position from which he could feed it. If it is a bird that has been weaned, the first symptom noticed will be a sort of convulsive fit which may be mistaken for the convulsions of avitaminosis B., **beri-beri.** The bird is discovered on the bottom of the cage, struggling violently. It is usually lying on its right side and is unable to regain its feet. The head is twisted far to the right, sometimes so far that the beak points upward and when the bird tries to get its beak down to take food, it loses its balance, which precipitates the convulsion-like struggle to regain its equilibrium. The bird is conscious at all times and has control of all the muscles of the body except those of the neck. Death follows from starvation.

In chronic cases there may be varying degrees of twist in the neck. In some very mild cases the bird never appears to be sick, performs all its normal functions and there is no noticeable twist in the neck. The head, however, is held awkwardly, thrust forward, neck bowed like that of a bull ready to charge. At night, if the bird is watched while it is going to sleep, it will be seen time after time trying to turn its head back over its shoulder to get it into the normal sleeping position. Some of these birds are able to turn their heads back and hold them there as long as they are conscious, but, as soon as they go to sleep, the head slips forward and falls between their feet. Eventually, the bird being able to do nothing else, adopts the habit of sleeping with his head hanging between its feet as illustrated in Figure 38. The onset of the illness is sometimes marked by a slight diarrhea which clears up without treatment within a few days. Asthmatic breathing of more or less severity is a rather common symptom of these chronically affected birds. Deaths, where they occur, are always the result of the bird's inability to care for itself, never the direct result of the infection.

---

* Note: Since the preparation of this manuscript has been completed, I have found among some of my old papers the article referred to on page 169. It appeared in the "Poultry Craftsman," May, 1931. It was written by A. J. Durant, Department of Veterinary Science, University of Missouri, and is entitled FOWL PARALYSIS—ITS CAUSE AND REMEDY.

It will be seen from the following excerpts from Dr. Durant's article that in discussing the disease in poultry in the text, my memory has played some tricks on me. It would be an easy matter to rewrite the text and correct the errors. I prefer to let them stand, however. I have not been very lenient with this gentleman in other places in this book (see LEU-KEMIA) and have no intention of being any more lenient in this section, so it would be manifestly unfair to suppress the evidence of my own shortcomings.

The following quoted passages are from the above-mentioned article:

"This disease is one which has affected poultry in practically the entire United States in the last few years. In Missouri, my own state, the disease is very prevalent. . . .

"The disease is characterized by the following common symptoms: (a) Paralysis of both legs. (b) Paralysis of both wings. (c) Blindness—in which the eyeball gradually turns gray. The pupil becomes smaller and smaller until it is finally closed over by an inflammatory growth of the iris. . . . (d) Wry-neck, the head twisting either to the right or the left, as in typical wry-neck. (e) There are other obscure symptoms which are not readily recognized and which will not be discussed in this article." To which I wish to comment that in the disease observed by me in canaries, where only the neck was involved, that the twist was always to the right; that birds over six months old were never affected. During my experiments with the disease there was one case of blindness in my flock, characterized by the formation of a gray opacity between the cornea and the pupil; but during the two years following the conclusion of the experiments there was a number of cases of blindness among birds to which infective materials had been fed during the experiments. To quote further:

"It appears to affect most birds from four to eighteen months of age and as a rule does not cause heavy losses in the flock.

"The cause of paralysis and blindness and the other symptoms of the disease is due to a diseased condition of the nerves supplying the affected parts. The affected nerve becomes swollen and yellow in color. These changes, however, are seen only in birds which have been paralyzed for several weeks. In the early stages or acute form of the paralysis, the nerve shows a reddening or hemorrhagic condition.

"The cause of the diseased condition of the nerves, and naturally the cause of the disease itself, is at present not known. There are two opinions in regard to this condition. One opinion is that the disease may be the result of parasitism (infection with worms or coccidia). The ones claiming this as a cause hold that inflammation of the intestines produced by these parasites results in the diseased condition of the nerves . . .

"The other opinion is that the disease is a specific one. That is, that it is produced by an unknown germ or element and is a distinct disease in itself and does not have any relation to parasitism."

In regard to these last two paragraphs, I wish to comment that I cannot see why it is necessary to consider these two opinions mutually exclusive. My conclusions, arrived at without the aid of microscopic equipment, indicate that the disease is a specific parasitic infection. Again quoting from the article:

"Since the cause of this disease is not known, it is difficult to give recommendations for the control of the disease. **There is no cure for fowl paralysis and not knowing the cause of the disease, control methods should be based on general sanitary principles.**"

I have underscored this last sentence for the purpose of contrasting the promise with the fulfilment—**FOWL PARALYSIS—ITS CAUSE AND REMEDY. We don't know what it is or what to do about it.** And that, my friends, is veterinary science at its best. The only worth-while suggestion offered for the control of the disease is, "If possible, the young chicks should be raised on grounds that have not been occupied by chickens for two years previously."

Since the completion of this manuscript, I have established the identity of the disease in poultry and canaries by feeding susceptible canary babies on green food from ground known to be contaminated with the droppings of infected chickens. The owner of the chickens reported some cases of wing and leg paralysis in his birds; the canaries developed the typical neck paralysis. The veterinarian he called in could suggest nothing more than **kill and disinfect.** At my suggestion the birds were removed from the contaminated ground, and the disease disappeared.

Morbid Anatomy. Examination of the visceral organs reveals no mascroscopic (capable of being seen with the naked eye) lesion not attributable to starvation. Cultures from the blood of living birds and fresh bodies remain sterile. At the time I was studying this disease I was not equipped for making minute pathological observations.

Experimentation. In 1928 I purchased a pair of cinnamon canaries from a breeder living in Missouri. They arrived in apparently good condition. The male was singing; the female was ready to breed. They were mated and raised some healthy chicks, but the male from the time of his arrival suffered from an asthmatic condition that bothered him more at night than in the daytime. He always slept with his head hanging between his feet. During the following winter he was caged with a large number of males. None of the babies he had fed and none of the birds he had been caged with developed symptoms of illness.

About this time I made up my mind to make a place in a concrete paved yard for growing greens and testing seed. This green food was for emergency feeding. Normally I had other arrangements for supplying my birds with green food, but in rainy weather these sometimes failed. No soil was available, so I used cage refuse which was mostly sand, waste seeds and bird droppings. I took a number of sacks of string beans and placed them in a corner of the yard and covered them with caged refuse. They rotted all winter. The next spring I spaded several pails of lime into this soil to sweeten it. The seed present in the cage refuse germinated and grew. The first plant to come up was rape. I was called upon to use greens from this plot only once in every two or three weeks.

The plants were pulled up by the roots, washed under a hydrant and fed .to the entire flock. And every time this was done every baby in the nests over fifteen days old developed within from three to five days the symptoms that have just been described. Old and very young birds remained well. Some of these babies had their heads twisted until the beaks pointed straight up. Some of the earlier hatched babies, birds between two and four months old, developed milder symptoms—some identical with those I had observed but not recognized in the old cinnamon male. It was only then that I realized that his way of carrying his head was something more than a habit. Realizing that I was dealing with a strange and probably infectious condition, I made blood cultures from all affected birds. They remained sterile. I fed washed and unwashed tops from this rape to the entire flock. The birds remained well. I fed washed roots from the rape to the entire flock. All susceptible birds developed the disease; the old and very young remained well. I gathered droppings from affected birds and placed them in the drinking water of birds of susceptible age. The susceptible birds remained well. I then fed these same birds on the roots of the rape, and they developed the disease. I took about 5 gallons of clean sand and had it roasted to almost a red heat. I placed this sand in a box, contaminated it with the droppings of affected birds, sowed it with rape seed, and fed the sprouted rape, roots and all, to babies of susceptible ages. They developed the disease.

I tried a number of different lines of treatment that had proven effective in bacterial septicemias. I was able to find nothing that had any influence, either good or bad, upon the course of the illness. Nothing I could do made the symptoms either better or worse. The degree of neck paralysis in all cases seemed to depend upon the severity of the initial attack, which in turn depended upon the density of the original infection and the susceptibility of the bird. Additional feeding of infective material did not make the condition worse. No improvement was ever observed to take place. Mildly affected birds remained in good health for about two years, but thereafter they developed a tendency to hypertrophy of the liver and digestive disorders. These experiments covered a period of over four years. The ground I had made remained infective at the end of that time—two years after the last bird droppings had been added to it.

Conclusions. I was forced to conclude that the causative agent was probably a parasite, protozoan in character, capable of an independent existence in the soil; that the parasite, once introduced into the body of a susceptible bird remained there throughout the life of the bird; that it was present in the droppings of affected birds in a form not directly infective; but that it underwent changes in the soil in the presence of growing greens that rendered it infective. That the disease cannot be considered contagious is evident from foregoing. In further experiments, carried out during the years 1940 and 1941, I have found that sulfanilamide is an absolute specific for this condition in canaries. The dose is 1/10 grain into the crop. It takes from four to six months for the bird to regain the use of the paralyzed muscles, but the actual infection is cured at once, from a single dose of the drug. Repeat doses are not necessary, and should they be given oftener than once per

week, might prove fatal. I killed several good birds in finding
this out, so be careful. Recent experiments on canaries have demonstrated that Sulfanilamide is an absolute specific for this condition. The dose for a canary is 1/10 grain into the crop. A single
dose of this size is sufficient to effect a complete cure, though it
may take the bird from four to six months to completely regain the
use of the affected muscles. A repeat dose of this size for a canary
is sure to prove fatal. For chickens the dose should be the largest
that can safely be given, which would probably be from 5 to 7
grains for a bird of three pounds to five pounds. The bird is caught
and the pill forced down its throat. Whether or not such birds
are subject to reinfection has not yet been investigated.*

FOWL TYPHOID. This is a contagious, septicemic disease of
chickens caused by Bacterium sanguinarium. It has been described
by Klein, Hadley, Moore, Dawson and others. The natural disease
is known only in chickens. Pigeons are susceptible to inoculation
with the causative organism.

Etiology. The organism responsible for fowl typhoid is a
plump, non-motile, Gram-negative rod which can be obtained in
pure cultures from the blood and organs of infected birds. It has
heavily staining borders and a lightly staining center and frequently occurs in pairs joined end to end, which gives the couplet
the appearance of a figure "8." This is illustrated in Figure 40,
from a section of the liver of a bird that died from fowl typhoid
and shows a capillary congested with blood and containing a clump
of organisms.†

Symptoms. These are the general symptoms of septicemic
diseases: The bird sleeps in the daytime, pays little attention to
food or its surroundings. There is generally a soft, thin, yellow
or greenish diarrhea. The droppings differ considerably from those
observed in cholera and diphtheria, being thinner and more mucid
in character; their color is lighter and brighter, too. The first

---

* **Note:** Some of the facts set forth in this discussion of fowl paralysis were
first published in a copyrighted article by me which appeared in the
"American Canary and Cage-Bird Life," Chicago, 1933. I believe that I
am the first to present any experimental evidence throwing light upon the
transmission of this disease.

† **Note:** For a complete description of this organism the reader is referred
to "Diseases of Domesticated Birds" by Ward and Gallagher, Macmillan
Company, or to the Biennial Report of the Bureau of Animal Industry
for the years 1895-96, in which Moore, laboring under the impression that
he was dealing with an outbreak of infectious leukemia, reported a thorough study of this organism. The paper is well illustrated and it is from
this source that the illustrations used in this section were obtained.

Figure 40.   **FOWL TYPHOID**

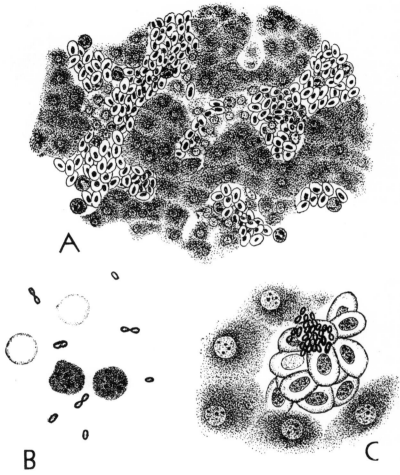

A, Section of liver from fowl. It shows the blood spaces engorged, and the considerable number of liver cells which have a thin or ragged border. Many of these appear to be separated from the adjacent tissue and to lie wholly within the blood spaces. Drawing made with a Zeiss apochromatic 16 mm. objective and compensating ocular No. 4.

B, Cover-glass preparation of the spleen of a rabbit showing the deeply stained periphery and light center of **Bacterium sanguinarium.** Also its appearance in pairs. Preparation stained with Loeffler's methylene blue.

C, A drawing from a section of a fowl's liver, showing capillary containing blood and a clump of the organisms. ($\times$ 2000.)

(After Moore.)

Figure 41.   **FOWL TYPHOID**

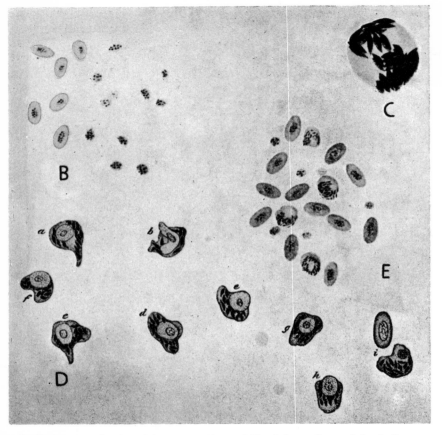

B, Red corpuscles found in preparations of blood from diseased fowl. Some of them take the eosin stain feebly, others not at all, and still others contain vacuoles. Many of these corpuscles are broken, the nuclei being either displaced or free. (× 1000.)

C, A very much enlarged leucocyte containing the spindle-shaped bodies. These bodies are highly refractive in the fresh condition.

D, A white blood corpuscle attacking a red one. Sketches made from a fresh preparation of blood from a diseased fowl. The changes illustrated in the different drawings occurred within a period of thirty-five minutes. The red corpuscle was not free from the leucocyte until the end, although it frequently became nearly so.

E, A drawing from a single field in a preparation of blood made from a fowl the day before death. (× 1000.)

(After Moore.)

symptom is an elevation of temperature which, before death, may reach 110 to 112 degrees F.

Morbid anatomy. The mucous and serous surfaces are generally pale, but there may be small areas of congestion or punctiform hemorrhages. There are no hemorrhages in the duodenum or the heart walls; the latter are pale and contain numerous small, gray, necrotic spots, both on its surface and throughout the muscular tissue. See A, B, C, Figure 42, which shows the macroscopic appearance of the heart, and E, Figure 42, which shows a section of one of the necrotic spots magnified about 1000 times. The spaces between the muscular fibers are filled with cells, granular matter and clumps of bacteria.

The liver is greatly enlarged and sprinkled with gray spots. In some cases the whole organ is congested; in others it is congested in bands. Figure 40 shows a section of a liver from a chicken that died of fowl typhoid. Note the congested capillaries and ragged borders of the liver cells. The magnification is about 1000 times. C, Figure 40 shows one of these capillaries magnified about 2000 times.

The kidneys are pale and streaked with reddish bands. The spleen is sometimes enlarged and dark colored, though this is not a constant lesion.

The number of red cells in the blood is greatly diminished, while the number of polymorphonuclear leucocytes is greatly increased. The proportion may be as high as 1:7 as against a normal proportion of 1:125. In Leukemia it is the mononuclear leucocytes that are increased and the proportion may be as high as from 1:5 to 1:2.

Moore observed the leucocytes attacking the red cells and destroying them, as illustrated in D, Figure 41. The cells that have been attacked become shadows and will no longer take the stain.

Treatment. I have found no report of the successful treatment of this disease. I have not treated the disease myself, but Mr. L. A. May, Reseda, California, who conducted a series of experiments with STROUD'S SPECIFIC, informed me that he had excellent results in the treatment of this disease with a mixture of one part STROUD'S EFFERVESCENT BIRD SALTS with three parts of STROUD'S SALTS NO. 1, administered in the drinking water in the proportion of one teaspoonful of salts to the quart of water. Reasoning from my own experience in the treatment of septicemic diseases I would expect better results from using one of these preparations unmixed. If called upon to treat this disease, I should advise that half of the flock be given one of these salts,

Figure 42. FOWL TYPHOID

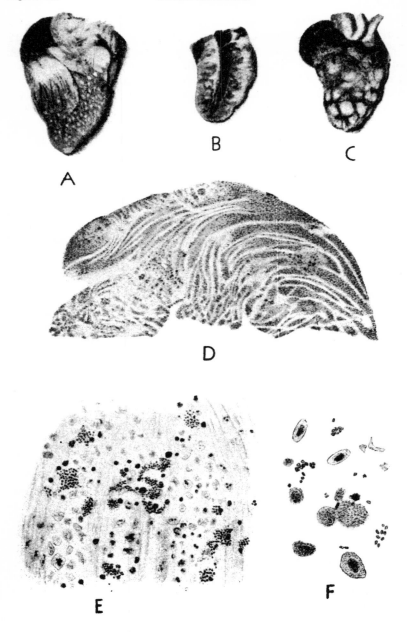

A

B

C

D

E

F

Figure 43.   **FUNGOID SKIN**

FAVUS IN CHICKENS

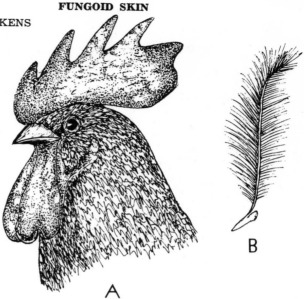

Freehand draw-
ings by the au-
thor, made from
memory.

A, The head of a
rooster, show-
ing white
patches on
comb and
wattle.

B, A body feath-
er from an
infected area,
showing piece
of attached
epidermis.

B

A

and the other half given the other, and that future treatment be
predicated upon the results obtained. Moore suggests the use of
quinine in doses of one to two grains per bird (adult chicken) and
the use of a 1:200 solution of sulphate of iron as drinking water.*

* Note: A 1:200 solution of copperas is obtained by adding one teaspoonful
of the green crystals to each quart of drinking water. Crystals that have
turned white from loss of water should be discarded, since their composition is uncertain.

Figure 42
THE LESIONS IN THE HEART

A, Drawing made from a heart of diseased fowl showing grayish areas or
points on the surface. (Natural size.)
B, Section of heart showing the grayish tubercles to extend through the
heart muscle. (Natural size.)
C, The heart of fowl which lived eleven days after inoculation. The surface
is covered with grayish tubercle-like projections. (Natural size.)
D, A section of heart muscle showing the grayish areas to be sprinkled
throughout the muscle. Drawing made from a section stained with
methylene blue and eosin. The grayish points consisting of round cell
infiltration with bacteria and stained blue in the preparation. Traced
with camera lucida. (× about 14.)
E, A drawing of a portion of one of the grayish points under high magnification with Zeiss apochromatic objective 2 mm., 1.30 N. A., and compensating ocular No. 4. Outlines traced with camera lucida. It shows
cells and masses of the bacteria between and surrounding the muscle
fibers.
F, A drawing from cover-glass preparation showing the bacteria. (× 1000.)
(After Moore.)

Figure 44. **GAPE**
GAPE WORMS

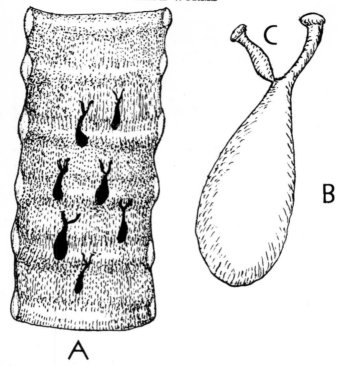

A

A, This sketch illustrates the way the worms appear in the split trachea of an infested bird.
B, The female worm.
C, The male worm.
What I spot for Shakespeare's PASSIONATE PILGRIM. It is too bad old Billy did not know about these worms.

FRACTURES. See BROKEN BONES.

FREESE'S DISEASE. Freese has described a septicemic disease of canaries caused by a Gram-positive, non-motile organism that is rod-like in shape, about .5 microns wide and 1.5 microns long. The organism thrives best with plenty of air but will grow without oxygen (Anaerobically). It can be obtained in pure culture from the heart blood of birds that have died from the disease, but it is sometimes found with difficulty in the blood of birds that have just died. When the examination is postponed for an hour or two the organisms will be present in great number and can still be obtained in pure culture, proving that they are not post-mortem invaders.

Cultivation. On agar at blood heat, colonies about the size of maw seed appear within 12 hours. They have a bright, shiny appearance, raised centers, becoming uniformly thinner toward the edges. Gray by reflected light, bright blue by transmitted light, they have the appearance of fine droplets of dew.

On gelatin, the colonies appear on the second day as fine, grayish-white points which show brown centers by transmitted light. Shortly thereafter a bright, transparent area forms around each colony, showing the beginning of liquefaction. Within five days from the time of seeding, the whole plate is liquefied.

In bouillon at blood heat, there is a uniform cloudiness after fourteen hours and the formation of a viscous sediment. After five days the cloudiness begins to disappear from the upper part

Figure 45. **GENERATIVE SYSTEM**
GENERATIVE ORGANS OF MALE BIRD

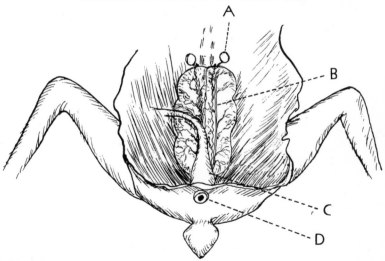

A, Testicles.
B, Kidneys, showing path of ureters and vasa deferentia. Compare this drawing with the one of the female organs under the heading, EGG STRUCTURE AND FORMATION.
The vasa and ureters are enclosed in the same stroma with the blood vessels.
C, Cloaca.
D, Vent.
Sketched by the author from memory.

Figure 46.   **GENERATIVE SYSTEM**
SECTION FROM THE TESTICLE OF A MALE CANARY

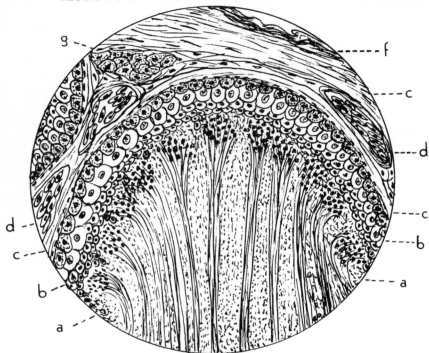

a, a, Spermatozoa developing in a tubule of a canary's testicle.
b, b, Germinal layers.
c, c, Stroma of the germinal tubule.
d, d, Blood vessels.
    e, Muscular stroma of testicle.
    f, Peritoneum.
    g, A clump of interstitial epithelial cells. These are the cells of internal
      secretion.

    Material fixed in mercury-iron solution and stained in toto with hema-
toxylin and eosin. Freehand drawing by the author, made with a magnification of 445 ×.

of the tube, and after fourteen days the liquid becomes entirely
clear. There is a thick, brownish-gray sediment in the bottom of
the tube. No pellicle is formed.

    On potato the growth appears in eighteen hours. The colonies
are grayish-white, prominent, sharply outlined and about the size
of maw seed. The growth forms a uniform layer along the needle
path.

    Milk is coagulated in fifteen hours at blood heat and in thirty-two hours at room temperature. Lactic acid is formed; but neither acid nor gas are formed in sugar media.

The organism will cause the death of canaries, sparrows and mice. Hens, rabbits and guinea pigs are insusceptible.

Symptoms. The symptoms of this disease are for the most part the general symptoms of septicemia. The bird carries its feathers loosely, has fever, is puffed up most of the time on the second day, but continues to eat and drinks more than usual. At times it has panting spells. There may be diarrhea. Freese describes as characteristic the fact that the sick bird will sometimes leave the perch and move about like a well bird, but it is rather common for sick birds, particularly fevered birds, to try to throw off their illness in this manner during the early stages of the attack; so this symptom is really of no diagnostic value. As the disease progresses the moments of activity become less frequent, and towards the last the bird sits in the bottom of the cage, its head turned back into its feathers. At times the breathing is very rapid. The bird continues to eat until within a few hours of death.

Morbid anatomy. The upper intestines are red and swollen.* The liver is either highly congested and enlarged or yellow and fragile. The spleen is usually normal, though in some cases it may be slightly enlarged.

Treatment. Having had no experience with this disease I can recommend no treatment other than the general treatments for septicemias.

FUNGOID SKIN. Birds are susceptible to mould infections of the skin that are in some respects analogous to the various types of ringworm afflicting man. There are undoubtedly several different varieties of fungi which attack the skin of different species of birds, but because only one of these has been closely studied and because the general treatment in all cases is about the same, I shall discuss the entire subject under this one all-inclusive heading.

Favus or White Comb. This is a disease of chickens caused by the fungus **Lophophyton gallinae,** which first attacks the comb and wattle (though it may later spread through the feathered areas), where it appears as small, white, downy-surfaced spots, firmly attached to the underlying tissue. Later the spots lose their

---

* **Note:** Freese does not say so, but I'd bet that the bird seeks a corner to sit in, sits on its heels with its tail touching the floor of the cage and its wing slightly drooped, to keep it from falling. These are the characteristics of dying birds; they are observed in almost all cases of acute, progressive illness.

downy appearance, become larger and thicker and scaly-surfaced; the adjacent spots coalesce. Scratching the spots causes them to shed fine white powder or mica-like scales. On the feathered areas a whitish crust is formed at the base of the feathers. The epidermial lining of the feather sockets are destroyed and separated from the underlying tissue, so that when the feather is pulled out—and all affected feathers come out without resistance—the entire socket lining and surface scale comes away, firmly attached to the base of the feather shaft. See Figure 43.

Etiology. The fungus causing favus can be grown by seeding agar containing one per cent peptone and four per cent glucose with bits of material from the comb lesions. The colonies appear as small, round, pure-white, downy growths on the surface of the media. When kept at room temperature the colonies remain white, but if kept at the temperature of 37 degrees C., they soon become a delicate rose color. The color diffuses throughout the media, which is said to be characteristic of this fungus. The infection is spread by contact. Inoculations may be made by rubbing the fungus from culture or infective material from other birds on the comb or wattle of the test bird. The period of incubation is fourteen days. Mice, rabbits and man are susceptible. So far as I know, other species have not been tested.

Fungoid skin in canaries. This condition has, so far as I am aware, never been closely studied. The lesions on the skin do not differ greatly from those occurring on the feathered areas of chickens, as just described, excepting that in this case the scales are yellow instead of white. As in the poultry infection, the feathers from the affected area are soon lost.

Treatment. These conditions are not generally fatal. Fowls have a tendency to recover from favus within from three to four months; and, while some birds have carried the disease for three or four years at a stretch, such cases are generally considered to be the result of a succession of reinfections. The skin lesions may be treated with carbolic vaseline, 1:10 salicylic acid ointment, 1:8 red oxide of mercury ointment or a 1:2 "cut" tincture of iodine. (The tincture may be cut either with alcohol or glycerin.) On canaries I have never used anything but straight tincture of iodine. One drop of saturated solution of potassium iodide may be added to each ounce of drinking water. This will increase the birds' resistance and aid them in throwing off the disease. Needless to say that the cages, houses and equipment with which affected birds have been in contact must be thoroughly cleaned. See IODIDES.

G

GANGRENE. This is the decay of any part of the living body. The tissue of the affected part usually turns blue. There are two kinds of gangrene frequently met with in birds. The first is the result of interference with the circulation; the second is the result of infection. Birds, because of their high body temperature, are not susceptible to ordinary wound infections but a gangrenous peritonitis is frequently met with. See BROKEN BONES; PERITONITIS; FEET.

GAPE. The condition called **gape** or **gapes** is the result of infestation of the trachea (windpipe) by a species of roundworm designated **Syngamus tracgealis,** which attaches itself to the mucous lining of the trachea and lives by sucking blood; and in doing so it sets up inflammatory changes and may block the passage to an extent that proves fatal. In some cases the worms invade the air sacs.

Description and life history. The female worm is red in color, from five-eighths to seven-eighths of an inch long, while the male worm is from three-sixteenths to one-quarter of an inch long. They are grown together in the act of continuous copulation, which gives them the appearance of a two-headed worm. Because the female has no way of discharging her eggs, they remain in her body until it becomes full and bursts. The body is then coughed up by the bird, swallowed and digested. The eggs pass on through the bird and out with the droppings, contaminating soil and water with eggs and larva. When the eggs or larva find their way into the body of a new host the young worms quickly make their way to the trachea, attach themselves to the mucous lining, and a new cycle of infestation is on its way. It has been shown that contaminated ground remains infective for at least one year.

Chickens, turkeys, pigeons, pheasants, peafowls, canaries, sparrows, finches, and probably most other birds are susceptible to infestation. There is a related species attacking waterfowls and infesting their air sacs, particularly those of young geese. Adult pigeons and chickens appear to be able to throw off the worms, resist the infestation, or tolerate the worms without any impairment of the general health. Where turkeys and chickens are kept in close association, the turkeys may be heavily infested while chickens remain practically free from infestation. Adult canaries

and sparrows show a high degree of resistance to gape-worm infestation, but unlike chickens and pigeons, those birds in which
the worms once gain a foothold—I probably should have said **mouth-
hold**—do not throw them off.

Symptoms. The symptoms of gape are unmistakable. The bird
carries on all its usual functions in a dull, listless manner. The
feathers are carried loosely; the breathing may be asthmatic in
character—especially noticeable at night—and the bird sleeps a
great deal in the daytime, which is probably to make up for its
broken rest at night. Every few minutes while at rest the bird
thrusts its head forward, opens its beak widely and works its neck
with a peculiar motion suggestive of an attempt to swallow something lodged in the throat. It is this characteristic motion from
which the disease takes its name, and it is so suggestive and characteristic that it can be recognized the first time it is seen, regardless of the species of bird affected. Sometimes the gape is followed
by a fit of coughing, after which a bloody froth may be noticed on
the edges of the beak.

Morbid anatomy. When the trachea is split open, the worms,
enveloped in a frothy mucous, will be seen adhering to its walls.
There may be yellow abscesses at the point of attachment. See
Figure 44.

Prevention and treatment. Prevention of gape in caged birds
is very simple. All one has to do is to see that their sand and green
food does not come from contaminated ground, from the neighborhood of a chicken yard or sparrow roost. The addition of a little
potassium permanganate to the drinking water has been recommended as a preventive measure in the handling of baby chicks.
Keeping the houses, equipment and grounds clean, or moving the
chicks to clean ground at frequent intervals, will aid in preventing
the spread of infestation. Young chickens should never be run
on ground that has been run over by turkeys. Where the birds
cannot be moved to clean ground, the soil may be treated to kill
the worms. Ward and Gallagher suggest that it be disinfected
by drenching it with one per cent sulphuric acid. Or chloride of
lime might be used, as suggested under the heading AVIAN DIPH-
THERIA.

A great many treatments—some stupid, most of them ineffective, and all of them dangerous—have been suggested for the removal of the worms from the trachea. The only one which I think
worthy of consideration where small birds are concerned is that

suggested by Klee, which consists of injecting a vermicide into the trachea. There are two ways of doing this: a fine, sharp canula (hypodermic needle) may be slipped through the skin of the neck and between the rings of the trachea; a blunt, curved canula may be introduced into the trachea through the mouth and larynx. In the treatment of small birds the first method is the best. The finest needle obtainable must be employed, and it must be very sharp, but given these conditions, it is best to make the injection through the wall of the trachea, since there is far less danger of inflicting fatal injuries on the bird. The syringe should have rings on the sides of the barrel, so that it may be handled with one hand and must be equipped with a graduated piston and locknut for controlling the dosage. Otherwise, there is grave danger of strangling the patient. For the adult chicken, the dose should be from 0.5 cc. to 1 cc. of whatever solution is used; for pigeons the dose is ¼ cc.; and for birds the size of a canary it should not be much over 1/100 cc. There are a number of solutions which may be used for this purpose. Klee recommends a five per cent solution of sodium salicylate. A 1:500 solution of potassium permanganate would be as effective as anything else. Other solutions that could be used are: one per cent borax; one-half per cent sodium chloride; one-half per cent carbolic acid; one per cent potassium chlorate; and 1:1000 copper sulphate.

Like other methods of treating gape, this treatment is dangerous. There are three ways in which it can result in the death of the bird: a carelessly manipulated needle may do irreparable injury; too much or a carelessly prepared solution may be injected; or the release of all the worms at once may block the larynx and cause death by strangulation. Because of the great size of the worms in proportion to the size of the trachea of a canary or other birds of comparable size, this last-mentioned danger is very great. It is a danger which must be faced, however. The only thing the operator can do to assist the bird is to release it the instant the injection is made; thus giving it a chance to put all of its power into the cough which follows.

GASTRITIS. This is any inflammation of the proventriculus or gizzard. See DIGESTIVE DISORDERS. The symptoms of acute gastritis are identical with those of obstruction of the gizzard—since, regardless of the cause of the inflammation, but as a direct result of it, the pyloric valve always becomes spasmodically contracted—thus producing obstruction even though no foreign body is present in the gizzard. This is especially true where the cause

of the inflammation is mouldy food or rancid seed. See ASPER-
GILLOSIS.

GENERATIVE SYSTEM. The male bird has two round or oval
testicles located in the abdominal cavity near the anterior (nearer
the head) border of the kidneys. In the male canary the testicles
are round and vary in size from that of a rape seed to that of a
large hemp seed. The mature rooster has oval testicles about one

Figure 47.   **GENERATIVE SYSTEM**

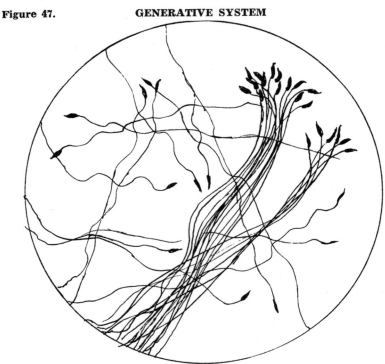

Spermatozoa in a smear from the testicle of a male canary. Notice the
extremely long flagula. Some of them are so long that they extend across
three 500 × fields. The length of the flagula of human spermatozoa is
about that of the portions of those two in the lower part of the field after
they have crossed the clump.

Preparation dried in air and stained with crystal violet. Freehand
drawing by the author, using 445 × magnification.

inch long and from one-half inch to five-eighths of an inch thick.
I once owned an old roller canary that was a wonderful breeder.
He was years past the age when most canary males are taken out
of the breeding room, but was still going strong. He was killed in

an accident and I found that he had a single testicle as large as a BB shot.* Each testicle is provided with a **vas deferens** (excretion duct) which leads to the uro-genital portion of the cloaca, where it ends in an erectile papilla provided with a plexus of nerves and blood vessels. The paths of the ducts follow closely .the paths of the ureters; but unlike the ureters, which follow straight courses, the courses of the **vasa deferniae** † are highly convoluted. Figure 45 shows the relative positions of the testicles, vasa, kidneys, ureters and cloaca. The branching lines on the surface of the kidneys represent the ureters. In the fresh specimen they are white.

During coition the chickens' vents appear to spread so that the erectile tissues of the male come into contact with those of the female. In canaries and finches the entire vent of the male is erectile and is inserted into the cloaca of the female. Some water-fowls, drakes and ganders for instance, have a single, well-developed penis which, after coition, can be seen hanging out—the drake's will drag on the ground as he gives himself a satisfied shake and waddles away. See Figure 45.

As a rule, only the left ovary and oviduct are developed, though exceptional cases of rudimentary development of the right ovary and oviduct have been observed. The structure and functions of the female organs have already been described. See EGG STRUC-TURE AND FORMATION.

GENTIAN. This is a bitter tonic from the roots of the plant **Gentiana lutea.** It comes on the market as a dry powder, a fluid extract, an alcoholic tincture and a compound tincture. The alcoholic tincture is of value in the preparation of bird tonics or may itself be used as a tonic. The dose for birds is one drop to each two ounces of drinking water—eight drops to the pint. Gentian is sometimes compounded with such substances as cascara, buckthorn, licorice, honey, etc. See CASCARA.

GIZZARD. See DIGESTIVE TRACT.

GLAUBER'S SALT, SODIUM SULPHATE. This salt comes on the market in large crystals containing ten molecules of water of crystallization and as a dried, white powder containing one molecule

---

* **Note:** I have found two of these birds since this was written. It is now known that such birds are natural females that have for some reason, probably disease, lost their ovary. Under these circumstances the rudimentary right ovary has developed into a testicle. In experiment ovariotomies about fifty per cent of the birds operated upon become males.

†**Note:** Both ducts. A rather silly way to form a plural, but if I did not use it someone disagreeing with my views might take it upon himself to publicly point out that fact rather than debase himself by stooping to argue with one such as I. Are you there, Durant?

of water. It is widely used as a laxative for birds and mammals. It is more pleasant to take and less drastic in action than Epsom salts, so widely used in human medicine. The dose for birds is one-half to one grain of the powder or a two to four-grain crystal to each ounce of drinking water. The solution should contain just enough salt to give it a slightly saline taste.

Once, when discussing bird medicine with a doctor, he said, "How it is that you fellows insist on giving Glauber's salt to your birds? Wouldn't Epsom salts be just as good? I asked a veterinarian the other day why it was he would not give Epsom salts to a horse and he just laughed at me. Why is it?"

I explained that Epsom salts is too irritating, is apt to do more harm than good, and then, too, that animals and birds are rather discriminating, that they will not take Epsom salts without an argument.

"Do you mean to tell me that you are more careful of your birds than we doctors are of our patients?"

"Certainly," I replied. "When a bird dies I cannot send a bill to his heirs. I am just out one bird. Then, again, man is the only animal that is fool enough to take anything that is suggested to him. If you put a poisonous solution of mercury bichloride before him without a label on it, he would be pretty apt to drink it and die. You can take all water away from a bird and fill the drinkers with a poisonous solution of mercury bichloride, but even though they are almost dying of thirst, the birds will not drink the solution. But, if you dilute the solution to a point where it is no longer poisonous, the birds will drink it as readily as they would pure water."

"Mmmm—they do seem to have a little sense at that."

Glauber's salt merits the preference shown it by birds and animals. Its one drawback is that it is not easily soluble in cold water. This difficulty is overcome by incorporating it in effervescent mixtures. Some of these mixtures are now widely used and no small part of their well-deserved popularity is due to the Glauber's salt they contain.

GLYCERIN. This is an organic base obtained from the decomposition of fats in the manufacture of soap. It is also manufactured from sugar by fermentation in an alkaline solution. It is a thick, syrupy, colorless liquid with a sweetish taste. It is soluble in water and alcohol in all proportions. Glycerin has been used in medicine as a laxative, but its principal employment is for the dilution of other drugs. It has the power of protecting tissue against irritants. For example, tincture of iodine cannot be used on mucous surfaces, such as the throat, without causing injury, but one of the best treatments we have for sore throat is a mixture of equal parts of tincture of iodine and glycerin.

Glycerin is also of value for softening hard tissues and is widely used in preparations for the skin.

Because of its power to withdraw water from tissue, glycerin is used as a preservative for organs intended for bacteriological examination.

In avian diphtheria, infectious bronchitis and some other conditions of the respiratory tract, the sick bird is forced to breathe through its mouth for days and weeks at a time which causes the surface of the tongue to become hard and dry and develop a tendency to split away from the softer tissue underneath, which causes the bird a lot of unnecessary suffering and makes eating almost impossible. This condition, called **Pip,** should be avoided by anointing the affected bird's tongue several times per day with an emulsion of glycerine and olive oil. The emulsion can be prepared as follows:

Take one-half ounce of glycerin; add about ten grains of egg-yolk powder; beat with a mechanical beater while one ounce of olive oil and fifteen minims of carbolic acid are being slowly added to the mixture, a few drops at a time. The beating should continue until a smooth, creamy emulsion is obtained.

GLYCYRRHIZA, Licorice. This is the dried root of the Spanish plant, **Glycyrrhiza glabra,** which, though it has no marked medical properties, is widely used in medicine in the form of an extract or ammoniate for the purpose of disguising the taste of unpleasant drugs. It is often used in conjunction with sugar, honey or syrup.

GOING LIGHT, Asthenia. This is a rather common and little understood condition of both poultry and caged birds. The most noticeable symptoms of **going light** are extreme emaciation, abnormal appetite, loss of pep and vigor. The bird is always hungry but seems to derive no benefit from the food consumed.

Etiology. I am not able to look upon this condition as a specific disease. The symptoms upon which a diagnosis of going light is based are common to a great many unrelated conditions. I am inclined to believe that the most common cause of these symptoms in caged birds is starvation—the use of food unfit for a bird to eat.

Extreme mite infestation, tapeworms, tuberculosis, and any number of other conditions which sap the bird's vitality and strength faster than he can build it up may produce these symptoms. But there are some conditions involving these symptoms to which no known cause can be assigned. In such cases we hide our ignorance behind the high-sounding word **asthenia.**

In teaching birds to do tricks, even where the utmost in kindness and patience is employed, they are subjected to considerable nervous shock. Many birds of a nervous temperament cannot stand this. They go into a decline and die. It has always been my opinion that such birds were suffering from shock-induced diabetes. And though I have found sugar in the urine of such birds, I have also found it in the urine of birds suffering from similar symptoms resulting from definite pathological causes, and I have not made the serieses analysis of blood and droppings necessary for the justification of a positive diagnosis of diabetes. My opinion, therefore, is merely an opinion, but it still stands. In several recent cases (1941) I have found degenerated areas in pancreas in which both the structures of internal and external secretion (those secreting pancreatic fluid and the islands of Langerhans) were obliterated. See drawing No. 6, Figure 56, under the heading LEUKEMIA.

Dawson has studied a similar condition in poultry and has assigned as its cause the invasion of the duodenum by a bacterium of the colon group. It was his opinion that the presence of the organism interfered with the process of nutrition—which is quite possible. He suggested the use of a calomel purge followed by a tonic.

There are many cases displaying these symptoms that do not respond to treatment and in which no specific cause can be found. It is noteworthy that such cases seldom occur in a well-cared-for flock. Therefore, it seems reasonable to suppose that most cases of going light are either the symptoms of some serious chronic condition or the result of some form of abuse or neglect. The more intelligent care the birds receive the less apt are such conditions to develop. There is a lot about these chronic diseases of birds that we do not understand. The answer to the problem presented by them is more study. Maybe this book will stimulate others into undertaking it.

GOUT. This is a nutritional disease resulting from a diet too rich in proteins and too lean in the salts and vitamins found in fresh green food and quickly follows the use of too much milk, milk products or egg food in the diet of caged birds. In one of my experiments I substituted moist bread for egg food for eighteen pair of breeding canaries. For nine pair the bread was moistened with water; for the other nine pair it was moistened with fresh milk. The milk-fed birds produced the most babies for the first two rounds; the babies were larger, feathered better and fewer of them were lost in the nests, but at the end of the two rounds, the old birds went out of breeding condition and seventeen out of eighteen old birds were showing symptoms of gout. About two-thirds of the old birds and practically all of the young of the milk-fed group developed soft moult the following fall. The males could not be gotten into song. The young were all extra healthy looking birds but something was missing. The old birds of the water-fed group continued in breeding condition over five rounds; seven of the nine hens refused to moult and became bald. In the entire season these birds raised almost twice as many young as those of the milk-fed group, but the young were smaller, scrubbier-looking birds. The males came into full song early but about half of them failed to moult their heads and necks and became bald. In another experiment cottage cheese was used instead of egg food. All of the birds fed on this item developed a very serious gout and none of them were of much value thereafter. See VITAMINOSIS A.

Symptoms. The liver and the abdomen become enlarged. In some cases the birds are emaciated and in others they are obese; but in both types of cases there is a retention of urates and uric acid in the system. The feet and joints become enlarged in varying degrees, exude a sticky fluid and are, therefore, always covered with dirt; they are tender rather than painful. Where only one foot is involved the bird will favor that foot and hold it up a great part of the time, but has no compunction about using it when necessary, and most certainly does not make the fuss over it that he would over a diphtheric sore or mosquito bite. The lesions seem to itch rather than pain and probably have little real feeling. I have seen gouty birds bite swollen toes to the bone and make no protest or show of pain as the amputation was completed. The droppings are usually soft and dull-yellow in color.

Treatment. The specific for gout is a newly discovered, complex organic compound called **cinchophen**. When mixed with sugar in the proportion of 1:10 and fed dusted on moist bread or other soft food, this drug will quickly reduce the swellings; the bird shows marked improvement from the very first dose; but it is a dangerous drug and must be discontinued as soon as the symptoms of the disease have vanished. The dose for a canary is not more than 1/10 grain per day.

The improvements gained by the judicious use of cinchophen must be consolidated by dietetic measures. If the case occurs during spring or summer, the best thing to do is place the bird in a large flight and feed it exclusively on milk-seed (the seeds of wild and cultivated plants and grasses in the milk stage of development) and green food for a while. Pepper grass, thistle heads, sunflower heads, all the seeding grasses and even broomcorn, kaffir corn or sweet or field corn may be used. A variety of such foods is better than a single item.

This subject will be further discussed under the headings VISCERAL GOUT and AVITMINOSIS A.

Once the gouty condition has been overcome, the bird must be kept in health by avoiding the dietetic errors originally responsible for the condition.

Cinchophen poisoning. Should cinchophen be administered in excessive doses or over too long a period of time, the bird will develop symptoms identical with those of one form of acute uremic poisoning. It loses control of its muscles, usually the muscles of one side of the body, which are subject to a slow, rhythmic, spasmodic jerking which continues for hours until the bird dies or recovers. The rate of these jerks is usually about one per second and all of the muscles of the affected side jerk in unison—the head shoots forward, the beak opens, the eye blinks, the foot jerks up and the wing jerks down against the side, which is least noticeable since the wing is carried against the side. See UREMIA. Cinchophen poisoning is quickly amendable to the same line of treatment suggested for the spasmodic symptoms of acute uremic poisoning.

GRAVEL. See DIGESTIVE TRACT.

HAND FEEDING. While the hand feeding of baby birds is more trouble than the resulting birds are apt to be worth, it is of advantage to know how to hand feed successfully. There are many cases where a fine nest of birds may be saved by tiding them over a day or two until they can be given to other birds to care for; there are also experimental results which can be arrived at by no other method.

Many methods of hand feeding canaries have been tried. One of the best is based upon the use of SPRATT'S COD-LIVER OIL CANARY FOOD and is carried out as follows:

A small bite of sweet apple or green food—dandelion leaves, spinach or tender cabbage may be used—is taken into the mouth and chewed to a fine pulp; then a little egg-yolk powder, ground bread, and SPRATT'S FOOD are added and the whole mass is chewed until it is reduced to a thick mush. It is then expectorated into a round canary egg cup and fed to the babies from the end of a match stick or toothpick. Day-old babies have been fed on this food and I have raised birds on it from the fifth day of life to weaning time. Where the birds are raised entirely by hand, a little sand and mineral food must be added to the food mixture once each day from the tenth day on. And it must never be forgotten that the food must always be fed warm. Nothing will do more to stunt the growth of a baby bird than a big cropful of cold food.

A method that has given me even better results is based on SCARLETT'S COD-LIVER OIL NESTLING FOOD. This food as it comes is unfit for feeding baby birds by hand, for it contains the hulls of ground seeds. I prepare it as follows: A thirty-inch strip of 16-mesh wire cloth is bent to form a trough. This trough is held at an angle of about 60 degrees and a pound or two of the nestling food is permitted to run down it by gravity. That part of the food which passes through the screen under these circumstances is fine enough for the smallest baby birds. This sifted food is mixed with an equal weight of ground bread, and to each pound is added one heaping teaspoonful of egg-yolk powder, one level teaspoonful of fine-ground and sifted mineral food, one teaspoonful of cod-liver oil and one tablespoonful of sifted alfalfa meal. This food does not need to be chewed. It is prepared for feeding by reducing it to the correct consistency with boiling water. It is fed from a match stick the same as the SPRATT'S FOOD

Wild nestlings are a source of many of our finest cage-birds, or they were until stupid laws * were passed against taking nestlings. Many of the birds that are used in naturalistic studies and to decorate our zoos come from the same source. In order to adapt them to cage life, they must be taken as babies and hand raised. The babies of the **hard-billed** species (all species living on seeds, grains, and digesting their food with sand or gravel in their gizzards. All other birds are called **soft billed;** they live on soft foods and do not use sand in their gizzards) may be fed exactly the same as young canaries, but better results will be obtained by reducing the richness of the mixtures suggested above by adding fifty per cent of fresh boiled potato as the food is mixed for feeding. A few insects or a few shreds of raw beef will help these wild babies considerably.

Soft-billed birds, robins, blackbirds, mockingbirds, etc., can be raised on a mixture of raw beef and boiled potato chewed up together with a little fine ground rape seed and cuttlebone. The rape should be ground fine, hulls and all, as these are rich in Vitamin B, which is the reason for adding this item to the mixture. Cod-liver oil, of course, is given as a source of Vitamins A and D. As the birds become older they may be fed bits of beef, banana and other fruits, live insects and prepared mockingbird food. Most of the persons who engage in the business of raising or feeding wild birds raise mealworms for them. This is the most reliable source of insect food that we have.†

Psittacine birds, particularly parrots, can be hand raised on thick corn-meal mush and bananas chewed together. It might be

---

* **Note:** I say stupid laws because they are just that. For every baby bird taken by a pet lover the very people who had these laws passed have killed thousands by their stupidity. I am speaking of the very persons to whom the wild birds are most valuable, the farmers. They whine about their insect losses; they cry for relief; they beef about the cost of insecticides and want the Government to supply them; and all the time they fence every bit of their land with barbed wire so they can plough the last foot of it. Thus, all nestling places for small birds are destroyed. In Europe where practically all agricultural land is fenced either with stone walls or hedges, bird trapping has been going on for a thousand years, millions of wild songsters have been exported, and there species are no nearer extinction now than they were in the beginning. If instead of making laws to discourage bird-keeping, our lawmakers would put a 25c tax on every acre of land fenced with wire, our wild songsters would have some chance of surviving.

† **Note:** A few years ago the Department of Agriculture had a study made of the life history and habits of mealworms. It was their idea to supply millers and elevatormen with the information necessary for the extermination of mealworms. The paper was in great demand. The demand did not come from millers, however; it came from birdmen wanting information on the domestic cultivation of these worms. Truth is always of value; the opinions of Governmental Bureaus are something else again.

wise to add a little mineral food, fine ground rape and cod-liver oil to take care of their mineral and vitamin needs.

In Europe many persons make their living and at the same time sign their own death warrants by hand-feeding squabs on grain chewed up in the mouth and forced into the birds in much the same manner in which their parents feed them. The death of the operator often results from aspergillus pneumomycosis—set up by the inhalation of fungus spores present in mouldy grain.

HAND WASHING. Though the hand-washing of birds is a practice which I think should not be encouraged, there are cases where it is necessary, where the sales value, show chances or even the life of a bird may depend upon it being successfully and efficiently performed; it should not be permitted to become a habit, however. The operation may be performed as follows:

Before beginning, the operator should bring the temperature of the room to at least 80 degrees F., and lay out in a warm, convenient place—on the door of a warming oven is as good a place as any—a number of towels, handkerchiefs or pieces of gauze of suitable size for the birds to be washed. For birds the size of a canary, a handkerchief makes a good drying cloth; for birds the size of pigeons, crash face towels are about right; for chickens, a turkish bath towel is not too large. Three vessels, pails, tubs or dishes, are filled two-thirds full of clean water at the temperature of 110 F. This is a little warmer than the bird's blood; it is not warm enough to feel uncomfortably hot to your elbow. A source of boiling water should be at hand so that as the water in the pails cool, its temperature can be adjusted by adding a little more hot water. A bar of Life Buoy soap that has been softened by standing in cold water is pressed into a shaving mug, covered with boiling water, permitted to stand for a few moments and then worked up with a shaving brush into a thick lather. When all of these preliminaries have been completed the operator is ready to begin the actual washing.

Hold the bird in the hand and dip it into the water up to its beak, ruffling its feathers with the other hand so that the water will reach the skin; then, beginning at the beak and working over the head and down the back, apply the thick lather and scrub the feathers with long even strokes of the brush until all dirt has been removed. The brush strokes should always be in the direction of the feathers and not too vigorous; otherwise the feathers will be injured. The tail is spread out on the wrist of the hand holding bird so that it is supported during the brushing. The wings are supported on the heel of the hand as they are brushed. The bird is dipped frequently during this brushing in order to note what progress is being made. When the back is clean the bird is turned over and the underside is done in the same manner. Then the bird is rinsed through the three waters until every trace of soap or soapy odor has been removed. It is then wiped as dry as possible, wrapped in one of the warm drying cloths and put aside to dry while the next bird is being washed. As each succeeding bird is washed and wrapped, each of those that have been previously washed is unwrapped and given a chance to shake itself and then rewrapped in another dry cloth. This is continued until each bird is dry enough to fly and to stand on the perch without shivering. Because hand washing takes all of the oil out of the feathers, the washed bird has a dull appearance and may fly with difficulty. There are two methods by which this difficulty can be partially overcome. The first is to incorporate oil in the soap used for washing birds, thus preventing it from taking all the oil out of the feathers; the second is to attempt to replace the lost oil by wiping the feathers with an oily cloth or by spraying them with an oil mixture.

To incorporate oil in the soap, shave up one bar of Life Buoy soap, placing the shavings in a dish and add four ounces of hot water; heat until the soap dissolves and then add two ounces of poppy-seed oil. Beat the mixture for a few minutes with an egg beater and while it is still hot, pour it into a large-mouthed jar. That part of the oil which is not incorporated with the soap will separate out as the soap cools. By removing and discarding the upper half inch of soap from the jar, the excess of oil is removed. The remaining soap will not take so much oil out of the bird's feathers as ordinary soap would.

To restore oil to the feathers by means of a cloth, place a little poppy-seed oil on a piece of soft flannel; fold this piece of oily cloth in a piece of clean flannel and place in a press overnight; then either of these two pieces of cloth may be used to wipe over the feathers of the washed birds.

Another way of restoring oil to the feathers is to mix three parts of absolute alcohol with one part xylene and an excess of poppy-seed oil. Shake well and let stand overnight in tightly corked flask. The excess of oil will settle to the bottom of flask and the top fluid is decanted into another bottle. Using a small atomizer, the washed birds may be sprayed gently with this solution. Care must be taken not to apply so much oil that the feathers are made gummy.

By spraying the washed birds slightly from an atomizer loaded with water, they can be induced to comb and oil their feathers several times per day for a while.

HEART. See CIRCULATORY SYSTEM; AVIAN DIPHTHERIA; FOWL TYPHOID.

HEMORRHAGES. A hemorrhage is any blood that has escaped from the veins, arteries or capillaries. A major hemorrhage is one involving the loss of sufficient blood to seriously weaken the bird or cause its death. A minor hemorrhage may be one of any smaller size down to a microscopic point.

The presence of hemorrhages, their location, distribution, size and general character, is often of the utmost importance in the diagnosing of bird diseases. In some cases they are the only lesions found; in others, the presence or absence of hemorrhages of a particular kind in a particular place may be the determining factor in the differentiation of two diseases of somewhat similar symptoms, but amendable to two diametrically opposed lines of treatment. In such cases careless observations are pretty sure to spell failure for your efforts at treatment. So it is a good plan to look for hemorrhages. A hemorrhage into a body cavity appears as an accumulation of blood; a hemorrhage into tissue appears as a red spot that cannot be washed off with water.

HEMORRHAGIC SEPTICEMIA. This is the name given to a large class of contagious septicemic diseases afflicting all warm-blooded creatures with the exception of man.* There may be a few other exceptions, but I am not aware of them. Cattle and kangaroos, sheep and shoats, canaries and condors, swallows and swans, rodents and rhinoceroses appear to be equally susceptible to diseases of this **group.**

I have used the word **group** in connection with these conditions with well-grounded reservations. Whether we are dealing with one disease or a whole group of closely related diseases when we discuss hemorrhagic septicemia is still an open question—more about this momentarily.

General characteristics. The spontaneous appearance of hemorrhagic septicemia as a complication of avian diphtheria has already been discussed as have been FOWL CHOLERA (hemorrhagic

---

* **Note:** Bubonic plague is now considered as being caused by a germ of this group. If this is so, even man is not exempt.

septicemia of chickens) and CANARY NECROSIS (thought to be
a hemorrhagic septicemia of canaries). The disease in cattle often
makes its appearance following shipment, exposure or hard driving
from one pasturage to another; in poultry it usually appears first
in birds of lowered resistance; in hogs this disease * is often associated with outbreaks of cholera.

Always a highly fatal disease, hemorrhagic septicemia is much
more rapidly fatal in some outbreaks than in others. It is more
rapidly fatal at the beginning of an outbreak than toward its end.
The first victims may fall dead without having shown previous
symptoms of illness. In later cases the disease may run an acute
course with well-developed symptoms and lesions; while, toward
the end of the outbreak, chronic cases appear. In some of the latter,
the birds hang on for weeks or months; in others they recover after
a short illness.

Symptoms and lesions. The symptoms and lesions of hemorrhagic septicemia naturally vary with the species of animal affected
and the duration of the illness. In acute cases there are the general
symptoms of illness: fever; increased thirst; decreased appetite;
weakness; and digestive disturbances, usually indicated by diarrhea. In hogs, in which the lungs are generally affected, there is
great weakness and rapid, shallow breathing; in cattle, large lumps
often appear on various parts of the body, caused by gelatinous
exudate deposited under the skin. In birds, the most common and
constant symptom is the presence of ochre-colored droppings. See
FOWL CHOLERA.

The two most constant lesions of hemorrhagic septicemia are
punctiform hemorrhages and a gelatinous exudate. In all species,
hemorrhages are found in the duodenum and usually in the heart
wall. See Figure 48. In cattle they are found in the fatty tissue,
particularly the fat around the kidneys, and there may be bloody
infusions into the body cavities. In hogs the lungs are hemorrhagic and pneumonia generally develops. In some outbreaks in
cattle and sheep the lungs are involved; in others the principal lesions are found in the intestines. The gelatinous exudate may be
found under the skin in cattle, in the pericardium or peritoneum
in birds, in the pleurae in hogs, in the thoracic and peritonial cavities in sheep, and regardless of species, some few cases will be found
where minute particles of this gelatinous material will be found
floating in the blood stream. The exudate into the serous cavities is
often accompanied by a bloody infusion. This gelatinous exudate is

---

* **Note:** Hemorrhagic septicemia of hogs is called Swine plague.

Figure 48.   **HEMORRHAGIC SEPTICEMIA**

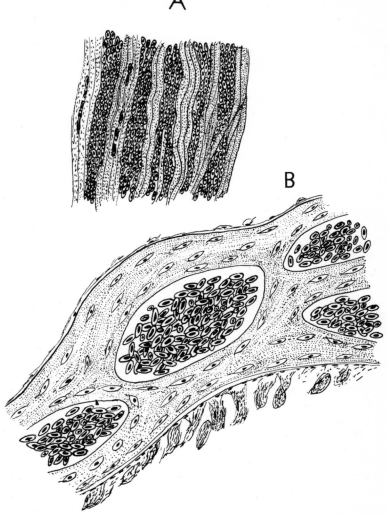

A, Section of heart muscle from a sparrow which died of hemorrhagic septicemia, showing the intermuscular spaces filled with blood.

B, Section of one of the bones of the head of the same sparrow, showing the bone sinuses filled with blood. This condition was found throughout the body. More than five thousand sections were examined and, literally, hundreds of thousands of small hemorrhages found. Very few of these were large enough to be seen with the unaided eyes.

not found in those cases where the periods of illness have been very short; where found, it is always a positive indication of hemorrhagic septicemia, which may be present either as a primary disease or a complication. Though differently located in different species, the lesions of hemorrhagic septicemia are so characteristic that once seen in one species they are easily recognized in another; once seen in a ten-gram finch, they become instantly recognizable in a ten-ton elephant.

Etiology. In all cases of hemorrhagic septicemia, examination of the blood reveals the presence of numerous small, oval, rod-like bodies which do not stain evenly with the ordinary aniline dyes. See Figure 37 which shows a blood smear and agar culture of this organism. Organisms cultivated from different species of animals vary somewhat in size, cultural characteristics and pathogenicity (the power to cause disease), but this is also true to an almost equal extent of organisms from different outbreaks in the same species and of strains from the same outbreaks cultivated for several generations in different environments. Organisms which cannot be differentiated from **B.** Pasteurella, the organism we are now discussing, are often found in the respiratory and alimentary tracts of healthy animals and birds.

Are all of these diseases in different species of animals and birds distinct, caused by similar but unrelated organisms, or are they identical, all caused by varying strains of one specific organism?

In support of the first view we have the clinical fact that when cattle and sheep or poultry and hogs are closely associated in the same pasture the disease may wipe out one species without affecting the other. The cattle may all die and the sheep remain well; the chickens may all die and the hogs be unaffected; or it may be the other way around. This appears to prove that we are dealing with two distinct conditions. So far, so good. But, we have equally well-authenticated cases where outbreaks of hemorrhagic septicemia in zoological gardens have run through from a dozen to a hundred species of animals and birds as unrelated as half-ounce finches and six-ton elephants. This appears to prove that we are dealing with a single disease to which all of these creatures are susceptible.

On the other hand, canaries and small finches are said to be subject to two distinct infections which are both classified as hemorrhagic septicemia. I think that this is an error in classification, however. There is nothing in the lesions or symptoms of canary necrosis which in any way remotely resembles the general symptoms and lesions of hemorrhagic septicemia in other animals. Therefore, it is my opinion that the organism of canary necrosis is not a true member of the hemorrhagic septicemia group. The differences in pathogenicity and virulence displayed by the organisms found in different outbreaks of hemorrhagic septicemia, are in no sense greater than the differences in pathogenicity and virulence of the fixed virus and street virus of rabies, and in this case we know the differences are the result of environmental influences—the passage of fixed virus through a single species of animals for many hundreds of passages, until it has become fixed for that species and lost its pathogenicity for all other species.

Treatment. For the treatment of all forms of hemorrhagic septicemia see the general treatment for avian diphtheria. The method of administration and the dosages are things that have to be worked out in each case, but the general principles are the same in all cases. To illustrate: the sick parrot cannot be given drinking water. It must be fed on a thick mush containing sufficient water for its needs. Naturally the medicine must be placed in the mush. See PSITTACOSIS. Mr. May, whose experiments with my treatment have already been mentioned several times, cured hemorrhagic septicemia in a hog by drenching it with a full pint of solutions containing a heaping teaspoonful of a mixture of STROUD'S SALTS NO. 1, and STROUD'S EFFERVESCENT BIRD SALTS in equal parts. He reported that nine hogs had been stricken and that eight were dead when he arrived. The ninth hog was unable to stand on its feet, eat or drink. Twenty-four hours later the animal was well. The same method could be used with cattle, but you would not drench a nine-foot tiger. The problem in every case is to administer the medicine in such a manner that the animal gets the effect. Dr. Herbert Sanborn, treating both diphtheria and cholera in pheasants, found that they would not eat the food or drink the water containing the medicine, so he injected it into their crops with a medicine dropper. The birds recovered.

HEMP SEED. The seed of Indian hemp is olive or greenish-brown in color, about three-sixteenths of an inch in diameter, and has a hard shell and soft, oily pulp, rich in proteins and oils. It is also rich in vitamins when fresh, and then has a pleasant, nut-like taste and odor. In small quantities, fresh hemp seed is one of the most valuable bird foods known. For the American breeder, however, that statement is in the wrong tense. A recently passed federal regulation requires the sterilization of all hemp seed sold in the

United States. I have recently run some tests on this sterilized seed and have found it utterly unfit for canaries to eat. The stimulating effects of good hemp on song and reproduction were lacking and there were several cases of serious poisoning among the birds to which this sterilized hemp seed was fed. So I want to make it perfectly clear right now that anything said either in this section or elsewhere in these pages about the virtues of hemp seed apply only to fresh, unsterilized hemp seed—most assuredly not to the rancid trash now on the market. The best way to overcome the deficiency in our birds' diets created by our ever-growing federal bureaucracy is to add two ounces of wheat germ oil to each 100 pounds of nestling and mating food used. See WHEAT GERM OIL. Ground sunflower seed is also a good substitute.

Because this seed is rich in the reproductive vitamin, an unlimited supply of it should be kept before the hens making eggs to insure a high percentage of hatchability.

For canaries and small finches hemp seed must be crushed, since they are unable to shell it for themselves. In crushing hemp, care should be taken not to grind up the hulls so that the birds cannot separate them from the meat of the seed, for the shells of hemp seed are rich in the drug **Hashish,** a narcotic poison.

The oil of hemp seed becomes rancid very quickly and what was formerly a valuable food becomes a deadly poison. For this reason hemp seed must always be used with care. I have fed fresh hemp to day-old canary babies without trouble, but even before our bureaucracy took a hand, there was very little hemp on the market which could be safely fed to birds under ten days old. If our experiments with wheat germ oil and the other new vitamin sources turn out as satisfactorily as preliminary tests lead us to hope, the bureaucrats will have done us a favor in the long run.

HOG CHOLERA. This can hardly be considered a bird disease, but because it is closely related to certain diseases of birds and is amendable to similar treatment—treatment of which I am the originator—and because a great many of the persons who keep birds and poultry also keep hogs, I think it is worthy of a brief discussion in this book.

Hog cholera is an acute, contagious, highly fatal, epizootic disease of hogs caused by a filterable virus. It was long thought to be a septicemic disease caused by an organism called **B. Suipestifer** or **B. salmonella** and considered to be identical with **B. paratyphosus B.** Dr. Salmon claimed to have produced typical cases of hog cholera by inoculating hogs with the organism just mentioned,

Figure 49.   **HOG CHOLERA**

LESIONS IN THE KIDNEY
AND INTESTINES

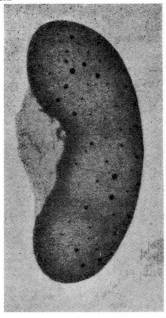

Fig. 2—Hog's kidney, showing
blood spots caused by cholera.

After Dorset & Hess, Bureau of
Animal Industry, 1917. Farmer's
Bull. 834

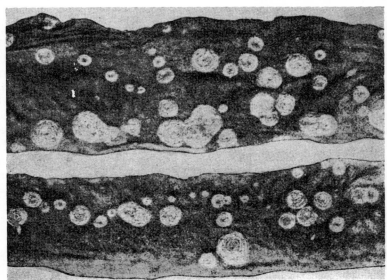

Fig. 3—Intestine of cholera hog, showing ulcers. (After Hutyra and Marek)

and B. paratyphosus B septicemia is undoubtedly a complication in a great many cases of hog cholera as it is in psittacosis and some outbreaks of avian diphtheria. Hog cholera is also often complicated with swine plague, which, as we have seen, is caused by an organism of the Pasteurella group, which is the most important of the secondary invaders in avian diphtheria.

Diagnosis. The sick hog has no appetite, hates to move, shivers and appears to be cold; and when forced to move about it walks with its back humped up as if suffering from a pain in the abdomen. It may die within a few hours or live a month or more. The most characteristic lesions are hemorrhagic spots on the surface of the lungs, kidneys and small intestines. These are red spots which look like blood-spatters but they do not wash off. In chronic cases there are found on the inner surface of the large intestine round, hard, yellow lumps called button ulcers. The presence of the hemorrhagic spots on the outer surface of the small intestines of a hog that has been sick but a short time or the presence of button ulcers on the inner surface of the large intestine of a hog that has been sick for some time are considered sufficient to establish a diagnosis of hog cholera. See Figure 49.

Treatment. This disease presents no problem which has not been solved in the treatment of avian diphtheria, fowl cholera, B. paratyphosus B infection, and canary typhoid. The exact line of treatment to use in any particular outbreak would depend to a large extent on the complicating organisms present in that particular outbreak, but in any outbreak one of three lines of treatment should prove immediately effective. The effervescent mixture alone, the effervescent mixture combined with an oxidizing agent, or the oxidizing agent alone should do the work in every outbreak. Which line of treatment to use in any particular outbreak would have to be determined by the results of treating the first three hogs to be taken sick with the three methods suggested. Hogs too sick to drink should be drenched and the dose should be one teaspoonful of the salts to the pint of water. Once one of the hogs shows improvement, flock treatment can be given by placing the medicine in all drinking water in the proportion of one teaspoonful to each quart of water used. See AVIAN DIPHTHERIA; HEMORRHAGIC SEPTICEMIA; CANARY TYPHOID; B. PARATYPHOSUS B INFECTION; and PSITTACOSIS.

HYDROGEN PEROXIDE. This is the oxidization product of water. It is sold in drugstores in the form of a three per cent solution. It is valuable in the treatment of several of the septicemic diseases of birds and may be administered in the drinking water in the proportion of from 10 to 25 drops to the ounce of water. The action is substantially the same as that of potassium chlorate and sodium perborate. See AVIAN DIPHTHERIA; APOPLECTIFORM SEPTICEMIA; CANARY TYPHOID; PSITTACOSIS; HEMORRHAGIC SEPTICEMIA; ANTISEPTICS FOR INTERNAL USE.

HUMERUS. This is the upper bone of your arm and the corresponding bone of a bird's wing.

ILEUM. This is the coiled intestine that connects the ascending loop of the duodenum with the upper end of the cloaca. Strange, but in birds this part of the intestines is seldom the seat of morbid changes, excepting those caused by intestinal parasites, of course.

ILIUM, pelvis. Strictly speaking, the ilium is just one of the three bones making up the pelvic arch, but usage has also established it as the name of the entire structure. The two other bones of the pelvic arch are the ischium and pubis. The hip socket sets at the junction of these three bones. See SKELETON.

IMPACTION OF THE CROP. This, a common condition of baby chicks, a less common though not unknown condition of older birds, is the result of the bird swallowing something that will not pass the crop—usually grass, clover heads or other fibrous material. If not relieved, this condition is fatal to chickens within a few days and to waterfowls within a few hours. In the latter case pressure on the trachea causes death from suffocation. Attention is usually called to the affected bird by its evident distress and the enlargement of the crop.

Treatment. The removal of the impacted material is the end to which all treatment must be directed. Sometimes this may be done by injecting a little warm water into the crop and working the impacted material out through the mouth. Clover heads can sometimes be fished from the crops of baby chicks with a buttonhook. In many cases, however, surgical treatment is indicated.

The feathers are plucked from the skin over the crop; an incision parallel to the grain of the skin and about three-quarters of an inch long is made in the skin; the crop is worked around until its top is opposite the opening in the skin; then it is opened, the impacted material forced out through the opening, the crop washed out with warm water and the bird released. By making the incisions parallel to the grain of the tissue and in such a manner that the one in the skin and the one in the crop wall do not come opposite each other, the necessity for sewing the wound and danger of adhesions between the skin and the crop are both avoided. Should the incisions be made opposite each other, they would have to be sewn separately with catgut and even then adhesions might occur.

Birds that have been operated on for crop impaction should be fed on soft mash for several days while the incisions are healing.

INCUBATION PERIODS:

Canaries, sparrows and finches................13½ days
Pigeons 18   "
Parakeets 20   "
Chickens 21   "
Pheasants, Guinea-fowls.......................25   "
Ducks, Peafowls, Turkeys.....................28   "
Geese 30   "

INDIGESTION. See DIGESTIVE DISORDERS; BALDNESS; MOULT; EGG FOOD.

INFECTIONS OF THE SKIN. See FUNGOID SKIN; AVIAN DIPHTHERIA.

INFECTIOUS BRONCHITIS, Fowl Flu.* This disease was studied in California, where it is quite prevalent, by George Kernohan— University of California, 1930, who apparently established beyond doubt its identity as a specific disease rather than a modified pox-virus infection, which, prior to his studies, many had thought it to be.

The disease appears to be a localized infection of the trachea and bronchi caused by a filterable virus that is in no way related to pox virus. Poultry and a wide range of wild birds are susceptible. The susceptibility of exposed birds seems to be almost 100 per cent. Fatalities may range from as low as two per cent in some outbreaks to as high as ninety per cent in others. The average mortality is from about twenty to thirty per cent. By what method the infection is spread is not known but entire localities have been swept by it in very short periods of time. Experimental propagation of the disease is accomplished by spraying the throat of a susceptible bird with material from the throat of a sick bird. The feeding of infective material does not always result in infection. No method of quarantine within a given poultry plant has been effective in preventing the spread of the disease throughout the plant. This suggests that the infective agent may be carried from bird to bird by contaminated air or flying insects, though this last does not appear to be very probable in the light of our experimental data.

Symptoms. The symptoms of fowl flu are identical with those

* **Note:** This disease would be better named if it were called **Contagious** or **Epizootic bronchitis.**

of the bronchial form of avian diphtheria. The bird has fever, sits on its haunches with head thrust forward, breathing rapidly through its open beak. The breathing becomes more rapid and shallow as the illness progresses toward a fatal termination. After three or four days, the symptoms may subside and the bird recover, or they may become progressively worse until the bird dies of suffocation.

Morbid anatomy. The morbid changes are confined to the respiratory tract. The mucous surfaces of the trachea and bronchi are covered with a thick, viscid exudate that interferes with the bird's breathing. In some cases, where the bronchi become plugged, pneumonic consolidations may be set up. The visceral organs are normal.

Treatment. Kernohan tested a number of prophylactic treatments for the throat and trachea. All proved ineffective.

In 1931, Mr. L. A. May, Reseda, California, made tests of STROUD'S SPECIFIC on birds suffering from this disease. Using a mixture of one part STROUD'S EFFERVESCENT BIRD SALTS and three parts STROUD'S SALTS NO. 1, he treated 156 pullets. He reported that the disease was controlled without losses.

Reasoning from Mr. May's results, I would suggest that in cases where STROUD'S SPECIFIC is unavailable, one teaspoonful of the following mixture be added to each quart of drinking water, which must, of course, be given in glass or crockery drinkers: one part CITROCARBONATE; one part SAL HEPATICA; three to four parts of sodium perborate. These salts should be mixed by weight and stored in tightly closed glass jars. The treatment should be given to the entire flock.

INFECTIOUS ENTRO-HEPATITIS, Blackheads of Turkeys. This is an infectious disease of turkeys, chickens and probably other similar species. Birds of all ages are susceptible, though the disease is most highly fatal to young turkeys, less so to young chickens, and rarely fatal to older chickens, which may serve as carriers. Infectious entro-hepatitis has been studied by Ward, Hadley, Smith and others.

Etiology. The causative agent of infectious entro-hepatitis is a protozoan parasite. There has been some dispute as to its exact nature. Smith described it as an ameba varying in diameter in fresh smears from eight to fifteen microns. Hadley contended that the amebic form was just one stage in the life cycle of a flagellate. Both forms are found in the material from the ceca of infected birds.* The flagellate has three anterior flagella and one posterior flagellum. The organism appears to be able to exist in soil for a year or more. Practically all young turkeys permitted to run on contaminated soil develop the disease. In the ground the organism exists in an encysted state (wrapped in a tough capsule), but when taken into the digestive tract of a young bird, the tough, resistant coverings are discarded and the active form develops. The parasites then invade the mucous lining of the intestines from where they are carried by the blood stream to the liver.

Symptoms. The symptoms of infectious entro-hepatitis make their appearance within four weeks of the time of exposure. In young birds the disease runs a rapid course; death occurring within a few days of the onset of the first symptoms. Adults show more resistance and may live for a month or more. Some of the adult birds recover. The affected bird becomes weak and unable to keep up with the rest of the flock in their daily foraging for food. The feathers are ruffled; the wings drooped; and there is a characteristic yellow diarrhea in which brown material is sometimes mixed with the yellow. As the disease progresses the head becomes noticeably darker in color, indicative of weakened heart action. This last is not an exclusive or constant symptom of this disease, but it is a very noticeable one and from it the disease takes its name, **Blackheads.**

Morbid anatomy. The morbid changes are confined to the liver and ceca. One or both ceca are greatly enlarged, the walls thickened, and the central space filled with a cheesy exudate composed of parasitic forms, mucous cells and debris. Sometimes blood cells are present. The entire length of both ceca may be involved or only a small section of one may be affected.

Round, yellow or greenish necrotic spots, varying in size from one-eighth to five-eighths of an inch in diameter, are usually found on the surface of the liver. See Figure 50.

Treatment. No recognized treatment for blackheads has so far been developed. One-third teaspoonful of crude catechu added to each gallon of drinking water is said to act as a preventative. It is used from the time the birds are placed on the ground until they are carried over the period of greatest susceptibility.

---

* **Note:** An **ameba** is a single celled animal that moves by stretching out and drawing in false arms from its body. A **flagellate** is a single celled animal that moves about by means of long threads attached to its body and called **flagella,** after the peculiar oscillating motion by which the organism moves.

** See Note Page 117.

Figure 50. INFECTIOUS ENTERO-HEPATITIS

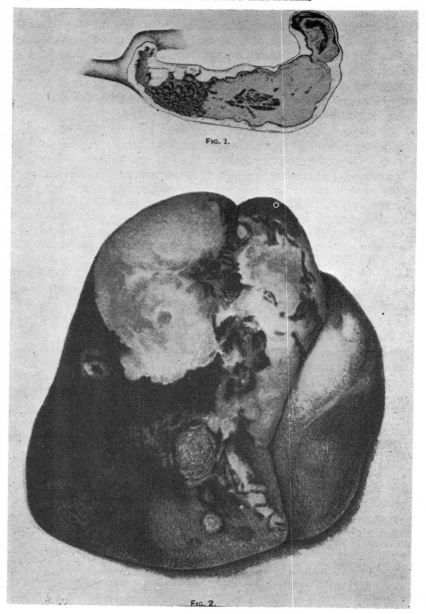

Fig. 1.

Fig. 2.

It was Hadley's opinion that the parasites are present in the intestines of all poultry; that the problem of control is one of resistance rather than prophylaxis. Assuming that there may be some truth in this view, and it is a well-known fact that resistance always plays an important part in the development of disease, I would suggest that in addition to the crude catechu, two teaspoonfuls of an effervescent saline be added to each gallon of drinking water. The water, of course, must be given in non-metallic drinkers. This will greatly increase the birds' resistance to disease, and there is no reason why they could not be kept on it from the time they are placed on the ground until they are sold. The only effect of this treatment that could be considered undesirable is the fact that it would make the young birds more active and less apt to put on fat.

INHERITED WEAKNESS. Many writers on bird subjects, particularly those conducting **question and answer** departments in the various trade journals, are wont to ascribe to **inherited weakness** any condition which they do not understand. This is such an easy way of covering their ignorance, and it has been so widely used that it has become a badge of ignorance. Any time that any so-called authority tells you that any condition found in adult birds is the result of inherited weakness, you can put it down that he does not know the first thing about birds.

This does not mean that inherited weakness does not exist. Stock can be weakened by poor breeding or over-breeding; it may be weakened to such an extent by the use of hothouse methods that it can no longer reproduce itself; but, under ordinary conditions of life, the inherently weak do not survive. Any adult bird with normal size, tight feathers, solid body, and normal vigor—or any bird that has ever been known to possess these qualities, can

Figure 50
ENTERO-HEPATITIS IN TURKEYS
Fig. 1. One cecum of turkey, cut open longitudinally. The middle portion of the tube is greatly distended and occluded with an exudate which is firm in consistency. The upper portion contains small stones which have passed down from the gizzard. The irregular thickening of the wall of the tube is shown by a faint line bordering the exudate. (After T. Smith.)

Fig. 2. Left lobe of liver of turkey (convex surface). The large yellow area in the upper portion of the figure represents a mass of dead tissue penetrating nearly through the entire thickness of the liver. On the right the pale grayish spot represents diseased liver tissue which is undergoing repair. Similarly, the spots in the lower portion of the figure correspond to diseased regions partly healed. Several other spots readily detected in the specimen could not be clearly brought out in the figure. The diffuse change, probably reparative, is shown along the lower margin. (After T. Smith.)

be safely assumed to be free from inherited weakness. When such a bird gets sick, do not blame the person who sold him to you, blame yourself; for the true cause of his trouble is certainly to be found in his environment—a deficiency or a poison in his food, a bug in his blood or in the cracks of his cage; a room too hot or too drafty will actually be responsible in 999 out of each 1000 cases of illness that are commonly ascribed to inherited weakness.

INJURIES AND ACCIDENTS. Birds, particularly the small flying birds with their keen curiosity and restless activity, get themselves into some queer situations and suffer some queer accidents. Most of their accidents are associated with faulty equipment, however, for which their owners are responsible. If there are two wires in a cage so close together that a bird can just get his head between them but cannot get it out again, some bird is certain to get his head caught between those wires and hang himself. If there is a sliding tray in the cage, sooner or later some bird will get his foot down behind it and break his leg.* If there is anything against the wall of the flight room, like a hung picture or feed box with a crack behind it that a bird may get caught in, some day you are certain to find a dead bird in that crack. If banded birds are kept in a screened flight and there is just one wire end projecting into the room, some bird is certain to get his band over that wire and break his leg. If there is an open-mouthed drinker into which a bird may plunge and drown, some day you will find a dead bird in that drinker. If the strings given to the hens for nest building are long enough for them to get tied around the bird's legs or neck, some birds are pretty certain to get tangled up and hang themselves. Sparrows are particularly apt to fall into accidents of this kind. The male sparrow carries the nesting material to the nest, and he is more on using main strength and awkwardness than he is on brains. He will pick up a string three feet long and fly with it. Canaries have more sense than to attempt that. The canary hen carries the nesting material and she will double the string in her beak until there are no trailing ends to string out behind her when she flies, but she is apt to get her feet wound up in it as she shapes the nest.

All the breeder can do in such cases is to use his best judgment to see that his cages and flights are so constructed that the possibility of accidents is reduced to a minimum. Anything he has over-

---

*Note:** This does not mean that sliding trays should not be used. On the contrary, they are the most practical cage bottom, but the back of the cage should be so constructed as to leave no crack in which a bird may get his foot caught.

looked the birds will find for him and, when they do, it is up to him to correct the condition.

Often the kindest thing to do for the victims of these accidents is to put them out of their misery. See BROKEN BONES.

A common cause of flight accidents is the failure of the breeder to trim his birds' claws often enough. See FEET, CARE OF. Screening flights with fine-mesh wire cloth in which birds can get their claws hung is another fruitful cause of accidents.

INSECT FOOD. The employment of live insects for bird food has already been mentioned in several places in these pages. Most of our domesticated birds, with the exception of pigeons and birds of the parrot family, are very fond of insect food. Canaries do not normally eat insects, because they do not come in contact with enough of them to learn what they are, but once they have tasted insect food they are very fond of it. I have used this fact to tame and train many canaries to do tricks. I would first teach the bird to eat flies and then offer it flies as an inducement for perfect behavior. Sparrows and finches do not have to be taught to eat insects. All they need is the opportunity. With no other insect food available, I have seen sparrows spend hours every day for weeks trying to learn to hawk flies.

I once kept a pet sparrow in a room infested with large black, roach-like beetles, some of which were almost two inches long. This sparrow's principal pastime was to sit on a radiator near the ceiling and watch for beetles. Every time he saw one he would swoop down and grab it. Then he would whip it on the floor until he had killed it, break up the shell by giving it a series of bites, and then, starting at the head, he would swallow it whole, though how he got some of them down was a mystery, and fly back to the pipes, his little crop sticking out like a balloon. One dark, cloudy day a small mouse ran across the floor. Down swooped the sparrow and he grabbed the mouse. I do not know which of them was the most scared. The sparrow threw the mouse about two feet into the air, jumped about that high himself and went back to his pipes like the devil was after him. The mouse did not waste any time getting away from that place either.

Live or fresh-killed insects are the only single item of bird food which contains all of the vitamins necessary to keep birds in health. "What about eggs from hens on free range?" you ask. If the eggs could be safely fed raw they would be just as valuable as insect food but, because canaries and chickens are subject to the same diseases, the use of raw eggs as bird food would be entirely too dangerous. The value of insects cannot be overestimated. I recently read of a Kansas farmer, who, seeing his crop being destroyed by grasshoppers, trapped a few tons of the hoppers, brought in a couple of carloads of young turkeys, permitted the turkeys to eat the hoppers, and then sold them at a better profit than he could have possibly made on his wheat crop.

The one great drawback about using live insects as food for cage-birds is the difficulty involved in securing a satisfactory supply. One remedy for this is the cultivation of mealworms. The canary breeder who will see that his birds each have several of these worms daily during the breeding season will never have to worry about clear eggs, weak chicks, and a number of other troubles that follow the use of a diet lacking in live food. See MEALWORMS.

INTESTINES. The intestines of birds consist of one large loop, beginning at the gizzard and returning on itself to the point of origin, called the **duodenum;** a long, closely coiled gut of smaller diameter called the **ileum;** two blind guts attached at the lower end of the **ileum,** called the **ceca** *; and a common pouch for the reception of discharges from the intestines, ureters and sex ducts, called the **cloaca.** For a fuller description of the intestines, see DIGESTIVE TRACT.

IODIDES. Minute quantities of iodides in the body are essential to life, growth and reproduction. The correct functioning of the glandular system, particularly the thyroid gland, depends upon an adequate supply of this substance. Note, please, that I say "iodides" not "iodine." Iodides are salts of the element iodine. Free iodine does not occur in nature; it is a poisonous substance suitable only for external use. All iodine used in the body is consumed in the form of iodides. Sodium and potassium salts are the forms most frequently occurring in nature, in food and water, and they are the forms most commonly used in medicine for the correction of iodide deficiency. In localities near the sea there is usually sufficient iodides in the food and water to supply all biological need. But this is not true of certain inland and mountainous localities. And in such localities all life—man, animals, birds and even fish, suffer from a condition which in man we call **goiter.**

All goiterous creatures become sluggish, usually obese and lose the power to produce normal offspring. Birds that are suffer-

---

* **Note:** Ceca are not present in some species, particularly the small seed eaters.

ing from iodide deficiency produce clear eggs, chicks that die in the shell or shortly after hatching. Those few that do survive are apt to be undersized and of little value. This deficiency can be quickly overcome by adding a little iodide of potassium to the drinking water. See MINERAL FOOD.

The iodides, belonging to a class of drugs called alteratives, are drugs which improve the general health without us being able to assign any logical reason for them doing so. When they are administered in small quantities over a long period of time they have a tendency to so improve the nutrition and functioning of the body that morbid conditions are thrown off. Iodides should probably be taken out of the alterative class, however, for we are coming to have a pretty clear understanding of the influence of the glands upon health and the influence of iodides upon the glands.

Iodides are secreted from the body very rapidly by the urine, skin, mucous membranes and are present in all the glandular secretions, but the secretion is not entirely complete. When iodides are administered in progressively increasing doses over a relatively long period of time it is possible to build up to a state of mild iodinosis in which the body is so saturated with the drug that it is present in all the secretion in quantities sufficient to exert a very destructive action upon the lower forms of life, particularly fungi and protozoa. Many stubborn infections can thus be brought under control.

To illustrate: I was recently confronted with a very stubborn micrococcus infection of the nasal sinuses involving eleven birds. There was a fluid discharge from the nostrils, asthmatic breathing, and in some cases the nostrils became plugged with puss and exfoliated (sluffed off, literally, no longer leaf-like) mucous cells. Swellings appeared above the beaks. When after several weeks these birds failed to respond to the usual treatments, they were placed in a single large flight cage and kept on the iodide treatment for four weeks. At the end of that time six of the birds were entirely well and only two of the eleven still showed active symptoms. The other three were in a convalescent stage. And by prolonged treatment, all of these birds were eventually cured. Prolonged iodide treatment is always indicated in long-standing, chronic infections. Care should be taken, however, to see that the dosage is kept within the capacity of the bird to withstand. In winter weather, two drops of saturated solution of iodide of potassium to each ounce of drinking water is not too much; but in summer, when the birds are drinking more water than usual, this amount has sometimes caused the death of large, heavily feathered canaries, while the lighter, thinner feathered varieties in the same flight are unaffected. This iodide treatment has been considered specific against chronic fungus infection, but I think that in "Anthroquinone" violet we now have an even more effective method of treating such condition. See ODIUM ALBICANS; ASPERGILLOSIS.

Iodinism. Iodides, when given in large doses, cause poisoning and death. The symptoms are those of shock and collapse, and are much more apt to follow the administration of a large initial dose of iodides than they are to result from repeated small doses. In fact, it is possible by repeated doses to build up the iodide content of the body to many times what it is in fatal cases following a large initial dose. The bird flutters to the floor in a state of complete collapse. It may die within a few minutes or it may live for as long as eighteen hours without regaining consciousness or muscular control. The body appears to be in a state of complete flaccid paralysis. For those birds that die quickly, nothing can be done; but those in which the symptoms are more gradual in their onset and less rapidly fatal may often be saved by administering into the crop 1/40 grain doses of cinchophen in syrup. Dissolve one five-grain cinchophen tablet in two hundred drops of water; add an equal amount of corn syrup; heat to almost boiling to melt the syrup and get an even mixture. Dilute this solution in the proportion of 1:5 with plain water and administer into the crop in ten drop doses every three hours until four doses have been given. Every hour or hour and a half between the doses of cinchophen, ten drops of water or water and syrup should be administered into the crop.* The theory back of this treatment is, first, to supply sugar to the blood to overcome the condition of shock; second, to supply water to the blood in order to dilute the iodide content; third, to re-establish the functioning of the kidney and eliminate the iodide from the body, and cinchophen was chosen for this purpose because it has a tonic effect on the kidneys and the involuntary muscles in general. Out of seventeen birds stricken with this condition on one occasion (the occasion when this treatment was born on the spur of the moment in the face of necessity) four died before any treatment could be given; two more died within the first hours; and one died during the night. The other ten were saved though one of them was in coma for more than eighteen hours.

---

* **Note:** The doses recommended are for a bird the size of a canary. For larger birds, larger doses would have to be used.

If available, minute doses of adrenalin * injected under the skin of the breast might be of value in overcoming the shock and collapse.

Should any bird to which iodides are being administered show any lack of muscular coordination, the drug must be discontinued at once. Sometimes a bird suffering from the first sign of iodinism will be mistaken for one with an injured wing. If the drug is discontinued at once, the symptoms pass off quickly.

IODINE. This is a solid, crystalline, non-metallic elementary substance formerly obtained by treating the ash of seaweed with concentrated sulphuric acid and subliming the reaction mixture. The iodine came over as a heavy purple vapor. Most of the iodine now found on the market is obtained as a by-product of the refining of chili nitrate. Pure iodine is not used in medicine. The tincture, which is a saturated solution of iodine in an alcoholic solution of potassium iodide, is a very valuable antiseptic for external use, especially in the treatment of skin infections. See FUNGOID SKIN.

IRON. The red coloring of the blood, the green coloring of grass and other growing plants, the yellow coloring of egg yolk and of some seed kernels are all due to the presence of certain closely related iron compounds. The function of iron in green leaves is the decomposition of carbon dioxide in the presence of sunlight and water vapor, the fixation of the carbon in the plant and the liberation of the oxygen. This is the **leaf** reaction.

In the reference works available to me I have been able to find nothing concerning the exact function of iron in the leaf reaction. The green pigment, **chlorophyl,** is a magnesium compound of a complex organic molecule, but the intensity of the green color is proportional to the iron content of the leaves, and in the absence of iron chlorophyl is not formed.

The reaction of iron in the blood is the exact reverse of the leaf reaction. Oxygen is absorbed from the air in the lungs and carried by the red cells to the tissue, where it undergoes combustion and is converted into carbon dioxide, which is carried back to the lungs by the blood cells and discharged. The very same energy that was absorbed from the sunlight during the first process is liberated in the second, and it is that energy which keeps our

---

* **Note:** The solution of adrenalin put up for human use is 1:1000 in physiological salt solution. To prepare a solution for use on a canary, one part of this human solution should be mixed with ten parts of salt solution, which give a solution of 1:11000. Of this solution from 1/10 to 1 minim should be injected under the skin, and the injection should be controlled by a locknut.

bodies warm. Without this reaction, which is possible only as the result of these special organic iron compounds, warm-blooded life would be impossible, since no other chemical element has the power of forming compounds having these properties.

When a sufficient supply of iron is lacking in the diet of any warm-blooded creature, that creature's body is unable to manufacture an adequate supply of red blood cells; those cells manufactured will be pale, smaller than usual and have little power of carrying oxygen; and, because the maintenance of the blood is the most vital of the body functions, the other iron containing tissues of the body, muscles and organs, will be broken down and their iron used in an effort to maintain the blood supply. The patient becomes pale, weak and emaciated. This condition is called **anemia.**

The canary that has an adequate supply of fresh green food always before it, that is given a little egg food occasionally, that has plenty of good fresh rape always in its seed cup; the chicken that has plenty of fresh, growing greens, a little meat and bone scraps in its mash, a chance to hunt a few bugs; the pigeon that has a liberal supply of red wheat and yellow corn in its diet and plenty of green food always available, are all pretty apt to avoid the condition we are now discussing. All birds are not that well treated, however. Many owners of cage-birds have the mistaken idea that a little apple or pale head-lettuce and a cup full of stale, package seed are all that a bird requires in order to remain in vigorous health. By the time they wake up to their error the health of their pet is apt to have been ruined beyond repair. Some poultrymen imagine that a high-production hen should be able to lay an egg every day on a diet of dry grain and a little cabbage and cannot guess what is wrong when the eggs fall off or the hen literally puts her body into the yolk. But wise poultrymen, when they notice that the hen's feet are becoming white, make it a point to add more iron to her diet in the form of meat and bone scraps and fresh, iron-rich green food—spinach, dandelion, alfalfa and lawn cuttings.

There are some owners of pet birds who actually have the idea that fresh green food is harmful to birds. If one of these persons could take the dropping from a bird that has been eating plenty of green food, break it up in a little water and examine it under the microscope, he would see that the cell structures of the leaves had passed through the bird without being broken up; but he would also see that all of those cells were colorless; that every particle chlorophyl had been extracted from them by the bird's digestive processes.

Birds that have been permitted to get run down or that have recovered from a severe illness are often reduced to such a weakened condition that they are unable to recover their strength on even the best diet. The iron in the diet does not do them any good because in their weakened condition they cannot assimilate it. In such cases iron tonics are indicated.

It was formerly thought that iron in organic form was the most suitable for combating anemia, but it has recently been demonstrated that organic iron is reduced to an inorganic form in the digestive tract before assimilation. For this reason, copperas is now replacing other iron salts in the treatment of human anemia.

IRON AND QUININE CITRATE—GREEN. This substance comes in greenish-yellow, transparent, deliquescent * scales having the bitter, characteristic, iron taste. This substance is a tonic, astringent and antipyretic. It contains 11.5 per cent of quinine and 13.5 per cent of iron combined to form quinine ferrocitrate. It also contains ammonia. There is a brown variety which contains the same percentages of iron and quinine, but as a tonic it is considered inferior to the preparation we are discussing. The dose for a bird is ⅛ grain to the ounce of drinking water. This preparation is used as a tonic and for the treatment of soft moult. It is often given to birds that are being pepper fed to fix the coloring matter in their feathers. While of less value than I.Q.S. in the treatment of acute illnesses or where a general stimulating tonic is needed, where prolonged administration is necessary, as in soft moult, it is preferable, since its continued use does not cause convulsions. Many breeders, with good reason, employ this salt as a general panacea. Some go so far as to give all of their birds a course of it before considering them in fit condition for the breeding room.

Effervescent I.Q. Citrate

I.Q. Citrate—green .... 2 parts
Sodium bicarbonate ....60 parts
Tartaric acid ....20 parts
Citric acid ....20 parts
Sugar ....64 parts

The citric acid is mixed with the bicarbonate of soda and permitted to thoroughly dry. It is then broken up and mixed with the other ingredients. The dose is from one to four grains to the ounce

---

* **Note: Deliquescent** substances are those which have the power of drawing water out of the air. When exposed to the air they either become moist or dissolve in the absorbed water and, therefore, must always be kept in tightly-stoppered bottles.

of drinking water—a good sized pinch to the ordinary cage drinking cup. This is one of the most valuable tonic preparations known to bird medicine. It is of value in the treatment of soft moult, as a tonic, and in the treatment of many serious bird fevers. Its greatest value seems to be that it increases the bird's natural resistance to infection. In one test I put 12 well birds and two birds suffering with avian diphtheria in each of two large flight cages. To the one group I gave the above preparation in all drinking water in the proportion of one heaping teaspoonful to each quart of water. The other group was left untreated. In all other respects these birds were treated exactly alike. All birds in the group drinking ordinary water developed the disease; only four birds of the group receiving the I.Q. Citrate solution as drinking water developed the disease. The birds were left exposed for one month, and during that time the trays of the cages were dumped twice each week, but the cages were not otherwise cleaned.

I.Q.S.—ELIXIR OF IRON QUININE AND STRYCHNINE PHOSPHATES.
This is a yellowish-green tonic with a pleasant, orange-like taste. In each 1000 parts, it contains the following:

Soluble ferric phosphate ....17.500 parts
Quinine .... 8.750 parts
Strychnine .... 0.275 parts
Phosphoric acid .... 2.000 parts
Ammonium carbonate, translucent pieces...... 9.000
Alcohol ....60.000 parts
Acetic acid ....28.650 parts
Ammonia water, distilled water and Aromatic Elixir to make up to 1000 parts.

This preparation is a very valuable iron tonic. Its use has been mentioned in a number of places in these pages. The dose for birds is from one to two drops to the ounce of drinking water. Whenever the larger dose is being administered the bird must be watched closely, and at the first sign of jerkiness of movement or nervous excitability the treatment must be discontinued for several days or a week. Otherwise, the bird is apt to go into convulsions from strychnine poisoning.

Note: Aromatic Elixir contains the following:
Compound spirits of orange.........................12 cc
Syrup ....375 cc
Purified talc ....30 grams
Alcohol and distilled water to make up to 1000 cc.
Note: I.Q.S. is put up by Parke-Davis & Company of Detroit.

WARNING. THIS PREPARATION MUST NEVER BE
ADMINISTERED DIRECTLY INTO THE BEAK. A
SMALL FRACTION OF A DROP IS SUFFICIENT TO
CAUSE THE DEATH OF A BIRD THE SIZE OF A
CANARY.*

ISCHIUM. This is one of the three bones making up the pelvic
arch. It is located posteriorly to the ilium and forms that part of
the pelvic lying between the hip socket and the lower part of
the spine.

---

* **Note:** All of these iron preparations should be kept in brown bottles, tightly
stoppered and away from the light. Otherwise they undergo changes
which render them at least useless and possibly dangerous. Never use one
of these preparations that has undergone a change in color.

Figure 51. **KIDNEY**
SECTION OF THE NORMAL KIDNEY OF A CANARY

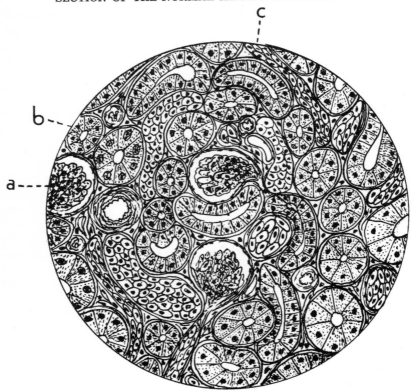

a, Glomerulus. Three are shown. These are the urine secreting organs.
b, Collection and convolution tubula.
c, Capillary.

Also shown are several small arteries and three tubules having squamous (flat) epithelium. These are more or less longitudinal cuts from the descending limb of Henle's loop, the lining of which differs from that of the rest of the tubes found in the kidney. Cut at right angles these tubules appear as small, oval or slit-like spaces. When cut at an acute angle the polygonal shape of the cells differentiates them from capillaries, which they somewhat resemble.

Tissue fixed in mercury-iron solution and stained in toto with hematoxylin and eosin.

Freehand drawing by the author, using 445 × magnification.

KEEL. This is a deep, sharp, bony ridge arising on the medial line of the sternum. Its function is to furnish attachment surface for the giant pectoral muscles—the breast muscles, which in flying birds are the most powerful members of the voluntary muscular system, since they are the muscles of flight.

KIDNEYS. A bird has two reddish-brown kidneys, each consisting of three lobes. They are set into cavities in the heavy pelvic structure, one on each side of the spine. Each kidney is drained by a ureter running along its ventral (towards the front) surface and emptying into the cloaca. The fragility and sensitiveness of a bird's kidneys is well illustrated by the protection nature has afforded them. The bony structure incasing them on all but the ventral side is the strongest of the entire skeleton, not excepting the skull. Figure 51 is a microscopic drawing from a section of a canary's kidney.

KIDNEYS, DISEASES OF. There are two common disease conditions involving the kidneys of birds. They are: **Chronic nephritis, yellow kidney, large fatty kidney** in which the prevailing lesions are fatty degeneration of the epithelial lining of the convolution tubes; thickening and round-cell infiltration of the glomeruli capsule; and hyaline degeneration of the glomeruli, occurring in the order named. See NEPHRITIS. And **Acute uremia, gray kidney,** in which functional suspension of the kidneys, resulting in acute uremic poisoning and death, is the sequel to the uriniferous tubes becoming plugged with crystallized uric acid. The white crystals in the plugged tubes give the kidney a gray appearance. For a complete discussion of this condition turn to the heading UREMIA.

LARYNX. This is a slit-like opening in the base of a bird's tongue. It is the mouth of the trachea. Unlike the mammalian larynx, the avian larynx is not provided with vocal cords. The seat of voice in birds is a box-like structure located at the lower end of the trachea and called the **Syrinx**.

LAXATIVES. Laxatives are drugs which have a mildly stimulating effect on the bowels, as distinguished from cathartics, which produce drastic bowel action. See CITROCARBONATE; CASCARA; etc.

LEG, BONES OF. Beginning at the hip, the first bone of the leg— the largest bone but not the longest, though it is the longest in man, is called the **femur**. The second large bone òf the leg, which extends from the knee to the ankle, is called the **tibia**. Between the femur and the tibia and located on the ventral side of the knee joint is a small bone corresponding to your kneecap and called the **patella**. Located dorsally to the tibia and extending half way from the knee to the ankle is a thin pointed bone which corresponds to your shin bone and is called the **fibula**. In some of the larger birds, swans, ostriches, etc., the tendons of this part of the leg are ossified and for the greater part of their length are ribbons of bone. The bone of the scaly shank, which is the first bone of the foot, is called the **metatarsus**. It is a long, round bone ending in a compound joint from which the toes radiate. Most birds have four claws, three in front and one behind. Woodpeckers, birds of the psittacine group, and possibly a few other species, have two claws in front and two in back. The back toe of the small perching birds has two bones, the two side toes have three bones each, and the central toe in front has four bones. These bones are called **phalanges**. There are a few walking birds, like ostriches, which have only two toes, both pointing frontwards. See SKELETON.

LEG, BROKEN. See BROKEN BONES.

LEAD POISONING. Lead plays a very large part in modern life. Lead arsenate is used as an insecticide for the spraying of garder. plants and fruit trees; the basic acetate of lead (white lead) enters into the composition of most paints; the chromates of lead are important yellow, orange and reddish pigments which may be found in paints which are otherwise free from lead (zinc enamels of a yellow, orange or green color may owe their color to the presence of lead chromates); and lead pipe and solder are widely used in plumbing (which, by the way, takes its very name from **plumbium, lead,** and literally means **leading)** and tinning.

Because this metal is relatively inactive, and because the effects of very small amounts of lead upon the human or animal system are often obscure and hard to recognize, we are apt to ascribe

Figure 52.   **LEAD POISONING**
SECTION OF THE KIDNEY OF A SEVEN-DAY-OLD CANARY CHICK
THAT DIED OF LEAD POISONING

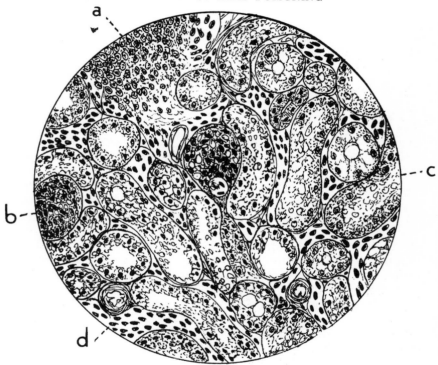

a, Area of dense infiltration.
b, Glomerulas, notice fat globules and cell nuclei.
c, Convolution tube. Notice that the cells lining all of the convolution and collection tubules are ragged, broken and contain round, open spaces. These spaces were filled with fat globules during life.
d, Interstitial spaces filled with stagnant blood. Only the nuclei of the blood cells can be seen, as the cytoplasm—cell body—has either been destroyed or fails to take the stain.
    Author's section. Tissue fixed in mercury-iron solution; stained in toto in hematoxylin and eosin; embedded in paraffin; cut on a hand mike, and mounted in balsam.
    Drawn freehand by the author, using a magnification of 445 ×.

those effects to other causes and overlook the part played by this dangerous and extremely poisonous substance.

In a recent article on this subject, Dr. Logan Glendening expressed the opinion that many of the human ills ascribed to premature old age—staggering gait; numbness of the fingers or toes; failing eyesight; chronic constipation; rheumatic pains; and a number of other symptoms commonly ascribed to advancing years, are often the result of chronic lead poisoning. And what is true of man in this case is doubly true of birds, since birds are far more sensitive to the toxic effects of lead than are humans. And the condition is so insidious that it is very difficult to recognize. This is illustrated by the following experience which recently occurred in my own bird room.

Some time ago I had a copper can made for cooking wheat for my birds. The can was used for some months without any illness appearing in my flock. I received from a friend two pair of prize-winning Yorkshires. These birds had no sooner arrived than they appeared out of sorts. Three of them moved with an awkward gait and flew so awkwardly that they were helpless in a large flight, and in the cages they would often miss the perches they were trying to hop to. They were all in good condition, otherwise, in breeding condition. But soon one hen went blind and one male developed digestive disorders which made it impossible to use him for breeding, even though he was still in full song. At about this time several nests of fine birds were lost. Babies in perfect health in the morning would be found dead in the evening. Post-mortem examination of these babies revealed no macroscopic (capable of being seen by the naked eye) lesions, and the deaths were attributed to food poisoning. Sections of the liver and kidneys examined microscopically revealed an extensive lipoid degeneration (a condition in which the tissue cells are broken down into fat globules). Figure 52 is a microscopic drawing from a section of the kidney of one of these babies. Notice the light circular spaces in the cells of the tubes and glomerali. These spaces were formerly occupied by fat, which was removed by the process by which the tissue was prepared for sectioning. Also see Figure 53.

The blind hen had to be killed. Abnormal bone growths were found in her pelvis, under the posterior lobes of both kidneys. All of her organs have not been sectioned yet, but the liver and kidneys were normal.

Then the male with the digestive disorder had an attack of convulsions very similar to those described as occurring in uremic poisoning, excepting that the jerking was somewhat slower and was accompanied by sufficient pain to cause the bird to cry out. He was treated for acute uremia. He was kept wrapped in a handkerchief for twenty-four hours and given warm water and diurol into the beak at frequent intervals. He was able to fly and eat at the end of 24 hours and was returned to the flight. He died in a convulsion six hours later.

Figure 53.   **LEAD POISONING**
LIVER SECTION FROM THE SAME BIRD MENTIONED UNDER
FIGURE 51

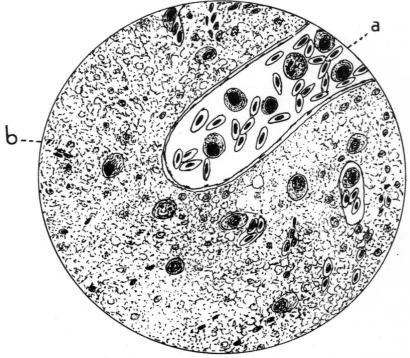

a, A hepatic vein showing an exceptionally good blood picture for fixed tissue. Notice the lymphocyte; polymorphonuclear leucocyte, and four large cells having round nuclei. These are probably plasmacytes, though it was impossible to positively identify them.

b, Liver tissue entirely destroyed. The contour of the strands can be followed only in fat globules and broken nuclei. The only cells taking a clear stain—the only ones alive at the time of fixing—are the leucocytes. In an older bird, having firmer tissue, the destruction would probably not be so complete.

Author's section and drawing. Drawing made freehand, using 445 × magnification.

The post mortem revealed some astonishing facts. The bird had died from a slow internal hemorrhage from one of the branches of the hepatic (pertaining to the liver) artery. The pressure of the blood had opened a path through the liver tissue along the course of the hepatic artery and escaped into the thoracic cavity. Had I suspected the true condition during life, the bird might have been saved by continuing to keep him quiet and feeding him. Undoubtedly, the strain of flying was responsible for the second spell of bleeding for it was evident that the bleeding had stopped while the bird was kept quiet. The most striking things observed, however, were the facts that the kidneys were generally healthy (they contained no macroscopic lesions, though they may contain microscopic changes. They have not yet been sectioned), while the liver was bright yellow in color and sclerotic, and the spleen was one-fourth normal size, soft in texture and almost transparent.

These changes in the liver and spleen suggested the possibility of metallic poisoning. A careful check of all food revealed that lead in the solder of the can I cooked my wheat in had reacted with the cooking wheat with the formation of white lead, which had penetrated the grains of wheat in contact with the solder. Only those grains were poisonous, and my old birds, which had been eating this boiled wheat for their entire lives, had probably detected something wrong with the leaded grains and refused to eat them. The new birds, eating this food for the first time, had probably lacked this discrimination.

I have reported this case just as it occurred in order to illustrate the different forms taken by the symptoms and lesions of lead poisoning and the ease with which they may be confused. Once the nature of the condition was suspected, it was a simple matter to check the possible sources of the metal.

Several other birds which have developed awkwardness of movement have been placed on iodide treatment — one drop of potassium iodide solution to each ounce of drinking water — and given bread and milk twice a day in addition to their regular diet.*

---

* **Note:** Minute quantities of lead may be detected by placing a drop of a solution or emulsion of the suspected substance on a microscopic slide, covering it with a coverglass, and then, while observing it through the microscope, placing a loopful of sodium or ammonium polysulphide at the edge of the coverglass, so that it will run under the coverglass. Practically all of the heavy metals, those of the copper, silver and iron groups, are thrown down as heavy, dense, black sulphides and the sulphide of lead is not acted upon by dilute hydrochloric acid, so the reaction of the sulphide is followed by placing a drop of hydrochloric acid solution on the slide and permitting it to run under the coverglass. In those cases where larger quantities of material are available these same reactions may be carried out in a test tube.

LEUKEMIA OF POULTRY.* This is a misnamed and little understood condition afflicting chickens, thought to be caused by a filterable virus, and in which there is a characteristic enlargement of the liver, spleen, and kidneys and marked changes in the blood and bone marrow. The disease is not known to occur in birds other than chickens, nor does there appear to be any relationship between the disease of chickens and leukemia in man. Pigeons, turkeys and guinea-hens are insusceptible to inoculation with morbid exudates from infected chickens.

Concerning the name, LEUKEMIA, the recent researches of Osgood and others have established beyond doubt that human leukemia is a malignant neoplasm (**tumor** or **sarcoma,** though these words leave much to be desired when applied to conditions of the blood) of one particular cell of the blood and bone marrow. The disease of fowls has many characteristics similar to those observed in human leukemia, but it lacks two most important features of the human disease: it is infectious and recoveries occur. There are no spontaneous recoveries from a true malignant disease. Actually, the disease of poultry most closely resembles infectious monocytosis of man and is in reality, a **leukosis** rather than a **leukemia.** I would suggest for it the name, CHICKEN MONOCYTOSIS, or, for those who cannot stand such a common word as **chicken** in the description of a disease, MONOCYTOSIS GALLINARUM.

Etiology. Several investigators have found protozoan-like bodies in the liver, spleen and bone marrow of infected chickens, but whether or not these bodies are of etiological importance remains undetermined. But, since the disease is transmissible by means of intravenous or intraperitoneal injections of cell-free filtrates of emulsified organs from infected birds, it is generally thought to be due to infection with a filterable virus. This does not entirely exclude the possibility that it is a protozoan infection, however, since rabies, which is generally considered to be a protozoan disease and which is identified by the presence of protozoalike bodies in the brain (the **Negri bodies)** has also been transmitted by cell-free filtrates.† It is not impossible that some protozoa with their multiple forms and complicated life histories, may in some phases of their existence exist as coccoid bodies small enough to escape microscopic detection and pass a Berkefeld filter.

Leukemia is readily transmitted by intraperitoneal inoculation

---

* **Note to Breeders:** You are not supposed to understand this paragraph. It is included for the benefit of some of my scientific friends and really does not mean anything of importance.
† **Note:** Ellerman and Bang, Centralbl. f. Bakteriol. 1908.

with the unfiltered emulsion of the liver of an infected bird. The period of incubation is from two to eight weeks; the duration of the illness may be from a few days to several months. Recoveries are few in number.

Symptoms. The disease usually runs a chronic course. There is dullness, emaciation, great weakness, and in some cases there is considerable enlargement of the abdomen. There is pronounced anemia, and the comb, wattles, skin, mucosa, and feet become very pale. The appetite is usually good. The blood is lighter in color than normal and has lost much of its clotting power.

Morbid anatomy. The liver may be greatly enlarged and congested, or it may be only slightly enlarged and sprinkled with white, punctiform spots. In some cases death results from hemorrhage from the liver, but usually the cut surface of the liver appears bloodless. Like the liver, the spleen is usually greatly congested and its pulp softened, though in some cases this organ may be only slightly enlarged and firm in structure.

The principal changes in this disease, however, are those taking place in the blood. The iron content of the blood is only about one-third normal as is the number of red blood cells, while the number of mononuclear leucocytes is increased from three to fifteen times normal. The ratio of red cells to white cells may change from 1:125 to 1:3 or even 1:2.

Treatments. Potassium iodide and iron tonics in the drinking water have been recommended. Should the disease take on epizootic proportions the sanitary measures recommended for avian diphtheria should be employed, but where the disease is sporadic in character, nothing more than the usual sanitary measures is required. Of course, the flock should be well fed and properly cared for. It is my opinion that in good care lies the secret of avoiding this condition in your flock. The causative agent appears to be of an extremely low order of virulence; since the disease cannot be transmitted by the ingestion or subcutaneous injection of infective material, it seems reasonable to believe that there is danger of its spread only among birds of greatly lowered resistance.

Pernicious anemia in man has many points of similarity to leukemia of fowls, and in that disease the feeding of fresh liver has recently been found to have a specific action. Liver is richer than any other tissue in organic iron compounds so, aside from any specific action, it should be of considerable dietetic value in all cases where the iron content of the blood is below normal.

For a detailed discussion of this disease the reader is referred to the biannual report of the New York State Veterinary College for 1915-16, in which Pickens discusses the literature and some original experiments on this disease in some detail. **Note:** In the September, 1938, issue of the American Canary Magazine, Drs. Durant and McDougle, Veterinary Department, University of Missouri, published an article entitled "Leukemia in Canaries," in which

Figure 54.　　　　　　**LEUKEMIA**

THE LESIONS OF LEU-
KEMIA AS ILLUSTRATED
BY PHOTOGRAPHS PUB-
LISHED BY DURANT AND
McDOUGLE

A, A line drawing from a halftone reproduction of a photomicrograph of a canary's blood. Magnification about 400 ×.

B and **D,** The spleen and liver of the same bird.

C and **E,** The spleen and liver of a normal canary.

These ink drawings were made by the employment of a scale of squares to the halftones, which had been reproduced by photographing through a 120 mesh screen. Any loss or inaccuracy of details results from the coarseness of the screen. The scale is probably of millimeters, though the good doctors did not take the trouble to say so.—Robert Stroud.

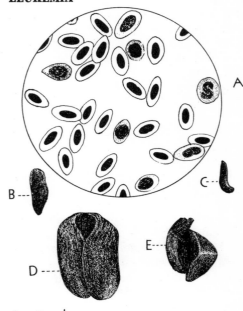

they described two exploratory laporotomies (an **exploratory laporotomy** is an opening of the abdomen for the purpose of examining the abdominal organs) on canaries, with their finding that the birds were suffering from **erythro leucosis,** although they do not take the trouble to define these words for their reader or explain how it is possible for a leucosis and a leukemia to be the same thing when one word presupposes malignancy and the other infection. (See Osgood's Atlas of Hematology.) The only evidence offered in support of their findings is reproduced in Figure 54.

This article had been press-agented in the bird magazines for several months prior to its appearance. I had been asked by a mutual friend of both myself and Dr. Durant to look for the article and to let him know what I thought of it. Frankly, I expected the article to contain some information really worth while, and here was the much touted article failing to even give an analysis of the blood picture or an explanation of the evidence upon which the diagnosis was based. I wrote to my friend and told him that I was surprised to find the work so poorly done. I was expressing my opinion of the written work, the article and the information it did not give. Concerning the laboratory work, I was not passing an opinion, but I might say here that according to the article one bird was killed by a bungled operation and two inoculation attempts failed because of bungled injections. I questioned the evidence offered in support of the diagnosis of leukemia because I had many times seen the same lesions and same blood picture in birds that I knew were suffering from other causes. And in the letter to my friend I explained how these lesions could be reproduced experimentally by the toxin present in spoiled egg food.

Some days later I received a marked copy of a newspaper published in Columbia, Missouri, containing the report of an interview in which Dr. Durant had given excerpts from my letter to the press and expressed his amazement that I, of all his thousands of readers, should have the temerity to question his findings, which were, of course, arrived at by the usual veterinary methods. My arguments, naturally, were beneath consideration. Whether or not Dr. Durant tried to communicate with me in any other manner, I do not know.

My friend, undoubtedly passing along the good doctor's explanation, pointed out that since the article was for the general reading of bird breeders it would have been impossible for it to have gone into the details of the diagnosis, since that would have been over the readers' heads.

I want to hereby inform Dr. Durant that I still question his diagnosis because he does not offer evidence enough to support it. I do not know what disease the birds had. It may have been leukemia; but I do know that I can reproduce the liver, spleen, and blood lesions described and illustrated in his article under circumstances which preclude the possibility of leukemia. I also wish to inform him that while I may have lacked some of his social and educational advantages in life, I have probably looked into the bodies of as many dead birds as he has and cured a hundred to his one, or to the one of any other man living. On the basis of the original researches reported in this book, particularly my work on avian therapeutics, I see no reason for standing in awe of the veterinary profession, which in its entirety has been able to find cures for but three bird diseases, and those it borrowed from human medicine.

When he can tell me how to differentiate his so-called leukemia from all other conditions known to canaries, or show me how to cure it, I will be glad to thank him and pass the information on to you. Until then, I give you his published data for what it is worth. And as a parting shot, I want to say that while it is unfair to criticize any man for an admitted error, if I could not inoculate a canary without killing it, not with a hypodermic, because I do not happen to have one, but with a drawn-out eye-dropper, I would be heartily ashamed of myself.*

History. The morning after she had laid the second egg of her second clutch of the season in 1937 a hen was found in a state of coma. She was on the nest. It was thought that the passage of the egg might have injured her kidneys and caused uremia. She was treated for uremia by administering diurol into her beak, wrapping her in a handkerchief and placing her in a warm place. After several administrations of medicine and water, her kidney functions were established and she came out of the coma and was returned to the nest. She did not lay the next day, and the egg laid on the fourth day had a rough shell, indicating possible inflammation of the oviduct. She sat on her eggs and raised her chicks. She raised two more nests of babies that year, and nothing could be noticed out of order with the eggs or babies, but the hen did not seem exactly well from that time on. She carried her feathers loosely and seemed sensitive to weather changes. Her breathing was very rapid and became more so as time passed.

The next season she raised five birds of her own and four from other hens, but none of the eggs in her last two nests were good. They had thin, light-colored shells, showing that there was some defect in her metabolism.

The next season she insisted on mating again, but none of the eggs she laid were any good, and she was only permitted to lay two clutches. She did, however, raise one nest of babies from other hens.

The following year she was too sick to even make an attempt to breed. She died during the summer of 1940. For the last year her symptoms had been those of chronic nephritis, but no line of treatment had done her any good. She seemed to get most comfort out of sunning herself against a 100-watt light, and she was permitted to do that all she pleased. During this last year of her life

---

* Note: Maybe canaries do have Leukemia or Lympho-sarcoma, but if they do, there are no points of resemblance between the case I wish to report and those cited by Dr. Durant.

Figure 55.

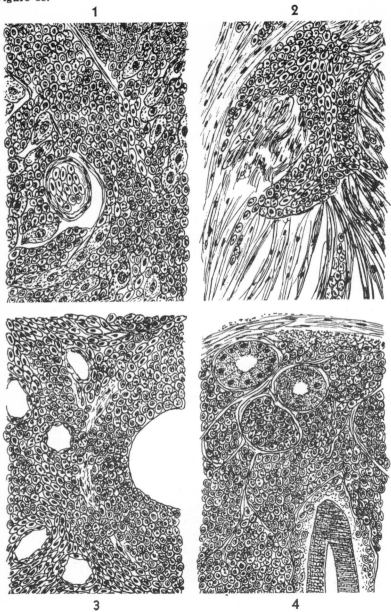

a number of studies were made of her blood. I was handicapped by lack of a counting chamber, however, so had to content myself with differential counts. Monocytes (cell 24—Figure 13) made up at least ninety per cent of the white cells (the counts varied from 80 to 94 per cent on different slides) and the average was about one white cell to six red cells. As the necessary reagents for the peroxidas stain were not at hand, I had no way of learning whether the cells were actually monocytes or myelocytes of the lymphatic series (myelocytes are marrow cells from which the blood cells are formed. They appear in the blood only in disease. See BLOOD).

Morbid anatomy. I was surprised to find few of the expected changes in the visceral organs. There was no extensive fatty degeneration of the kidneys. The liver was about normal size, but its edges were pale and bloodless. The spleen looked normal. The lungs were but slightly off-color and had a faint speckled appearance. As the true nature of the condition was not suspected, the bones were not saved for study.

More than 2000 sections were made and studied and Figures 55 and 56 give eight drawings of some of the most characteristic changes found.

No. 1.   This is a section from the liver and shows part of a hepatic vein and the spaces between the strands of hepatic cells densely packed with lymphocytes, or, at least, small round cells. Cells show great variation in size and mitotic figures are very numerous. Healthy red blood cells are seen in the mist of these round cells and not separated from them, as if they were passing through unlined channels cut in the cell masses. This is characteristic of sarcoma.

No. 2.   This section shows an infiltered foci in the heart muscle. The general character of the lesion is identical with that shown in section No. 1.

No. 3.   Section from the lung showing a condition which might be called advanced interstitial pneumonia; but please notice that there is no cell debris. The bronchus shown on the right side of the drawing is almost two-thirds obliterated by close-packed cells lining its inner wall.

No. 4.   This is a section of the duodenum and shows most of the glandular elements entirely replaced by the infiltering round cell, others undergoing degeneration, probably from being cut off from their blood supply, and still others in

Figure 56.

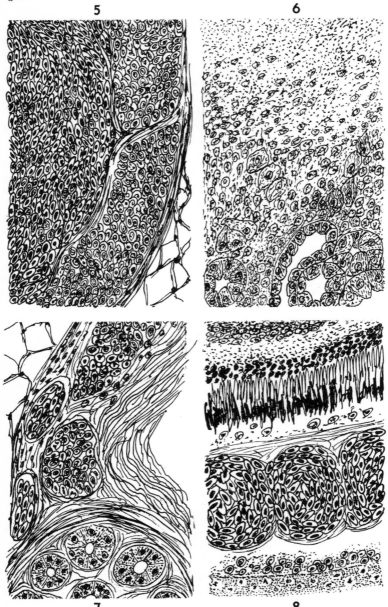

almost normal condition. At the point where this section was made, only about one-third of the circumference of the gut was involved. The rest was normal.

No. 5.   This is a section of a blood vessel. Notice the newly formed false stroma, walling off infiltering masses of round cells. Just beyond the ends of these false stroma the two types of cells were in direct contact.

No. 6.   This is a section of the pancreas taken from a large, necrotic area. Just beyond the lower edge of the drawing the tissue was almost normal, but the organ was liberally sprinkled with these necrotic areas.

No. 7.   This drawing was made from a section of the small intestines, which were themselves almost normal. It shows infiltration into the mesentry (the plexus of veins, nerves, lymphatics, and connective tissue making up the structure that carries absorbed food from the intestines to the liver). This condition was typical of the entire structure.

No. 8.   This section is from the eye and shows infiltration of the ganglion layer; infiltration below the pigmented layer; greatly congested sub-retinal capillaries; and an infiltration between the capillaries and the cartilage. The capillaries and the two lower infiltrations were drawn out of scale in order to make the drawing fit the space available. The two lower infiltrations were at least four times as thick and dense as shown, and the capillaries were twice as large as shown.

Tissue for these sections was fixed in mercury; stained in toto with hematoxylin and eosin; impregnated with paraffin, and mounted in balsam. Drawings were made with 4mm. objective and 10x. ocular.

LEUCOCYTES. See BLOOD.

LICE. See FEATHER LICE.

LIME. Calcium oxide is used in making whitewash, which is best prepared by slaking the amount of lime to be used in from five to seven times its own weight of water. Then for each ten pounds of lime used take one pound of rice flour and one pound of good wood glue; boil the flour with enough water to make a thin paste; soak the glue in cold water for several hours and then add it to the boiling paste; stir until the glue has melted and become thoroughly mixed with the paste. The paste is then mixed with the slaked lime, and enough water is added to bring the whitewash to the desired consistency. Some persons are of the opinion that adding one pound of common salt for each pound of lime used will make the whitewash set harder and faster. Some poultrymen add crude carbolic acid or coal-tar disinfectants to the whitewash.

LIME. Calcium carbonate is the principal constituent of egg shells, oyster shells and lime rock. It is an important constituent of all mineral foods. See MINERAL FOOD; EGG, STRUCTURE AND FORMATION.

LINSEED. Flaxseed. This is a flat, tear-shaped seed with a brown husk. It is not quite so long or wide as a grain of wheat and much thinner. This seed is raised principally as a source of linseed oil for painting. In small quantities linseed is a valuable food for birds. This is especially true during the moulting season, for it gives the feathers a high gloss. It is sometimes fed to cattle and horses to give the coat a gloss, too. And, because it is a cheap source of protein food, mealcake (residue from the oil presses) is sometimes used as a substitute for more expensive proteins. Its continued use has an irritating effect on the kidneys that will eventually ruin the health of the animal or bird eating it. I have not met with this condition in pet birds, however, probably because they are fed only the more expensive seeds and those only in small quantities.

LIVER. The liver of a healthy bird is a large, dark, reddish-brown organ located in the right upper division of the abdominal cavity, just above and to the right of the gizzard. It is attached to the spine and receives a large blood supply through the short hepatic artery, which is a branch of the descending aorta. It is the greatest of all glands and some of its manifold functions are:

The manufacture of bile; the storage and chemical conversion of sugars; the storage of vitamins and other substances necessary to health; the chemical conversion of the proteins of foods into forms suitable for use in the body; the chemical conversion of poisons resulting from cell activity or absorbed from the intestines into less harmful substances before passing them on to the kidneys for elimination; the elaboration of hormones essential to the correct functioning of other organs, particularly one that has something to do with maintaining normal blood pressure. It is actually a great chemical laboratory standing at the main portal of the body, guarding that portal against the admission of harmful substances, regulating the admission of needed materials, and reprocessing those materials to make them more suitable for bodily consumption.

Bacteria invading the body are often isolated in the liver and walled off. There they may cause abscesses from which the individual may recover; but, had they entered the blood stream, they might have set up a septicemia from which there would have been no recovery.

The right lobe of a bird's liver empties its gall into a gall bladder; the left lobe empties its gall directly into the duodenum.

The changes which take place in the liver during the progress of a disease are often of considerable diagnostic value. They are frequently the determining factor in the differentiation of one disease from another. For illustrations of the liver see APOPLEC-TIFORM SEPTICEMIA; AVIAN DIPHTHERIA; CANARY NE-CROSIS; CANARY TYPHOID; COCCIDOSIS; FOWL TYPHOID.

LIVER AS FOOD. In the last section mention was made of the fact that certain vital substances are manufactured and stored in the liver. Among these is a substance that has the power to reduce blood pressure; another that has something to do with certain forms of anemia, since the presence of liver in the diet will cure the condition; a third which prevents pellagra, and a long list of others.* Liver also has a very high food value, being rich in proteins, fats, animal sugar, salts, and iron. It is low in indigestible material.

If we could always keep our birds under the conditions they were accustomed to in the wild state, many of the ailments with which this book deals would be unknown. If we could only approach that condition by feeding them a limited but regular supply of live insects, they would often thrive better than they do. One reason we do not always give our birds the things they need is that we do not always know what those things are. That our ignorance of this subject is colossal is demonstrated by the fact that we do not know why a linnet kept in captivity † loses the rose tint

---

* **Note:** It might be interesting to feed raw beef liver to birds suffering from so-called leukemia.

† **Note:** Recent experiments with the fertile hybrid of the canary and the black-hooded siskin, experiments which are still in progress, have convinced me that the red pigmentation in the feathers of many birds is the result of the presence of a particular kind of lipochrome which is yellow at the time it is deposited in the feathers, but turns red under the influence of direct sunlight. My experiments and observations indicate that this change in color from yellow to red is the direct result of the action of ultra-violet light on the pigment in the growing feathers. Vitamin D in the diet has no influence on the formation of red pigment in the feathers. I believe that this is the first time this phenomenon has been observed. More will be said about it under the heading RED CA-NARIES.

from its breast; why mockingbirds in captivity mate and hatch their young but do not raise them; why sparrows kept in captivity and fed on canary seed have a tendency to throw white feathers. It is evident that these birds do not get something that they need, something that they enjoyed in the wild state. What that something is we do not know. With these thoughts in mind I have fed canaries small amounts of liver with results which I think justify further experimentation.

Canaries given liver once or twice each week during the breeding season appear to do a little better than the birds fed on egg food alone. The old birds seem less apt to fall into moult or breeding exhaustion; the young appear to be a little more vigorous. As all of the birds were well cared for and giving good results, the differences noticed were not striking.

The best method I have found for preparing liver for cage-bird food is to boil it with the ground wheat (see EGG FOOD), and then granulate it by pressing it through a piece of wire cloth. The blood vessels and strings of connective tissue that will not pass through the cloth are thrown away. The granulated liver is mixed in with the other ingredients, just as granulated egg would be mixed in making egg food. If desirable, raw liver could be prepared in the same manner. Care would have to be exercised to see that the food did not spoil and poison the birds, however.

WARNING. Liver is rich in amo acids (the acids of which complex proteins are formed). Two ounces are sufficient to feed one hundred canaries or finches, and the use of more would certainly be harmful. It can be fed raw in chunks to breeding sparrows and jays, but it should never be fed to the strictly granivorous birds—pigeons, parrots, etc.—for in their case it will set up a skin irritation resulting in the loss of feathers. If fed too often or in too great quantities it will cause the same condition in canaries, and its continual use will certainly be followed by the development of gout. This warning applies to man as well as to birds. Liver once each week is of benefit to human health, but its more frequent consumption is distinctly harmful and is certain to be followed by the development of gout.

LIVER LESIONS.

Enlarged hypertrophy. The liver is enlarged in so many diseases that this lesion alone can mean nothing unless it is of some particular character or associated with other lesions which give it meaning. A greatly enlarged, necrotic liver in which the envelope and connective tissue have been destroyed may indicate avian diphtheria. In a parrot it is indicative of psittacosis.

An equally enlarged liver in which the envelope is intact and unclouded may indicate bacillary white diarrhea in a baby chick. In a canary it may indicate canary typhoid, B. paratyphosis B infection. In the first of these two diseases there may be yellow bands or lacings visible through the outer covering.

A greatly enlarged liver surrounded by the blood from a major hemorrhage may indicate food poisoning, apoplectiform septicemia, B. paratyphosis B infection. If the blood is pale and unclotted it may indicate leukemia. If the organ is dark in color and its envelope destroyed, it may indicate diphtheria or psittacosis.

Shrunken. Atrophy and softening of the liver may result from a lessened or interfered-with blood supply. This is often caused by a partial thrombosis of the hepatic artery in the pox form of diphtheria and in B. paratyphosis B infection. In such cases the edges of the liver are bloodless and transparent.

Yellow. An enlarged yellow liver is a lesion of septic enteritis of cross-bills—a disease of canaries and finches.

Spots. Spots or nodules in or on the liver may be of considerable diagnostic value in canary necrosis; tuberculosis; coccidiosis; apoplectiform septicemia; infectious entro-hepatitis and leukemia.

This is not a complete list. The object of this is just to give you an idea of what to look for. The spots may vary in color from almost white to almost black; they may be on the surface of the organ or scattered through its mass; they may be large or small; round or irregular in shape; firmly attached to the surrounding tissue or walled off from it and easily detached. In each case all of these details must be considered in connection with the symptoms, other lesions and the history of the outbreak. To illustrate:

The liver lesions in canary necrosis and tuberculosis are almost identical, but one is a chronic disease of older birds; the other is an acute disease attacking birds of all ages. The livers in canary typhoid, B. paratyphosis B infection are similar, but the bowel symptoms are equally dissimilar. In almost every case the liver lesions alone might suggest from two to half a dozen diseases, and it is by eliminating them one at a time that the final and correct diagnosis is arrived at.

It is not difficult for the bird breeder or poultryman to make

himself familiar with these liver lesions. All that he has to do
is to examine carefully the liver of every bird that dies or is killed.
Soon he will become so familiar with the appearance of the normal
liver that any abnormality will stand out like a headlight in a fog.

LOSS OF WEIGHT. See GOING LIGHT; APOPLECTIFORM
SEPTICEMIA; TUBERCULOSIS; LEUKEMIA.

LUMPS. This is a condition found in the heavy types of exhibition
canaries. It is not met with in rollers or the common types of
canaries, nor is it met with in other species, so far as I am aware.
Professor Tom Hare * of the Royal Veterinary College, London,
has studied this condition and has suggested the name **Hypopterbosis cystica.** In this work, however, I think that the simpler,
more descriptive, and better known appellation, **Lumps,** is preferable.

This condition was unknown in England until comparatively
recent years. Professor Hare states that he has found isolated
references to it in English bird literature dating back as far as 1911.
T. Johnson, a well-known English breeder and exhibitor, states that
to his certain knowledge the condition made its appearance in
England in 1921 and that all strains of English canaries now affected
can be traced to three bird rooms where breeding for size, **double
buffing,** has been extensively practiced for many years.

In most cases the first lumps make their appearance during the
baby moult, which occurs when the bird is about four months old;
though there are cases where the lumps do not make their appearance until the bird enters the adult moult at the age of about sixteen months. If untreated, the lump may grow to considerable
size—the size of a hickory nut or walnut. The affected bird shows
no signs of illness other than the presence of the lumps and the
handicap they place in the way of it taking proper care of itself.

Morbid anatomy. On general inspection the cyst appears to
be an abscess filled with yellow pus, but, when opened, it is seen
to contain a yellow, cheesy material partly made up of immature
feathers. Dr. Hare demonstrated that the lesion is actually an
anatomical maldevelopment, a feather follicle located below the
epidermis (the surface of the skin); in plain language, **ingrown
feathers** describes the condition. Though the feathers are not
ingrown in the sense that they grew back into the skin, they orig-

*Note: Professor Hare's findings are reported in "Cage Birds," London,
October 31, 1931. I am indebted to J. Tomlinson, Stafford, England, for
most of my information concerning this condition and for copies of Dr.
Hare's paper.

inated there in a group of misplaced epidermal cells. This is illustrated in Figure 57. The only difference between the lump and the normal feathers is that the feathers forming the lump have lost contact with the surface of the skin. If the cyst is opened and the matter forced out, the wound will heal and the bird becomes apparently well until the next moulting season; then the lump will reappear. Sometimes the birds will open the lumps themselves by pecking the epidermis away. Hare has shown that the lining

Figure 57.   **LUMPS**
DIAGRAMMATIC ILLUSTRATION OF THE DEVELOPMENT
OF THE LUMP

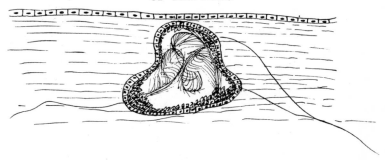

After Tom Hare, Cage-Birds, London, October, 1931

of the cyst is composed of misplaced epidermal cells and that so long as those cells exist below the surface of the skin the lump will reappear at each succeeding moult.

Etiology. Lumps is undoubtedly an hereditary condition brought about by inbreeding along lines intended to increase the size of the bird and the thickness of its feathers—by double buffing and double cresting (mating buff to buff or crest to crest. See BALDNESS). Johnson has pointed out that inbreeding alone cannot be considered an etiological factor in the development of lumps, since some of the most closely bred strains of canaries in England, bred on conventional lines (yellow to buff; crest bred to crest), have remained consistently free from this defect. He further points out that these correctly bred strains have not been able to make the records for size and feathers attained by the birds of those breeders who have been willing to sacrifice physical perfection for show points.

Treatment. As previously mentioned, the cyst may be opened; its contents pressed out; then, when the wound heals, the bird will be well for another year. Hare has suggested the destruction of the inner lining of the cyst by burning it with silver nitrate. He has found that lumps so treated do not reappear, but that the off-spring of such birds are pretty certain to be affected with lumps. Johnson disapproves of this treatment, contending with considerable

Figure 58.   **LUNGS**

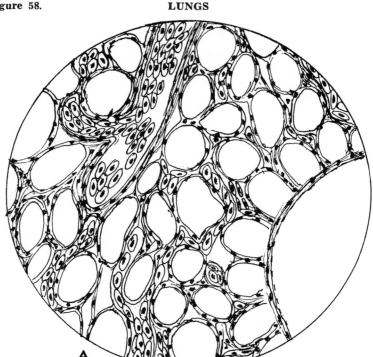

A, Section from the lung of a healthy canary killed in an accident.
(Continued on page 249)

justification that this only tends to keep the defective birds in the breeding room. He thinks that all lumpy birds should be de-stroyed. If this were done, it is reasoned, the condition could be stamped out within two years.

LUNGS. Avian lungs are considerably smaller than mammalian lungs in relation to the size of the body. Mammalian lungs have to perform the whole task of aerating the blood; avian lungs have the assistance of an extensive and complicated system of air tubes and air sacs. See AIR SACS; RESPIRATORY SYSTEM.

Healthy lung tissue is pale pink in color, of porous structure and will float in water. See Figure 58.

Figure 58 (Continued)   **LUNGS**

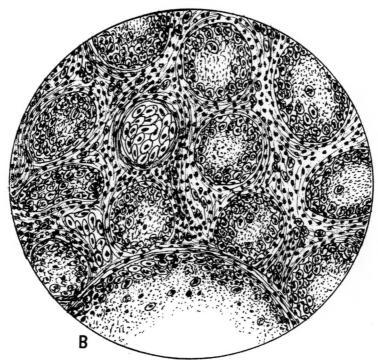

B, Section from the lung of a sparrow found in the last stages of the bronchial form of avian diphtheria. Notice that all of the air spaces are entirely plugged and that there has been considerable infiltration of the interstitial tissue. This bird had undoubtedly been sick for some time.

Sections and drawings by the author. Magnification about 400 ×.

Congested lung tissue may be light red, dark red or purple in color, depending on the age of the condition. It retains its porous structure and will float in water. See Figure 59.

The tubercular lung—something rarely seen in birds—contains yellow nodules (lumps) of cheesy material varying in size from mere points to the size of rape seed in birds the size of canaries. In larger birds the nodules might be larger. The larger of these nodules are encapsulated and easily separated from the surrounding tissue, which may or may not be inflamed. When the contents of these larger nodules are rubbed between the fingers or two microscopic slides, it is seen to contain a gritty material.

Hemorrhagic lung tissue is studded with bright-red or dark-red spots where the blood has escaped into the alveoli (air cells). It will still float. Hemorrhages into the lungs are usually followed by the development of hemorrhagic pneumonia, however.

Figure 59.   **LUNGS**

SECTION OF THE LUNG OF A PIGEON SHOWING
TRAUMATIC CONGESTION

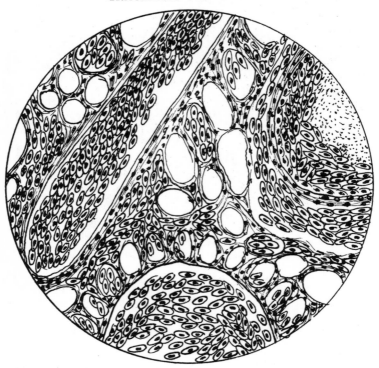

Notice the extrusions of blood cells into the air cells and interstitial spaces. The bird was choked and the congestion resulted from the choking. Author's section and drawing. Conditions the same as in Figure 58.

Pneumonic lung tissue may be of several kinds. In sporadic pneumonia the pneumonic spots are red or brown in color, have a liver-like appearance, are thinner than the surrounding tissue, and each spot extends straight through the organ from its ventral to its dorsal surface. This condition is called **red hepatization** (meaning **red and turned liver-like).**

At the time of death in bronchial pneumonia associated with avian diphtheria, the pneumonic lesion usually occupies most of the central area of each lung—Figure 58. In some cases, only the tip of the lung above the bronchus will remain unaffected. The spots are gray in color and much thicker than the surrounding tissue, but the sponge-like structure is retained, even though the alveoli are plugged to bursting point with morbid exudate. This condition is called **gray hepatization.** When the bird is killed early in the attack, the lungs may be found in a state of red hepatization, but it is one that differs considerably from that observed in sporadic pneumonia. The spots are browner, thicker than the surrounding tissue, and have a dull, rather opaque appearance, while those of sporadic pneumonia are translucent. In neither case will a plug from the pneumonic area float in water.

In interstitial pneumonia the lung is uniformly thickened and may be flecked with brownish spots which do not extend through the organ from front to back. In some cases the appearance is so near normal that the lesion is apt to escape notice. This condition is rarely seen in canaries.

In some of the acute septicemic diseases, gray, yellow or greenish spots may be found in the lungs, resulting from foci of infection or pulmonary thrombi (clots in blood vessels) developing during the course of the generalized infection.

LYE. Lye, true lye, the kind your grandmother used to extract from the wood ashes from the big fireplace and use for making soft soap, was composed principally of potassium carbonate. It has long since been displaced as a general cleaning agent by the cheaper, purer and more powerful sodium hydroxide, of which most lye now sold consists. This product is also sold under the name **caustic soda.** It is manufactured by the electrical decomposition of common salt. A boiling solution of from one to five per cent sodium hydroxide is one of the most powerful and thorough cleaning agents known. It will destroy life of all kinds, dissolve all kinds of organic matter— including fats, oils, gums, proteins and the protective covering of bacterial spores. It will remove all kinds of filth; but it will also remove the paint from your cages and the skin from your hands. A drop of it splattered into the eye will cause blindness.

LYE SOAP. This is the familiar, yellow laundry soap which is sold everywhere. It is made by dissolving resin in a boiling so-

lution of sodium hydroxide, and then combining the resulting product with a soap made from sodium hydroxide and fat.   Sometimes
petroleum products are incorporated in its composition.   A strong
solution of lye soap has most of the virtues of a lye solution and is
free from some of its more disagreeable features.   It is safe to
handle.

LYMPHATICS.   See CIRCULATORY SYSTEM.

MALARIA. Though a rare disease among domesticated birds, excepting pigeons, avian malaria is said to be a rather common disease among wild birds. The parasite—a hematozoan which is very similar to the parasite of human malaria—invades the red cells, where it grows at the expense of the cytoplasm (the material of the cell body) until it reaches such size that the cell wall is ruptured. There are both male and female forms. The male form, when observed in a blood cell, has an elongated nucleus; the female form, observed under the same circumstances, has a round or oval nucleus. Both male and female forms are often seen in

Figure 60.　　　　　　　　**MALARIA**
HEMATOZOA OF AVIAN MALARIA. After Neumann

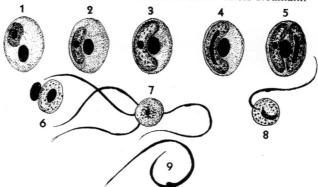

1, 2, 3, Development of male parasite in the blood cell of a pigeon; 4, female parasite; 5, cell containing both male and female parasites; 6, parasite after the rupture of the cell, notice nucleus still clinging to it; 7, male parasite swimming free in the blood; 8, female cell in the blood plasma in the act of being fertilized by a flagellum from the male; 9, free flagellum. Magnification 1500 ×.

the same cell. The free-swimming male is flagellated. Fertilization is effected by a flagellum becoming detached from the male and entering the body of the female cell. The different forms assumed by this parasite in the blood of a pigeon have been ably illustrated by Neumann. See Figure 60.

Notwithstanding that many species of wild birds are said to harbor these parasites without noticeable evidence of illness, in some species the infection is said to cause a mortality of ninety per cent.

Treatment. I know of no experiments throwing light upon the treatment of this disease. It appears to me, however, from the similarity of the infection to the disease in man that quinine would be indicated. The dose, of course, would have to be established by experiments. It is possible that the effective dose would be one approaching the limit of tolerance. It might be necessary to determine the quinine tolerance for each species by experimenting on uninfected birds.

MALES. In most species of birds the sexes can be differentiated by their secondary characteristics—such as plumage, spurs, comb, song and stance. In some of our domesticated birds—canaries and pigeons, for instance—inbreeding has so muddled these characteristics that it is often impossible to tell the sex of a bird that is not in breeding condition. Canaries that have finished the baby moult, this also applies to pigeons, can usually be differentiated by build and stance. Song is always an infallible guide to the sex of canaries, providing the birds are in full song. There are singing females, however, and it may be hard to tell the difference between one of these and a male that is out of song. See BREEDING CONDITION; WHEAT GERM OIL.

MANSON'S EYE WORM. This is a small round worm parasitic in the eyes of birds. Although a great many species of eye worms have been found in the eyes of wild birds, only one species, **Oxyspirura** mansoni, is said to commonly attack the eye of domesticated birds. The worms are about one-half inch long and about one-fiftieth of an inch in diameter at their thickest part and tapering towards the ends.

The only worms that I have ever found in the eyes of a canary are much smaller than those just described. They were white, not over one-eighth to three-sixteenths of an inch long and so thin they could just be seen with the naked eye. Had their color matched that of the tissue, it would have been impossible to have seen them with the naked eye. Only one case has come to my attention in the eighteen years I have been constantly associated with canaries.

Symptoms. In some cases the worms do not appear to cause the bird any inconvenience; in others they may cause complete destruction of the eye. The bird is noticed constantly scratching at the affected eye. The eye becomes inflamed; there is a watery discharge and later, as the inflammation spreads to the surrounding tissue, a white, cheesy exudate appears. If neglected the entire eye as well as the ocular sinuses become involved, and the sight may be destroyed.

Treatment. This is not a difficult condition to treat. As said above, only one case has come to my attention, and that was years before I had run onto any mention of the condition in bird literature. I washed the bird's eye out with a strong solution of sodium perborate. Among the methods that have been recommended for the treatment of this condition in poultry and zoological birds the following are simple and are said to be effective: a saturated solution of borax or sodium bicarbonate or a two per cent solution of creolin may be used to wash the eye out. If an ointment is preferred, one per cent iodoform, one per cent carbolic vaseline or two per cent yellow oxide of mercury may be employed. They are probably equally effective. In fact, a drop of olive oil introduced into the eye would probably be as good as anything else.*

MATING. With most of our domesticated birds it is only necessary to put healthy, vigorous males and females of suitable age together, give them a suitable place for nest-building, suitable material for a nest, suitable food for egg-making, and leave them alone. They will do the rest. Of course, they must have an environment suitable to their natural habits. Canaries and most finches build open nests in the wild state and they still prefer open nests in captivity. They require plenty of light. If the nests are not well lighted, a good many of the babies are going to be crippled because the hens, not being able to see well in dim light, are going to bite their toes off by accident while cleaning the nests. Sparrows and parakeets build dark nests in the wild state and they prefer dark boxes to nest in in captivity. Sparrows will build open nests if a suitable site for a closed nest is not available, but they prefer to nest in a box with a hole in it just large enough for them to go in and out. Given an open site and plenty of straw, they will make heroic efforts to roof the nest over. Each breeder should study the requirements of his particular species. When discussing a disease, I try to give you, first, a digest or summation of all the authoritative literature I have been able to find on that subject supplemented by and interpreted in the light of my own experience, but to attempt to do this in respect to all of the habits of birds would take us too far

* **Note:** All insects and most worms find any kind of oil or grease deadly. It kills the insects by plugging the holes through which they breathe. How it kills the worms, I do not know. Many of the parasitic worms do not breathe, however.

afield. In such matters I am able to speak only for the species with which I have had personal experience.

There are many methods of handling canaries. Each breeder thinks that his method is the best. They all seem to get birds with more or less difficulty. My method is as follows:

Breeding method. My males and females are wintered separately in a cold room. The females are free in a large flight. The males are caged in groups of from ten to twenty in flights consisting of from three to six breeding cages, with their ends removed, hung in a row. My breeding birds never see a small singing cage in their entire lives. My room is so cold that I can count on at least five per cent of the females being lost with uremia or nephritis each winter.* I usually feed them a little soft food daily all the year around, but there is very little egg used in the soft food during the fall and winter. It usually consists of boiled wheat, ground bread, a little cod-liver oil and sometimes a little prepared nestling food. About six weeks before I am ready to mate my birds I add egg powder and crushed hemp † seed to the soft food. Of course, all the birds have all the green food they care to eat every day of their lives. The seed in the flight is fed in large creeps holding a month's supply for a couple of hundred birds and I usually keep only about thirty hens through the winter.

The time of mating depends a lot on the birds and the desires of the breeder. I have mated my birds as early as January. I do not say that I would not do that again. I might if the conditions appealed to me, but I usually do not mate my birds before the first or middle of March. I like to see the old birds with their beaks black from eating fresh green food and the babies with their little crops black with plenty of good dandelion and chickweed. That tells me they have a chance to grow up into big, husky youngsters. A good start in life means less trouble later on.

A week or two before I intend to mate my birds, my breed cages are all washed, sanded and made ready for occupancy. They are hung on three rows of nails driven into the wall—two nails for each cage. For a general arrangement of the equipment, see

---

* **Note:** I could easily stop those losses, but they are natural and normal. If the room was warmer and less well ventilated there would be fewer losses from the cause mentioned; actually, I could avoid all deaths from these causes but I might have a whole flock in soft moult when the breeding season came around. Birds that cannot stand a reasonable amount of cold and draft during the winter are not the kind I want to breed from.
† **Note:** I did, in the past, add crushed hemp to my soft food. For the present I am using wheat germ oil and trying to learn all I can about the new synthetic vitamins and hormones in the hope of eventually working out a system which will give better results than hemp ever gave.

CAGES. The nests and nest boxes are washed; the bottom of each nest box is fitted with paper, which will catch the droppings from the baby birds later on; the nests are put in place; and the whole is powdered with pyrethrum powder. The boxes are hung over the openings in the cage fronts; nestling material, seed cups, water cups, and mineral food cups are placed on top of each cage. To

Figure 61.   **MATING**
BREEDING RECORD

MATED - - - *Mar. 1st*
MALE - - - - - - *W74*
FEMALE - - - - - *Y39*
LAID - - - - - *Mar. 9th*
SET - - - - - *13th*
OFF - - - - - *26th*
EGG - - - - - - - - - 5
HATCH - - - - - - - 4
BIRDS - - - *W93-4-5-6*
REMARKS

the front of each cage is attached a card holder into which fits a small card upon which the following information can be recorded: date of mating; male's band number; female's band number; date the first egg is laid; date of setting; date of hatch; number of eggs; number of birds hatched; number lost; band numbers of the babies—arranged as shown in Figure 61.

In the space for remarks are noted the changes of babies or eggs from nest to nest. These cards are later filed and become a permanent record of the year's breeding operations; though another record is kept of the babies, showing the parents, hatching date, band number, color, marks, sex and final disposition of each bird raised.

The birds are then caught, paired, placed together and permitted to go to work. This is done at night. They are not held in separate compartments during any period of acquaintance. If both birds are in breeding condition and do not have other mates in the room, there will be no trouble. If the birds are not in breeding condition as determined by vent inspection, they are not mated. It is only upon very rare occasions that I have to separate birds to keep them from injuring each other.

For the bodies of their nests, I give my birds lawn cuttings and shredded-up burlap, cut so the strings will not be more than four inches long. When the body of the nest is completed, I give them cotton to line it with. This cotton is the best grade of surgical absorbent cotton and just enough is given to line the nest. It is fastened by sticking it under one of the rails of a door and closing the door on it, so that the birds cannot drag it all over the cage—for you know the hen has to shred it up into little bits in order to line the nest with it. If too much cotton is given, some hens will spoil an otherwise perfect nest by stuffing it so full of cotton that there will be no room for the eggs.

When the eggs come, the first three are taken away and replaced by nest eggs. For the first nest they are replaced on the evening of the day on which the third egg was laid, but thereafter they are replaced, according to how many eggs the hen lays, on the evening before the last egg is laid—hens laying five eggs do not get theirs back until the evening of the fourth day. By this method all of the young birds should hatch on the morning of the 14th day of incubation, reckoned from the date on which the eggs were returned. The eggs that have been taken from the nest will require 13½ days to hatch, but that last egg will hatch in an even 13 days. This gives the babies an equal chance for life.

From the time the birds are mated until the last egg is laid, they are given all the soft food they will use, but the minute the last egg is laid no more soft food is given until the 12th day of incubation and the cage is always resanded on the day the last egg is laid so no crumbs of egg food will remain on the floor for the birds to peck at. The male is never taken out. Any male that proves untrustworthy in the breeding cage is disposed of. See BREEDING BIRDS; BREEDING CONDITION; SEX BREEDING.

MATING SEASON. Although it is possible to breed canaries in every month of the year, best results are obtained by breeding them only during the natural spring breeding season, March to June, the same time the sparrows do their breeding. Many of the wild finches that are used as cage-birds and for mule breeding do not come into breeding condition until May and then raise only two nests of babies. Parakeets that have been brought to this country from the antipodes breed in the fall and winter and moult in the winter and spring. This habit is said to persist for several generations.

MAW SEED. This is the seed of the opium poppy. It is a small blue seed, the meat of which is rich in oil and protein and contains no opium. There is a small amount of opium in the hulls, however, though not over 0.12 per cent. Canaries and small finches will shell maw seed given to them in bulk. Most maw seed, however, is fed mixed in soft foods and under these circumstances many of the seeds will be swallowed whole. Weanlings, too, usually swallow this seed whole, which makes it of considerable value at weaning time, since at this time young birds often swallow things which upset them and cause diarrhea. The small amount of opium in the maw seed is just sufficient to allay the resulting intestinal irritation. All birds are very fond of maw seed, and it is indispensable in the diets of some of the small finches. Rancid maw seed, like rancid hemp seed, is very dangerous, but the keeping qualities of maw seed are vastly superior to those of hemp seed.

MEAL-WORMS. There are two varieties of meal-worms used for bird food. Both are common as grain pests, and differ principally in color and breeding habits. See Figure 62. The worms are the larvae of a beetle about seven-eighths of an inch long which makes its home in places where grain is stored. The light or yellow variety (so-called because the worm is lighter in color than that of the other variety) makes its appearance about May or June; the beetles of the darker variety make their appearance about a month earlier. After the beetles have laid their eggs they disappear and are not seen again until the following year. The eggs soon hatch out into young worms which attain their greatest size in about three months, though they do not go into the pupa stage until the following spring.

The full-grown worms are about three-sixteenth of an inch thick and one and one-quarter inches long.

Propagation. At one time it was the habit of bird fanciers to gather their worms from the neighborhoods of flour mills and granaries, but for some years these worms have been an established article of commerce, purchasable at almost any pet shop. At the time this is being written, they are selling for about three dollars per pound. For that reason, many breeders will find it profitable to raise their own worms.

Figure 62.

MEAL WORMS

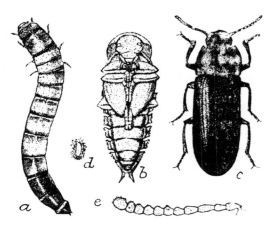

a, larva; *b,* pupa; *c,* female beetle; *d,* **egg with surrounding case;** *e,* antenna. (All except *e* **about twice natural** size; *e* greatly enlarged.) (Courtesy **U. S. Dept. of Agriculture.**)

To do this, make a box about five or six feet long, eighteen inches wide and twenty inches deep; cover the floor of the box with wooden cleats about one-half inch thick and one inch wide and placed about three inches apart, running crosswise of the box. A number of strips of burlap are cut sixteen inches wide and two inches shorter than the inside length of the box. The first strip of burlap is placed on the bottom of the box, and the one-inch margin around its edges and the cleats on the bottom of the box will permit

Note: For a complete description of the two principal varieties of mealworms, see "Stored Grain Pests," Farmer's Bulletin 1260, U. S. Department of Agriculture.

free passage to the worms and beetles. Over this burlap is placed about two inches of bran; then another strip of burlap is placed in the box and another layer of bran put on top of it. This second layer of bran is made about one inch deep. This is continued, a strip of burlap and an inch-deep layer of bran, until the box is from one-half to two-thirds full of layers of bran and burlap The top of the box is fitted with a tight cover of wire cloth and a second tight cover of muslin—these are to keep the beetles and young worms from escaping.

The beetles or worms are placed in the box; a banana skin or apple core placed on top of the bran; the tops fixed into place; and then the box is put in a warm place and left alone, excepting that once each week it is opened and a fresh apple core or banana skin is placed on top of the bran—these are to provide moisture for the worms. Too much moisture must not be given and those foods which are given with this end in view must never be permitted to become mouldy, since in that condition they would be fatal to the worms.

After the worms hatch, they may be transferred to storage boxes which resemble the breeding box, excepting that they are only about one-third as large. By keeping these boxes in warm or cool places it is possible to accelerate or retard the development of the worms to such an extent that full-grown worms will be available throughout the year.

Man undoubtedly consumes thousands of tons of these worms in flour and meal. Whether they do him any good or not, I do not know, but they are undoubtedly the best food known for breeding birds. They are in such great demand that the breeder who raises a surplus will have no trouble in disposing of it through pet shops, and he may earn enough from his worms to pay a large part of his birds' food bill.

MEGRIMS. This is the name applied to a peculiar kind of headache in man. Moore applied it to a form of B. paratyphosus B infection of pigeons in which there is formation of an exudate in the subarachnoid spaces over the brain, and in which the birds display all the symptoms of a frightful headache. These symptoms are so realistic that they can be recognized by the observant breeder the first time they are seen. The only reason why the affected bird does not hold his head in his hands and moan is that he has no hands. See B. PARATYPHOSUS B INFECTION.

MERCURIC CHLORIDE, mercury bichloride, corrosive sublimate.

This salt, a powerful disinfectant and germicide, is used in hospitals for the treatment of wounds and the sterilization of the hands. The advantage of its high germ-killing power is partially offset by the facts that its continual use is injurious to the hands and that it will corrode metal instruments. It is employed in solutions of 1:1000 to 1:10000. Although this salt is highly poisonous to man and animals, Gallagher has shown that an adult chicken can withstand a dose of two grains without displaying any symptoms of poisoning. He has also reported keeping an entire flock of chickens on a 1:6000 solution of mercury bichloride as drinking water for eighteen days without any of the birds showing symptoms of mercury poisoning. No other water was given. The flock to which this treatment was given was suffering with cholera. The effect of the drug upon the control of the disease was not mentioned in the account to come to my attention. I have not used this salt upon canaries.

METHYLENE BLUE. This substance, one of the more common coal-tar dyestuffs, has the formula $C_{16}H_{18}N_3SCl$, and is used in the arts for dyeing fabric, making ink, blueing clothes, etc. It is used as a biological stain for staining the nuclei of cells and bacteria; it does not, as a rule, stain cell cytoplasm. It is used in medicine as an anodyne, antipyretic and urinary antiseptic. It has been employed in the treatment of rheumatism, malaria, cystitis, pyelitis, carcinoma, black-water fever, diabetes, neuralgia and gonorrhea, but it is no longer used in any of these conditions. While they probably would not admit it to their wives, most of my older male readers will remember the "Blue bullets" so famous and widely used thirty years ago, the active ingredient of which was methylene blue. It is now employed in human medicine principally as an antidote for carbon-monoxide and cyanide poisoning, for which purpose a one per cent solution in sterile salt solution is injected into a vein. Why methylene blue acts as an antidote for these poisons is something we do not understand.*

Under the headings DIGESTIVE DISORDERS; NEPHRITIS;

---

* **Note:** None of these dyes are found on the market in chemically pure form. In fact the expression **Chemically pure** (C P) is more of a hope than an actuality. Purity is always relative, never absolute. Some of the grades of dyestuff found on the market contain poisonous metallic compounds among their impurities. Only those grades that are labeled "U.S.P. MEDICINAL" are fit for internal administration. The dye used in the experiments to be described presently was HARLECA brand, U.S.P. Medicinal Methylene Blue; dye content, 85 per cent; manufactured by Hartman-Leddon Company, Philadelphia, Pa. I cannot say that the results described would follow the use of any other grade of dye; they most certainly would not follow the use of cotton or Easter-egg dye.

and UREMIA, I have mentioned the difficulty involved in arriving at a correct diagnosis in certain digestive and urinary disorders, and the fact that the treatment of such conditions was greatly hampered by the resulting uncertainty. Birds have lived for years suffering from digestive symptoms and a dull-yellow, pasty diarrhea, becoming progressively more emaciated, without the breeder being able to determine the true nature of the trouble until they were killed and examined internally; then it has often been realized that had it been possible to determine the condition of the organs during life it would have been possible to save the bird. Every breeder has such birds, and usually he gets disgusted with them sooner or later and chokes them. I am no exception. Rather than choke mine, however, I experiment with them. The one drawback to such experiments, however, is the uncertainty of the diagnosis, which robs the results of value. These facts should be borne in mind in connection with what is to follow.

I recently carried out a number of experiments on the color-feeding of white canaries, and naturally, I did not use my best birds for the first experiments. Among the birds selected were several that were suffering with symptoms which could have been referred to either the digestive or urinary tracts. In none of these cases had I been able to establish a positive diagnosis, though in some cases the condition had been present for more than a year. Soon after these birds were placed on methylene blue, I noticed that the bowel symptoms had cleared up. The females became more lively and the male began to sing. Gradually the ailing birds put on weight and were restored to normal health and vigor. Realizing that I might have found something of value, other ailing birds were tested, and some of these I had sound reason for believing were suffering from kidney disorders resulting from exposure. All but two recovered. These two died later and were found to have been suffering from chronic nephritis, which throws some doubt upon correctness of the diagnosis in the other cases.

Preparation. Add two and one-half grams of medicinal methylene blue to sixty cubic centimeters (about two ounces) of water, shake well at frequent intervals for several days, and then let the solution settle until the supernatant fluid becomes clear.* In using this solution care is taken not to shake the bottle, and only the top of the fluid is picked up by the medicine dropper.

Dosage. Canary cage drinkers hold from twenty to forty cubic

---

* **Note:** Because the solution is very dark it is hard to see through that contained in the bottle. This difficulty is overcome by picking up a few drops in a medicine dropper and holding the dropper to the light.

centimeters. An eye dropper usually delivers from fifteen to twenty drops per cubic centimeter. The experiment was started by administering five drops of the dye solution to each drinker of water, and the dosage was increased until twenty-five drops of dye solution were being added to each drinker; that is, one drop of dye solution to each cc of drinking water.

Later, in treating sick birds, I started the courses with six drops of dye solution to each drinker and increased the dose, one drop every second day until the birds showed marked signs of improvement or symptoms of poisoning.

Toxicity. In all cases the administration of methylene blue caused slight diarrhea. This was more noticeable during the early stages of the treatment than later. The first sign of toxemia is indicated by shortness of breath. There is a decrease in the number of red cells in the blood. No birds became seriously ill during or directly following the experiments with this dye. In no case was the dosage carried beyond one drop of dye solution for each cubic centimeter of water used.

Action. Methylene blue appears to act as an antiseptic in the urinary and digestive tracts. Only part of the dye is absorbed, and that portion is eliminated through the kidneys; the rest of the dye is eliminated through the bowels. During the treatment there is a noticeable drop in the number of bacteria in the droppings. As the treatment progresses the birds develop a resistance to the absorption of the drug and their urine becomes lighter in color.

MINERAL FOOD. As has been already mentioned several times, birds require minerals in larger quantities than are to be found in their ordinary diet. Their greatest need is for calcium carbonate. Their blood and droppings are both rich in calcium salts, which appear to play some important part in the elimination of waste products. Large quantities of calcium carbonate are also used in the manufacture of egg shells. All poultrymen and bird keepers have learned that they must give their birds some form of mineral food. The simplest form is ground limestone; the more complex forms follow more or less closely the formula to be given below. Many bird keepers keep a piece of cuttlebone in the cage for the birds to peck at—for, in addition to calcium carbonate, it contains minute quantities of phosphates, chlorides, iodides, bromides and fluorides. No! That is a lie! They do not give their birds cuttlebone because it contains these elements; they give it to them because someone told them to do so. It does contain these necessary elements, however, and in most localities it serves all requirements. Most poultrymen find that their chickens do well on a mixture of steamed bone meal and ground oyster shells.

Once, some years ago, I lost a lot of canaries because of iodide deficiency. I then turned my thoughts to the development of a perfect mineral food, one that would contain all of the mineral elements which might be deficient in the birds' diet. The following formula meets these requirements:

Ground oyster shells ....60 per cent
    (Sterilized egg shells may be substituted)
Steamed bone meal........................38 per cent
Sodium chloride (common salt)................02 per cent

To each 100 pounds of the above mixture add two ounces of potassium iodide; one-half ounce of zinc sulphate; one-half ounce of copper sulphate; one-eighth ounce of nickel sulphate. All of these substances are dissolved in a pint of hot water which is then sprinkled over the mineral mixture, which is mixed until it is uniformly moist throughout. This is done to assure a uniform mixture. When the mixture has dried it may be stored in cans or bags. I keep such a mixture before my birds at all times.

MITES. I have no idea how many kinds of mites attack birds. Some attack the feathers; some attack the skin; some invade the air sacs; some invade the connective tissues; some bore under the scales of the feet; and some suck the blood of their host.

The blood-sucking mites and bugs, which include the common bedbug; his relative, the nestbug or bluebug; the chicken tick; and the red mite, live on the blood sucked from the bird during the night. The tick may hang on the bird during the daytime, but the others all leave the body of the bird during the daytime and hide in cracks, where their breeding operations are carried on. Their favorite places of residence are in nesting material and the cracks of the nestboxes and because of the warmth received from the body of the sitting hen, they are enabled to breed very rapidly and in great numbers. They come out only at night, if there are but a few present, but soon they become so numerous and bold that in the darkness of the nest they will feed on the babies both day and night. Is it any wonder that the mothers sometimes quit their nest or that the babies are found pale and lifeless, every bit of blood having been sucked from their bodies.

Feather mites have been discussed. Some mites, more or less closely related to the feather mite, invade the air sacs, bore into the skin and live on the connective tissue and work their way under the scales of the feet. Only the latter variety is of any considerable importance; it will be discussed under the headings SCALY-LEG; FEET, CARE OF.

The control of mites does not present a problem of any considerable magnitude where an intelligent system of cleanliness is adhered to. They must be controlled, but a few of them in the bird room is nothing for the breeder to have a fit about. Neglected, they do great harm, but great harm may also be done by the employment of drastic, ill-advised, or poorly-thought-out methods of extermination. I know that in my early days as a bird keeper I probably killed more birds through my fear of mites than were killed by the mites. Now, a bushel basket full of mites could be dumped into my bird room without causing either me or my birds one moment's trouble. My regular cleaning system would care for them before they had any chance to do any harm. More will be said on this subject under the heading RED MITES.

MOSQUITOES. Under the heading FEET, SWOLLEN, I had something to say about mosquitoes and the sores they cause on the feet of young birds. They are the worst pests with which we have to deal, since their presence is very apt to be overlooked. They often suck enough blood from young birds to kill them in a single night, the birds being found in the morning hanging from the perch, head down, dead—and this can happen to vigorous young sparrows four months old. The young bird is afraid to leave the perch during the night, and its only defense is to kick at the mosquitoes with its free foot.

It is only the foot that the bird is standing on during sleep that is attacked by mosquitoes, for they do not like to get themselves mixed up in the bird's feathers. The worst they can do in the case of older birds is to drill between the scales, but they often drill right through the scales on the feet of young birds, and after the mosquitoes quit feeding, the blood continues to flow until large clots are formed. These wounds cause bad sores which heal slowly. Often the toe is lost. Old birds realizing the attack of the mosquitoes is more to be feared than the bumps resulting from blind flying, will quit the perches and flutter to the floor, where they protect their feet by sitting on them.

The breeder who wants to know whether or not mosquitoes are bothering his birds needs only to go into his bird room at night and sit quietly in the dark and listen. If there are mosquitoes, he will soon hear a peculiar stamping of feet. The sound is not easily described but once heard, it is easily recognized. It is caused by the bird kicking with the free foot at the mosquitoes feeding on the foot it is standing on; it sounds something like the sound of **two dots—dash—two dots** as sounded on a telegraph instrument. If the breeder will locate the stamping bird and suddenly turn a flashlight on its feet, he will see the mosquitoes. I have seen as many as six of them crowded around the foot of one canary.

Protection. The first protective measure is to screen all doors and windows with a 16 or 18 mesh wire cloth. If the room is to contain flying birds which have access to the windows and doors, the screen-frames must be covered on the inside with ¾ inch chicken netting and on the outside with the fine wire cloth, for otherwise some of the birds would get their feet caught in the fine wire and break their toes.

Even with the room screened, during the mosquito season the breeder should make a habit of going into his bird room at night and listening to his birds. If they are bothered by mites he will hear the champ of their beaks and the whir of their wings as they comb and shake their feathers.

Any time the birds are restless at night the room should be thoroughly sprayed the next morning.

MOUTH. See DIGESTIVE TRACT.

MYCOSIS. This is a term applied to lesions resulting from infection by pathogenic fungi (moulds) as, **pneumomycosis,** a mould infection of the lungs; **dermatomycosis,** a mould infection of the skin. See ASPERGILLOSIS; FUNGOID SKIN.

NAPHTHALENE. This is a coal-tar hydrocarbon with the chemical formula $C_{10}H_8$. Most moth balls were once made from this substance, which is a powerful insecticide.* Naphthalene is used in medicine as an antiseptic, antidiarrheac, anthelmintic, and antipyretic—which simply means that it stops the growth of germs, checks diarrhea, destroys or expels intestinal worms and lowers body temperature.

Naphthalene comes on the market in several grades. The purest grade is pure white and has the strong, characteristic odor of moth balls. This is the only grade that should be used in the bird room. Inferior grades are yellow or brown in color.

This substance has a wide range of uses in the bird room. It is invaluable for preserving stored seed, keeping it free from insects. Whenever I get new seed supplies, I mix a handful of moth balls through the contents of each 100-pound sack.

There is no better substance for keeping the nests of chickens and pigeons free from lice and mites. One or two moth balls may be thrown into the nest with the eggs or thrust down into the nesting material. The heat of the hen's body will evaporate the naphthalene, which will then penetrate her feathers and the nesting material, reaching the hiding places of both lice and mites. Several writers have suggested the use of naphthalene in the nests of canaries. I have tested this idea with the following results: One moth ball placed in a canary's nest with the eggs will kill the chicks in the eggs within twelve hours; will kill eight-day old chicks in the nest within sixteen hours, but not in twelve hours; will make the hen dopey and groggy, but will not kill her—as a rule she has sense enough to leave the nest about the time she is so far gone that she can no longer fly or cling to the perch. A very small pinch of naphthalene powder sprinkled on the lining of the nest pan or mixed in the nesting material will keep the nest free from mites without harming the birds. Not more than two grains should be used, and it should be placed as far away from the heat of the hen's body as possible. I prefer to use pyrethrum.

The poisonous effects of naphthalene are fatal only in those

---

* **Note:** Some of the moth balls now on the market are made from a naphthalene derivative, rather than the hydrocarbon itself, and I have no information concerning the physiological properties of these. I have, however, found them satisfactory for the preservation of stored seed.

cases where the administration is continued up to the point of death. They disappear quickly when the bird is given plenty of fresh air.

In order to have plenty of good nests for making changes, I save all good, unsoiled nests. These are placed in a tight-topped can containing a handful of moth balls. The fumes make the nest mite-proof. These nests must be aired and warmed for at least one hour before using. I usually hang them on an electric light.

Naphthalene has been used in human medicine for the treatment of chronic inflammation of the intestines, catarrh, intestinal worms, typhoid, cholera and chronic bronchitis. It is eliminated from the body through the skin, respiratory tract, and in the urine. I have not tested this drug in the treatment of birds suffering from acute, contagious diseases; but it will lower the body temperature, relieve some stubborn cases of intestinal inflammation, cure some colds and throat ailments, and remove intestinal worms.

For internal administration in cases of colds, etc., it is mixed with sugar in the proportion of 1:100 and given on soft food in one or two grain doses; for worms the dilution used is 1:20. The dosage remains the same. For larger birds the dose would have to be increased proportionally.

Naphthalene is sometimes fed to poultry on the theory that it will not only keep them free from worms but will be secreted by the oil gland and thus louse-proof the feathers. I have not found this of value in the handling of cage-birds. Where large numbers of birds are kept in a large flight which cannot be effectively deloused, a little naphthalene in the bath water will go a long ways toward keeping lice and mites off the birds. All birds will not use the bath, but those that do so will be kept free of the pests. Two teaspoonfuls of a saturated solution of naphthalene in pure grain alcohol is added to each gallon of bath water. The naphthalene is precipitated in fine flakes which remain in suspension. Full feathered birds will suffer no ill effects from bathing in this solution, but moulting birds will sometimes be blistered on their naked spots. The injury is seldom very serious, however.

I once ran some comparative tests on naphthalene and quassia infusion in the bath water, to see which was the most effective for delousing birds. In order to arrive at a sound basis for comparison I caught the entire flock once each week and removed all of the louse-eaten feathers. By counting the number of feathers removed each week and dividing that number by the total number of birds in the room I arrived at an index of infestation. The birds were considered 100 per cent infested at the beginning of the test. Quassia infusion was first employed for three weeks; then naphthalene was used for five weeks. The results were:

Quassia—No reduction in the extent of infestation when used daily for three weeks. In fact, the density of infestation increased considerably during the test. The infusion was made by steeping quassia chips in hot water. I have been told since that I should have used cold water. In any case, the results were negative.

Naphthalene—30% reduction in infestation at the end of the first week; 50% reduction at the end of second week; 65% reduction at the end of third week. There was no reduction beyond the third week; the birds that used the bath were free from lice, those that did not were more heavily infested than ever.

The room was not sprayed or otherwise cleaned during the course of the test.

I have found that a spray made from a saturated solution of naphthalene in kerosene is very effective against red mites. It can be used around full-feathered birds without harming them, if care is taken not to spray the mixture directly on the birds, but moulting birds are apt to be blistered by the fine drops of oil in the air coming in contact with the unfeathered areas of their bodies. There is nothing to be gained by mixing one's own spray, however, since there are so many cheap, harmless and effective sprays on the market.

Warning. Naphthalene fed to chickens can be tasted in the eggs. For internal use only the best grade of pure white naphthalene should be employed. Overdoses of this drug may produce coma and death.* The drug has a narcotic reaction. The bird to which an overdose of naphthalene has been administered becomes dopey and droopy and acts very much like a person to whom an overdose of morphine has been administered. It should be put in a warm, well ventilated place, where it will usually recover. Even those cases where the bird has fallen into coma before being discovered can be prevented from resulting fatally by administering heart stimulants—ten drops of a warm water containing I.Q.S. in the proportion of three drops to the ounce may be administered into the beak.

---

* **Note:** I have seen hopheads eat moth balls to break a morphine habit.

NASAL CAVITY. Below each nostril, which is a small opening in the upper margin of the upper mandible, there is a short tube which communicates with a slit-like opening located on the medial line of the hard palate. Above this opening in the roof of the mouth the cavity is divided by a bone and cartilage septum. On each side of the head, connecting with the nasal cavities at their lower extremities by means of a short, curved tube, there is a cavity known as the **suborbital sinus,** which receives the drainage from the eye through the lachrymal duct. Since these cavities do not drain by gravity, they are very apt to become affected during attacks of cold, roup or any other infection involving the nasal passages. In such cases they become plugged with exudates for which there is no natural avenue of escape. The eyes water and the feathers around them become matted with tears; swellings appear above the beak; and sometimes the pressure of the exudates will be so great that it will force an artificial opening in the front of the head; at other times it is necessary to open the swelling and establish drainage in order to relieve the pressure on the eyes.

In some cases of sinus infection the entire nasal cavity may become plugged with a cheesy exudate which is largely composed of exfoliated mucous cells in various stages of degeneration. This exudate has to be removed by digging it out through the nostrils with a thin looped wire. The cavity is then irrigated with a solution of boric acid or sodium perborate. It may take a week or more of daily treatments to clear the passages out sufficiently for the bird to breathe through them. The inflammation is then treated with NASAL OIL. The eyes should be treated with mercuric ointment. See ANTISEPTICS FOR THE EYES.

NASAL OIL. Rx

Camphor	1.5 cc's or gr's.
Menthol	0.3 cc's or gr's.
Eucalyptol	0.5 cc's or gr's.
Methyl salicylate	0.8 cc's or gr's.
Pine-needle oil	1.0 cc's or gr's.
Cassia	0.8 cc's or gr's.
Ephedrine alkaloid	1.0 cc's or gr's.
Petrolatum liquidum to make up to	100.0 cc's or gr's.

I have found this prescription valuable in the treatment of nasal infection. See ASTHMA.

NASAL PARASITES. The oral and nasal cavities of water fowls, and sometimes their eyes, esophagus, larynx and trachea, are attacked by small leeches. Megnin has recommended an irrigation with two per cent sodium chloride to effect their removal.

Chickens, pigeons and probably a number of other birds are sometimes attacked by a mite, called **Rhinonyssus**, which invades the nasal passages causing coryza (a watery discharge from the nostrils) in old birds and sometimes death in baby birds. There is no better treatment for the removal of these pests than the NASAL OIL described in the previous section. For large birds a drop of oil may be placed in each nostril with a medicine dropper. The bird should be held with its beak pointing upward for a few moments, so that the oil will run back into the remote cavities. Small birds are treated by dipping a fine wire or an inoculation needle (this is a piece of number 24 platinum or nichrome wire fitted in a glass handle and used for inoculating cultures) into the oil; drawing it quickly across the lip of the bottle containing the oil, to remove any large drops; and then holding it in a vertical position with its lower end resting on the bird's nostril. The surplus oil will trickle slowly down the wire and into the nostril without coming in contact with the skin or soiling the head feathers.

NASTURTIUM. This is a garden plant with soft, succulent leaves and stems and large, bell-shaped, red and yellow flowers. The leaves and stems have a sharp, biting, but pleasant taste. Small cage-birds are very fond of this plant and will eat all parts of it. The pigment of the red flowers will color the feathers of moulting canaries. See COLOR FOOD.

NEMBUTAL ANESTHESIA FOR CANARIES. Dr. A. J. Durant, the same gentleman to whom I pay my respects under the headings FOWL PARALYSIS and LEUKEMIA, has described two abdominal operations upon canaries in which this substance was used as the anesthetic. Of its use he says:

"The use of nembutal for canaries is the same as for large animals; that is, 1 cc to each five pounds of body weight. Because of the small size of the canary (19 to 24 grams), however, it is necessary to dilute the nembutal by measuring out .04 of a cc of nembutal solution, then adding .36 of a cc of sterile water. One-tenth of this diluted nembutal to a 24 gram bird will produce approximately complete anesthesia. However, in some cases the amount has to be varied a little, depending on the size and condition of the bird. The anesthetic is injected subcutaneously. Injections are made with a one cc all glass tuberculin syringe and a 27 gauge needle."

You will notice that the gentleman is speaking about some kind of solution, but he does not take the trouble to say what strength it is.

Page 416 of Merck's Index, 1940 edition, lists, "Pentobarbital Sodium, Nembutal, Embutal, Sodium Ethyl—(1 methyl-butyl) bar-biturate.

White, odorless, slightly bitter, crystaline powder. . . .

Use: As other barbiturates. Dose: 1½ grains; preanesthetic sedative, 3 grains; rectally for analgesia, 5 to 6 grains."

No standard veterinary doses are given. Gould's Dictionary, 1937 edition, lists the drug for human use and gives the dose as 2 grains. It does not list it for veterinary use nor mention any standard solution to use for the production of anesthesia; it does, however, say that injection of the drug is considered dangerous.

Since these two books are the latest and most authoritative works we have on the uses and dosages of drugs in both human and veterinary medicine, it seems that no standard solution for the administration of this drug exists, and the good doctor has again been guilty of passing out incomplete and useless information. And these are not out of date books, doctor!

NECROSIS. This is the destruction of functional tissue by poisons, caustics, or by the causative agents of disease. See CANARY NECROSIS.

NEPHRITIS. This, as the name indicates, is any inflammation of the kidneys. The type of nephritis to which birds are commonly susceptible is identical with Bright's disease in man, a chronic fatty degeneration of one or both kidneys.

This condition is not described in any literature on birds to come to my attention. It is hard to believe that a condition so common could escape observation, but that is evidently the case, since all books describing the symptoms of this condition attribute those symptoms to other pathological changes which, by the way, do not occur under the circumstances described as contributing causes. I have observed this condition in canaries, finches, sparrows and blackbirds and have reasons for believing it to be of common occurrence in all species of birds, both wild and domesticated. The only reason I can see for this condition escaping observation is the fact that most bird keepers are too lazy to perform post-mortem examinations, and that veterinarians are too prone in such cases to follow book teaching rather than their eyes. That the condition is very common is illustrated by the fact that canary breeders, poultrymen, and in one case a veterinarian, in their letters to me have described dozens, if not hundreds, of case histories that could apply to no other condition, still not one of them ever suspected that the affected birds might have been suffering from kidney disorders.

Etiology. In all cases of chronic nephritis to come to my attention there has been a history of exposure or chilling associated with the appearance of the first symptoms. In the cases of some blackbirds, the bodies of which were sent to me for examination, there was also a history of metallic poisoning, resulting from the administration of medicine in metal drinkers. In many cases of chronic nephritis in canaries the condition develops following recovery from an attack of acute uremia. I have observed other cases in which the disease was chronic from the onset. The condition is more prevalent among females than males, and is sometimes associated with ovarian tumor.*

Morbid anatomy. The kidneys are usually enlarged to from two to three times normal size. They are smooth, glistening and bright yellow in color. Usually both kidneys are equally involved, though there are cases where only one kidney or a single lobe is affected. Such cases are only observed, however, where death is from other causes, since any bird with as much as one of its six kidney lobes in good condition will not die. The organs are bright yellow in color, swollen, glistening. The blood vessels stand out as bright red lines, but the ureters are invisible—in the normal kidney the ureters and their larger branches stand out as bold white lines.

Figure 63 shows a section from the cortex of a canary's kidney well advanced in the degenerative process. The bird had been sick for about a year. It will be noticed that while the glomerulus shown at the top of the field, at (a), has a tuft that is completely degenerated, the tuft of the glomerulus in the center of the field is almost normal and is still functioning (notice the blood cells); there is some granular matter between the tuft and the capsule, and the capsule is considerably thickened, however. It will also be

---

* **Note:** It may be that one reason for the greater prevalence of this condition among females is the fact that male canaries are more valuable than their sisters and are apt to receive better care and be guarded more closely against exposure and drafts. But it may be that the females have greater resistance to the effects of exposure, for far more males than females die of acute uremia.

noticed that the cells of the convolution and collection tubes are broken and degenerated and that the tubes are filled with fatty and granular material, (b,b). Some of the areas normally occupied by capillaries are filled with connective tissue, (c,c).

The urine contains epithelial cells in various stages of degeneration, casts, fat globes, albuminous matter, urates in much smaller quantities than normal, uric acid crystals, and crystals of inorganic salts. Epithelial casts are sometimes found, but usually

Figure 63. **NEPHRITIS**
LESIONS OF CHRONIC NEPHRITIS IN A CANARY

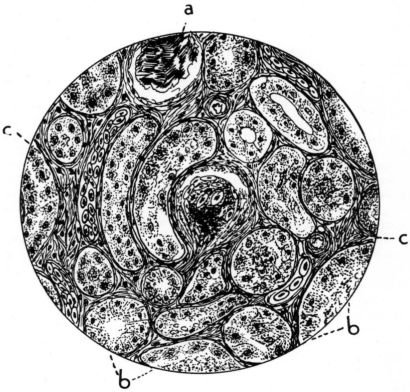

A section from a canary's kidney magnified about 600 ×.
a, a degenerated glomerulus; **b, b,** plugged and degenerated convolution tubes. Notice the irregular, broken appearance of the cells. **c, c,** areas where connective tissue has replaced tubulas or blood vessels. It will be noticed that the walls of the glomeruli, and of the tubes, too, for that matter, are considerably thickened.
Drawing by Robert Stroud.

the material is so badly broken up that they are not easily identified. The urine of birds in the advanced stages of chronic nephritis
gives a reaction for both sugar and albumen.* It is regrettable
that the discharge from inflamed intestines also contains albumen
and may, in some diseases (diphtheria for one), contain urates.

Symptoms. A bird in the early stages of nephritis appears to
be but slightly out of condition. The appetite is good, but the
digestion seems to be poor and the voided material usually contains a lot of fluid. The bird loses its taste for seed, but will eat
large quantities of soft food and green food. If seed alone is given
to these birds they will shell more of the seeds than they swallow—
a common trait of birds suffering from digestive disturbances. The
sick bird may sleep a little in the daytime, but this is not a usual
symptom during the early stages of the illness. On warm days
these birds appear as healthy and lively as any bird in your flock.
They love to sit in the sun. As the disease progresses the bird
sleeps in the daytime, acts constantly cold and loves to snuggle
up against an electric light and sleep. I have found that by placing
a 100-watt light in my cold flight, so arranged that the birds can
cluster around it, the number of cases of uremia and nephritis are
greatly reduced. All of the birds, sick and well alike, love to get
right under the light and let it beat down on their backs, directly
above the kidneys. The sick appear to be greatly benefited by this
self-administered treatment. I have had some of them live for as
long as two years. Sooner or later, however, a spell of cold weather
gets them and they are found dead or dying.

As the illness progresses the symptoms of indigestion become
more pronounced. The feces becomes dull-yellow in color and of
more or less pasty consistency; the urine becomes thinner and
more transparent than normal, of stringy, viscid consistency. It
contains considerable albumen and is very irritating to the tissues
of the vent and cloaca. The bird whips its tail after each passage.

---

* **Note:** The test for albumen is performed by dissolving or emulsifying the
droppings in a little water; filtering the emulsion; then, after adding a
drop of hydrochloric acid to the filterate, bringing it to a boil. If albumen
is present, it will be thrown down as a white powder. If there is only a
trace of albumen, the filterate will become cloudy or milky in appearance.
The test for sugar is performed by adding ten drops of the filterate to ten
cc of boiling Fehling's solution, which is made as follows: dissolve 36.64
grams of cupric sulphate in 200 cc of distilled water; dissolve 80 grams of
sodium hydroxide in 600 cc of distilled water and add 173 grams of Rochelle
Salts. Mix the two solutions and add enough water to make up to 1000 cc.
If sugar is present in the suspected urine in abnormal quantities, and if
not more than five times their weight of water has been used to emulsify
the droppings, ten to twenty drops of the filterate should be sufficient to
cause the boiling Fehling's solution to turn a bright, brick red.

The feathers around the vent become fouled and have to be removed to keep them from blocking the opening. The female vent often protrudes to such an extent that she might be mistaken for a male. There is progressive emaciation; the bird becomes very weak, passes into a coma and dies.

Differential diagnosis. It is impossible to recognize all cases of nephritis during life. The symptoms of other chronic conditions, such as aspergillosis of the abdominal air sacs, streptococcus infection of the gall bladder and gall duct, tuberculosis, atrophy of the spleen, and at least a half-dozen distinct disorders of the digestive tract present symptoms closely resembling those of chronic nephritis. Where there is a history of chilling or exposure directly

Figure 64. . **NEPHRITIS**
BIRD URINE

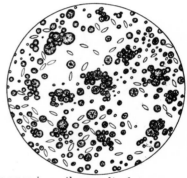

Fresh normal urine from a canary magnified about 600 times.

The preparation is made by emulsifying a small amount of the urine on the slide with a drop of water and then placing a cover-glass over it and examining at once. The round bodies are the only ones observed upon the first examination. They are composed of uric acid and urates. The small almond-shaped crystals of uric acid do not appear in normal urine as it is voided, nor do they make their appearance as the undiluted urine dries. They appear rapidly as evaporation takes place from the diluted emulsion, however. They are the forerunners of much larger crystals which make their appearance in the urine of birds suffering from acute uremia as the result of exposure.

preceding the appearance of the first symptoms, or where the chronic symptoms followed an attack of acute uremia, the breeder is justified in assuming that the bird is suffering with nephritis and treating it accordingly.*

I have found, however, that when a loopful of Gentian violet— a 0.5% solution to which two drops of normal sodium hydroxide solution has been added for each 100 cc—is permitted to run under

* **Note:** Since completing this manuscript, I have carried out some investigations with the view of developing methods of diagnosing chronic nephritis in canaries and other birds during life. To this end, Figure 64 represents the microscopic appearance of normal bird urine. I had intended to include at this place a microscopic drawing from the urine of a bird suffering from nephritis, but mature consideration convinced me that it would be of little value. The morbid changes that are of diagnostic value are usually so obscured by deposits of uric acid and urates during the early stages of the illness that they are identified with great difficulty and are of little diagnostic value.

the coverglass under which an emulsion of normal urine is being observed, crystalization of uric acid and phosphates takes place with the formation of crystals like those shown in Figure 65; but in the case of urine from a bird suffering with chronic nephritis the crystals take the form shown in Figure 66. It will be noticed that in the one case the crystals have sharp angles and edges and in the other case all of the angles and edges are rounded. In normal urine there is little or no debris left after the crystalization; in abnormal urine there is considerable debris, it remains on the plan of the surface of the microscopic slide, however, while the crystals form on the under surface of the coverglass. Not being in the same plan, they are not visible at the same time; thus Figure 66 is actually two drawings—one made in the plan of the under surface of

Figure 65.   **NEPHRITIS**

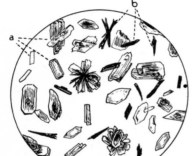

CRYSTALS RESULTING FROM TREATING NORMAL BIRD URINE WITH A SLIGHTLY ALKALINE SOLUTION OF GENTIAN VIOLET

a, crystals of uric acid and urates; **b,** crystals of phosphates.

Magnification 300 ×.

Drawn by Robert Stroud.

the coverglass and one made in the plan of the upper surface of the slide.

Treatment. It is possible that some birds recover from this condition. But since there is no way of proving that the recovered birds were or were not suffering with nephritis, it is impossible to say that any particular line of treatment is of value. I have used diuretics and urotropine, potassium iodide, chinosol, cinchopen, and methylene blue. See UROTROPINE; CHINOSOL; DIUROL; UREMIA; METHYLENE BLUE. I have taken birds in a state of complete coma in acute uremia and brought them back to health and years of care-free existence; but, still, I cannot offer a line of treatment which may be depended upon to clear up this condition.

The most effective of our kidney antiseptics is urotropine, but it is a very dangerous drug where birds are concerned, and its administration requires considerable care.   Dissolve one 5-grain urotropine tablet in four ounces of water.   Place the ailing bird in a cage by itself; arrange a glass plate under the perch upon which the bird sleeps, so as to catch the droppings for examination; then

Figure 66.   **NEPHRITIS**

CRYSTALS RESULTING FROM TREATING THE URINE OF A BIRD SUFFERING FROM CHRONIC NEPHRITIS WITH GENTIAN VIOLET

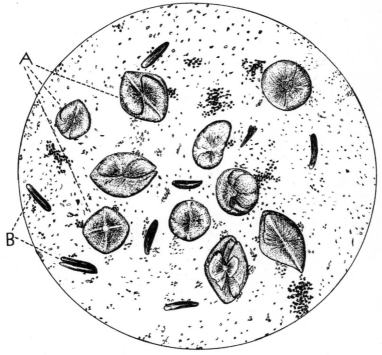

a, Uric acid and urates; **b,** Phosphates.
Magnification 300 ×.
Drawn by Robert Stroud.

administer the urotropine solution in the drinking water, starting at a single drop to the ounce of drinking water and increasing the dose gradually, studying the effect upon the droppings each morning, searching carefully for the presence of blood.   At the first appearance of blood or blood cells in the urine the dosage of urotropine solution should be reduced by one-third to one-half and

Figure 67.   NERVE TISSUE

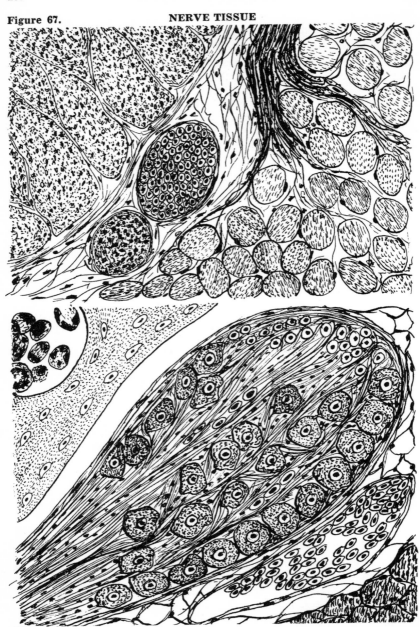

Figure 68.

continued at that figure for several months. This experimental treatment is necessary in every case because some birds suffering with nephritis drink enormous quantities of water while others drink very little, and an overdose of this drug will cause fatal hemorrhages from the kidneys.

On bright sunny days the bird should be carried out into the sunshine for an hour or so; on chilly days he should be permitted to warm himself by an electric light. The diet should contain plenty of egg food, plenty of green food, and a good tonic-seed mixture. Under this careful treatment many suspected birds will recover. Some, of course, will die; and when their bodies are opened and the breeder sees those large yellow kidneys he is apt to feel that all of his efforts were just so much lost motion.

NERVOUS SYSTEM. The central organ of the nervous system,

Figure 67.

This plate illustrates the four kinds of avian nerve tissue found outside of the brain and spinal cord.

Cranial nerve. Filling the upper left-hand corner of the upper drawing is a small segment of the optic nerve of a sparrow. Notice that the bundles of non-medullated fibers are enclosed in a single stroma from which trabeculae separating the bundles ramify into and throughout the nerve. In mammals the cranial nerves are composed bundles of medullated fibers, each bundle of which is enclosed in its individual stroma, but in birds this construction is reserved for the spinal nerves.

Spinal nerve. Of the two large oval bodies directly below and to the right of the optic nerve is a transversely-cut spinal nerve. The dark body entering the drawing from the top is a spinal nerve cut longitudinally. It supplies the voluntary muscular bundles, cut transversely, filling the right side of the field.

Sympathetic nerve. The smaller of the two oval bodies directly below the optic nerve is a sympathetic nerve. In structure it is similar to the optic nerve, but takes a much deeper stain.

In the lower drawing, beginning at the upper left-hand corner, we have a clump of myelocytes in a small marrow cavity in one of the spinal processes; next, the bone; and separated from this by a small open space is a spinal ganglion composed of motor cells and medullated fibers, beyond which is a vein and small bundle of voluntary muscular fibers.

Sections from the eye and spine of a sparrow. Tissue fixed in a mercury-iron solution; demetalized and decalciumized in acidulated iodine solution; stained in hematoxylin and phloxine, in toto; imbedded in paraffin and cut on a hand mike. Differentiation takes place as a natural consequence of the dehydrating process.

These tissues stain by this process as follows:

Optic nerve, general color, pink or lavender; fibers blue and brown; connective tissue dull, pale yellow; nuclei almost black.

Spinal nerves, all structures varying shades of rich blue.

Sympathetic nerves, brown; fibers, black.

Muscular tissue, reddish-brown; striations, brownish-yellow.

Myelocytes: chromatin, deep purple; cytoplasm, pale yellow, blue, and pink; granules can be seen but do not take distinct colors.

Bone, pearl-gray.

Blood cells, chromatin deep blue or black; cytoplasm, rich orange-pink.

Drawings made with the 4 mm. objective and 10 × ocular.

Author's sections and drawings.

the brain, has already been described. Arising at the base of the brain and extending throughout the entire length of the spinal column and into the coccygeal vertebrae, the spinal cord sends out nerve trunks, the fibrils of which reach all parts of the body. These nerve trunks are grouped in pairs and pass out of the spinal channel through small openings between the vertebrae. In the cervico region of the spine (between the shoulders) there is an expansion of the spinal cord called the cervico-dorsal plexus. Its function is to supply nerve impulses to the wings. It is here that all of those split-second, minute adjustments and coordinations necessary to flight are effected. Nerve channels from this plexus also serve the organs of the pectoral region (the chest), heart, lungs, etc. There is another expansion of the spinal cord in the sacral region (between the hips) which is called the sacral plexus and from which arises the nerve trunks serving the legs and abdominal organs. Each spinal nerve arises from two roots. The ventral roots, those arising on the inner side of the cord, are made up of motor nerves; the dorsal roots, those arising from the outer side of the cord are made up of sensory fibers. See BRAIN. Figure 68 is a microscopic drawing of a section of the spinal cord of a canary. Figure 67 shows types of nerve tissue seen outside of brain and cord.

As in mammals, the sympathetic nervous system supplies fibers to all of the organs and the blood vessels. These nerves control the automatic functions of the various organs, such as the beating of the heart, digestion, the secretion of glands, etc., and they are distinguished from the spinal nerves microscopically by the fact that fibers of the spinal system are usually medullated (inclosed in thick sheaths of fatty material) while those of the sympathetic system are non-medullated; that is, their sheaths consist of thin, close-fitting membranes.

NERVOUS TWITCHING. A spasmodic twitching or jumping of all of the muscles on one side of the body at constant intervals of from one to ten seconds is a symptom of cinchophen poisoning and of some cases of acute uremia resulting from sudden, severe chilling. See UREMIA. In both cases diuretics are indicated. A general twitching of all of the nerves is a symptom of AVITA-MINOSIS B. Sudden spells of spasmodic jerking which last for only a moment may indicate APOPLECTIFORM SEPTICEMIA. More pronounced attacks may be the result of strychnine poisoning. See I.Q.S. This symptom can also indicate a slow internal hemorrhage.

THE PRINCIPAL FEATURES OF THE SPINAL CORD OF A CANARY
(as it appears when stained with hematoxylin and eosin)

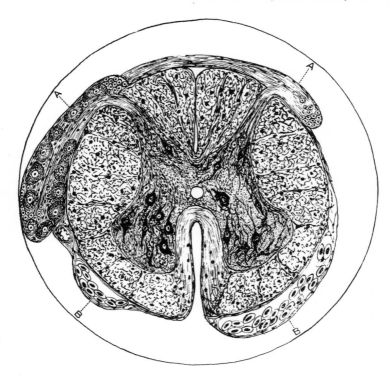

The two horns in the upper dorsal half of the drawing are known as the **dorsal root fibers.** They communicate with plexuses located just outside of the cord. Just the edges of these are shown at A.A.

The gray matter of the cord is collected into the large cross-shaped mass in the center, and the large dark masses contained therein are the motor neurons.

The lighter, coarse-grained tissue making up the outer part of the cord is composed of nerve fibers and **neuroglia** (supporting) cells. No nerve cells are found in this "white" matter.

In the lower part of the drawing, outside of the cord, are shown two small blood vessels supplying the **pia mater**—the inner covering of the cord, B.B.

Note.—Drawn from memory by Robert Stroud.

NEST, DAMP AND FOUL. When young canaries or other young nest-raised birds are fed on stale or mouldy food they develop a thin, watery diarrhea which makes the nest damp and foul and causes the breast feathers of the hen to become matted, giving her the appearance of having been sweating. This condition is called **nestling diarrhea**; it is sometimes miscalled **Sweating hens.** This last name, of course, is a misnomer, since hens do not sweat. Birds have no sweat glands. See NESTLING DIARRHEA; ASPERGILLOSIS.

NESTING MATERIAL. The nesting material supplied to birds in captivity must be of such a nature as to meet the requirements of the particular species and to enable them to build strong, well-ventilated nests. For canaries and small finches, burlap and lawn cuttings make an ideal combination for the building of the nest bodies. The burlap is cut into four-inch squares and unraveled. When burlap alone is used the nest lacks body and shape and is poorly ventilated. When grass alone is used the nest will lack strength. Canaries are very fond of long-stapled cotton for lining their nests—just how fond of it they are is illustrated by the following experiment:

Take a bunch of young canary hens that have not been mated before, have never built nests or seen any cotton. Put them in a large flight room. When they are all in breeding condition put the males in the flight and give the birds nest boxes and material for building the bodies of their nests, but nothing to line them with. Wait until several of the hens have their nests ready to line; then take a chair and book, go into the flight and sit down to read. I am assuming that you are using birds which have been little handled and are normally wild, wild enough that they would not think of coming near you. Now if you will stick a piece of cotton on your shoulder, on your head, or hold it in your hand, it will not be long until several of the little ladies are down there fighting over it, just as if you did not exist.

Some of the smaller finches prefer deer's hair for making the bodies of their nests; some of the larger ones will use a lot of straw.

Parakeets are partial to bark fibre. They like nothing better than a few bunches of willow switches, from which they will strip the bark themselves. After shredding the bark they fold it up and tuck it into their feathers, so that no one can see them flying home with it. Wise little creatures.

NESTLING DIARRHEA. You may notice that the breast feathers of a canary hen are damp and matted, as if she had been sweating while hovering the young. Of course, hens do not sweat. The damp, matted condition of her feathers is the result of a thin, viscous diarrhea present in the young birds. If the nest is examined it will be seen that the young are very thin and weak and look half starved; the nest will be found to be damp and foul-smelling. If the hen is watched closely it will be seen that she is suffering with a grayish, stringy diarrhea. This condition is called nestling diarrhea, and it results from the use of stale, mouldy or rancid food, or from the hen picking up bits of spoiled food from the floor of the cage or taking poisonous material into her system while cleaning the nest.

Should any of the babies be breathing in a spasmodic manner, it will mean that they are suffering with Aspergillosis, and the only hope of saving them will depend upon the administration of "Anthroquirone" Violet. See ASPERGILLOSIS.

Treatment. Place a pinch of STROUD'S SALTS NO. 1,* in the drinking water. Give the babies a clean, warm nest, and be sure to see that the food is O.K. Remember that it is much better to take all egg food away and give the hen a piece of moistened bread, a boiled potato, or an ear of sweet corn—many nests have been saved by such foods—than it is to continue to feed a doubtful mixture.

Should there be nothing wrong with the food and should the babies have escaped aspergillus infection, medication of the drinking water for a single day will be sufficient to clear up the condition. No medicine can correct the effects of the continuous use of spoiled food, however.

NODULES. These are cysts, lumps, occurring in various parts of the body during the development of certain diseases. In many cases they are walled-off areas of infection; in some cases they are the result of irritation set up by parasites, as in the case of some intestinal worms; and in at least one case, that of AVITAMINOSIS A, the nodules are the result of a morbid physiology unrelated to infection. In making post-mortem examinations, nodules in any part of the body should be searched for and studied closely. They may be found in the breast muscles, B. PARATYPHOSIS B INFECTION; the intestines, CANARY NECROSIS; TUBERCULOSIS; TAPEWORM; the liver, CANARY NECROSIS; TUBERCULOSIS; LEUKEMIA; ENTRO-HEPATITIS; COCCIDIOSIS; and

---

* **Note:** If STROUD'S SALTS are not available, add a pinch of sodium perborate or ten drops of commercial peroxide of hydrogen to each ounce of drinking water.

a number of other conditions; the heart muscles, FOWL TYPHOID; the throat, CANARY NECROSIS; AVITAMINOSIS A; the lungs, TUBERCULOSIS, rarely. In most cases where nodules are found in the liver they are also found in the spleen. This is not a complete list; it is given simply for the purpose of emphasizing the importance of lesions of this nature and the locations in which they are to be looked for.

NOSTRILS. See NASAL CAVITY; RESPIRATORY SYSTEM.

NUX VOMICA. This is the dried, ripe seed of the plant **Strychnos nux vomica, L. Loganiaceae.** It contains strychnine, brucine, igasuric acid, and proteids. The name, **nux vomica,** means **stops vomiting,** and is applied to this drug because it has the power to settle the stomach and stopping vomiting. It is also a powerful stimulant for the heart and other muscles, and acts by increasing the force and frequency of the impulses sent out by the brain and spinal cord. When given in small quantities over a considerable period of time it improves the circulation, and this in turn improves the appetite and the nourishment of the body, with a resulting improvement in the general health. This is called **tonic action.** The stimulating dose for a bird is about five drops of tincture of nux vomica to the quart of water; the tonic dose for a bird is about two drops of the tincture to the quart of water. It is sometimes cooked in oatmeal or **Cream of Wheat** for administration. The dose is the same as when given in water. I prefer to use a strychnine tonic. See I.Q.S.

Nux vomica is found on the market in several preparations, of which the alcoholic extract is the strongest. The fluid extract is about ¼ as strong as the dried alcoholic extract; the dried aqueous extract is about the same strength as the fluid extract. The alcoholic tincture is about ⅕ as strong as the fluid extract, about 1/20 as strong as the dried alcoholic extract. The doses mentioned above refer to the alcoholic tincture. Should the bird show signs of extreme nervousness or convulsions, the administration of the drug must be discontinued at once. See STRYCHNINE.

OBESITY. Fat, and more fat, the fervent prayer of the producer of market poultry, is anything but desirable in songbirds. The overfat male cannot sing; the overfat female cannot breed; but, because most songbirds are kept in small cages permitting little exercise, and, because they usually have fattening foods constantly before them and are allowed a much longer eating day than any bird enjoys in the wild state, the caged bird has a hundred chances to put on fat for every chance he has to work it off. Is it any wonder that he is apt to become so fat that he can neither sing nor fly; in fact, he often gets so fat that breathing becomes a great difficulty. Fat crowds and presses upon all the organs and permeates his muscular and organic tissues until it has placed a burden upon him which leaves little vitality for song or resistance against disease. As Mr. C. C. Mulligan, with his wonderful patience, used to say over and over again, "But, Madam, an overfat bird is not a healthy bird." *

Hens wintered in cold flights and fed liberally on soft food put on a heavy layer of fat during the winter. This is a necessary protection for their bodies; it enables them to withstand the cold and exposure and renders them much less susceptible to kidney disorders. Most of these birds will discard their excess fat as they come into breeding condition in the spring. Once in a while, however, we find a hen that will not come into breeding condition that continues to lay on fat in spite of anything the breeder seems able to do. If he starves her down to correct weight, she is certain to become ill. In some cases this condition may result from the burden of fat that so cramps the vital organs that the bird is unable to carry on the activities which would burn it up, but most of these cases, in my opinion, are the result of abnormalities in the functioning of the ductless glands, particularly a sluggishness of the thyroid.

Really, though, it is the caged singer that suffers most from excess fat. These are not abnormal birds to start with, but through

* **Note:** In the descriptions of the organic changes found associated with various diseases, mention has often been made of a pathological condition which is called **fatty degeneration.** It should be understood that there is no relation between body fat and fatty degeneration of organs. In the latter case the birds are usually in a state of extreme emaciation. The expression is derived from the fact that in connection with certain disease conditions, the organic cells are broken down and their materials converted into fat globules.

lack of exercise, insufficient green food, and a diet far too rich in fats, they are often brought into a state which is really pitiful. I have never been able to understand why it is that the average pet owner has such a morbid fear of feeding his bird fresh green food, and then will permit it to constantly overeat on fattening food.

Treatment. The caged singer should be returned to the flight room if possible. He should have all the green food he can eat and few of the more fattening seeds, such as hemp and niger. He should be caught and inspected for fat once each week; and, if overfat, his eating day must be shortened. Remember that the eating day of the sparrow outside your window during the period of the year when he is not converting excess energy into feathers or babies is not over seven hours, and he has to get out and hustle his food, withstand cold, rain and storm, and sometimes has his food supply entirely cut off by snow. Does that indicate that it is necessary for the protected canary, with all his food in the cups before him, to eat from six o'clock in the morning until ten or eleven at night?

The best way to shorten the eating day of a caged bird is to put him in the dark for a few hours every day. This can be done by placing the cage in a dark room or by covering it for a few hours each day with a black cloth. This darkening method is preferable to attempts at removing all fattening foods from the diet, since such practices only unbalance the diet and ruin the bird's health. This darkening method is used by all roller breeders in training their singers. By using it you can reduce your bird and at the same time make him a good night singer. If he is put in the dark at eleven o'clock each morning and kept there until six or seven in the evening, he may then be permitted to stay up until the time the family goes to bed, say at ten or eleven P.M.

Overfat hens, or males for that matter, that are intended for breeding purposes can often be reduced by putting an effervescent saline in their drinking water for several weeks, using one teaspoonful of the salts to each quart of drinking water. There is nothing better for this purpose than STROUD'S EFFERVESCENT BIRD SALTS, but any of the preparations described in this book will give good results. See IRON AND QUININE CITRATE; CITRO-CARBONATE, etc. Any of the effervescent salines put up for human use may be employed; they are all about the same.

Another good way to reduce birds and bring them into song or breeding condition is to give them a course of the iodide of potassium treatment—one drop of saturated solution of iodide of potassium to each ounce of drinking water for three or four weeks. This treatment is always beneficial to hens that are intended for breeders, because it peps up their glandular reactions, and it is invaluable for reducing those overfat hens that cannot otherwise be gotten into breeding condition. They should be caged alone; given their regular diet for not more than eight hours' eating time each day; given all the green food they will eat at all times; and darkened for at least sixteen hours out of each twenty-four. If this treatment does not remove the excess fat, the eating day should be still further shortened. When these birds are down to normal weight they should be placed in larger cages and receive a small, daily supply of soft food containing a little wheat germ oil.

Some of these birds that are overfat because of sluggish thyroid activity can be reduced by treatment with thyroid extract, which is mixed with sugar in the proportion of 1:1000 and dusted on soft food in such amounts that the bird will actually get not more than ⅛ grain of the mixture. While this method sometimes succeeds after all others have failed, it is considered of little value. Such birds can be maintained in a state of vigorous health only by frequent dosing, and there is every reason for believing that some of their young will inherit their defect. It is best to choke them and use nothing but strong, vigorous stock in the breeding room. Which brings me to a thought I probably should have expressed before. I am interested in saving of birds as a scientific proposition. I want to put them in vigorous health; I want to prevent as much suffering among them as possible; but that does not mean that I would use a defective bird in my breeding room. There may be some justification for the human doctor filling the world with misfits, though I doubt it, but there can be no excuse for the bird doctor imitating him.

OBSTRUCTION OF THE GIZZARD. Foreign bodies, usually seed hull, sometimes find their way into the gizzards of birds and there set up inflammations which cause a spasmodic contraction of the pyloric valve. An acute indigestion is set up and the bird usually dies within from four to thirty hours. Sometimes the obstruction can be removed and the bird saved by withholding all other food and giving the bird water, olive oil and sweet-apple pulp. See DIGESTIVE DISORDERS.

ODIUM ALBICANS. This is a fungus which attacks the mucous lining of the mouth and throat of both animals and birds. Sometimes it invades the crops of birds. Children are very susceptible to this infection. The disease process set up by this organism is called **Thrush.** There are reports of this condition in chickens, pigeons and turkeys. And while I have found no mention of it as a disease of canaries, it is really rather common among neglected birds, particularly those that have had to live under unsanitary conditions for long periods of time and have been shipped about a lot, which is the case with birds that have been imported from Europe and Japan. The organism is easily recognized in smears from the mouths and throats of infected individuals.

Figure 69.   **THRUSH**
OIDIUM ALBICANS, THE ORGANISM OF THRUSH, FROM THE
THROAT OF A CANARY

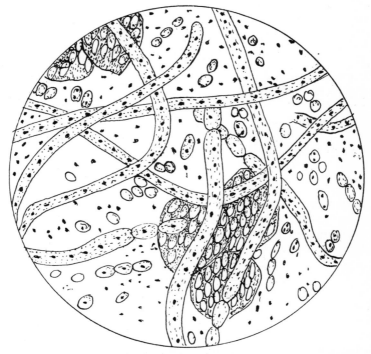

The large dark masses are epithelial cells. Notice the construction of the threads and the endo-spores.
Magnification about 500 ✕.

The smear is taken by twisting a small pellet of cotton around the end of an inoculating needle, rubbing the pellet over the infected area, and then rubbing it over the center of a microscopic slide. Figure 69 gives some idea of the microscopic appearance of this organism.

Morbid anatomy. Grayish white or yellow patches appear on the mucous membranes of the mouth, throat or crop. These patches grow without causing inflammatory changes in the underlying tissue. In some cases they block the opening of the trachea, causing death by suffocation; in others the infection may cause debility and death by interfering with digestion and nutrition.

Treatment. Larger birds may be treated by washing out the mouth and crop with a strong solution of STROUD'S SALTS NO. 1, or with boric acid. The mouth lesions may be painted with a 1:1000 solution of mercury bichloride or a ten per cent solution of iron chloride or copper sulphate.

Small birds are best treated by internal administrations. STROUD'S SALTS NO. 1, three grains to the ounce of drinking water; potassium iodide, two drops of saturated solution to the ounce of drinking water may be used. Four or five days' treatment with "Anthroquinone" Violet, one milligram per day for each gram of body weight should clear up the condition. See IODIDES; ASPERGILLOSIS. I have recently had very good results in the treatment of this condition, particularly where it has invaded the cleft in the palate, by swabbing the affected area with a few shreds of cotton that have been dipped in tincture of merthiolate, the red solution the doctor swabs your belly with before cutting out your appendix.

OIL GLAND. Located in the pygostyle, that fleshy structure that supports the tail feathers, are two glands having a common duct which end in a nipple located just about the root of the tail. These glands secrete a waterproofing oil with which the bird dresses its feathers. By pressing the nipple between the mandibles, the bird draws a little of this oil into the beak and then applies it to the feathers as they are combed through the beak. Birds living in the wild state get their feathers wet frequently; so they never neglect to comb and dress them. Birds in captivity which are permitted to bathe daily do not neglect to oil their feathers, either. But where birds are not permitted to bathe, they sometimes get into the habit of neglecting to oil their feathers, and the unused oil may become thick and obstruct the oil duct.

OIL GLAND OBSTRUCTION. As has just been mentioned, birds that are kept in close confinement and given no opportunity to bathe, sometimes neglect to oil their feathers. Now it happens that the oil secreted by the oil glands belong to a class of substances known as **drying oils,** as distinguished from **fixed oils.** Drying oils have the property of absorbing oxygen from the air and changing from fluids to solids. When the bird fails to dress its feathers at regular intervals, the unused oil in the oil duct absorbs oxygen from the air and becomes hardened. The hardened oil obstructs the duct; and, since the gland continues to secrete oil at a uniform rate, the pressure of the oil in the glands increases until it sets up an inflammation in the surrounding tissues. This phenomenon is identical with that of the formation of a blackhead in your own skin, with the difference that in your case the oil glands are very small and scattered all over your body while the entire surface of a bird's body, excepting the head, must be oiled from a single gland.

Treatment. By massaging the oil duct between the tips of the fingers it is sometimes possible to work the plug out. Sometimes the hardened plug can be dug out with the blunt end of a needle, or with a loop of fine wire, much on the same order as you dig wax from your own ears. Some books have recommended the destruction of the gland by puncturing it with a red-hot needle. I often wonder where some persons get their ideas, and getting them, how they manage to escape homes for the feeble-minded. To say that such treatment is uncalled for is putting it too mildly; it is stupid, idiotic, sadistic and probably originated in a diseased mind, but it has been passed on by many otherwise thoughtful writers. The only possible outcome from such a treatment is prolonged suffering and death. Though the bird probably will not die at the time, it will surely die during the next moult, for without a functioning oil gland, it would be unable to clean the quill-like coverings from the new feathers and the feathers could not develop normally. The plug can often be softened by repeated application of olive oil or xylene in minute quantities. The oil is applied with the tip of an inoculating needle. See NASAL CAVITY. By keeping a bath constantly before the bird it can be induced to apply the necessary massaging, once the plug is softened enough to remove.

OLIVE OIL. This is a pale yellow oil pressed from ripe olives. It has been mentioned dozens of times in these pages and will be mentioned dozens of times more before we reach the end. Its one great virtue is the fact that it is harmless. It will not blister the skin; it will not irritate the digestive tract. Birds require a certain amount of fat in their diet, and it is usually present as a natural constituent of the foods they eat. There are cases, however, where birds are fed on old seeds, which are not spoiled, but which have lost their oil. Such birds may become constipated. The correct treatment would be to put in a supply of new seeds and food, but where this is impossible, the condition may be helped considerably by administering a little olive oil and giving the bird plenty of green food.

Pepper-fed birds, because of the large amounts of pepper they are forced to consume, are apt to become constipated. To avoid this, it is the general practice to add olive and cod-liver oils to the pepper food. Some breeders advocate the use of as much as four ounces of oil to each pound of pepper.

OPIUM. This is the dried milk of the unripe poppy. It contains a large number of alkaloids, the chief of which are morphine and codeine. Tincture of opium is a basic constituent of many valuable prescriptions. See CASCARA. It is a ten per cent solution of opium in alcohol. Standard paregoric is a 1:250 solution of opium and contains 0.12 gram of opium to each 30 grams (30 grams is about one fluid ounce; 0.12 gram is about two grains), together with camphor, benzoic acid, oil of anise, and glycerin. The correct dose of paregoric for a bird is from three to five drops to the ounce of drinking water. Paregoric is employed in the treatment of intestinal conditions. Should a sedative be required, the cascara prescription is preferable. Uusually the only sedatives and narcotics needed in the handling of birds can be supplied by feeding maw seed or the stalks of fresh lettuce. See MAW SEED.

ORANGE OIL. This is a light yellow oil pressed from the fresh rinds of **Citrus vulgaris** and other citrus fruits. It is a flavoring material and is sometimes used in the preparation of bird medicines.

OVARY. This is a small, silver-white or cream-colored organ, triangular in shape, attached to the spine at a point just above the anterior edge of the left kidney in female birds—it usually overlaps the left kidney to some extent. When inactive, the ovary is smooth and glistening; when active, its surface is broken by clusters of developing ova of various sizes, which cause it to resemble a bunch of grapes. See EGG STRUCTURE AND FORMATION.

In a healthy ovary the ova are either round or oval in shape; in a diseased ovary they may sometimes be angular. See BACILLARY WHITE DIARRHEA.

OVIDUCT. See EGG STRUCTURE AND FORMATION.

OXALIC ACID. This is an organic acid made from treating wood sawdust with strong alkalies. It is valuable for cleaning glassware, since its strong affinity for lime causes it to remove all scaly deposits at once.

Warning. Oxalic acid is a dangerous poison. Should it ever be taken by accident, large quantities of chalk should be administered at once. This will neutralize the acid and render it harmless.

OXYSPIRURA MANSONI. This is the hard way of saying MANSON'S EYE WORM.

P

PALATE. Birds have no soft palate resembling that found in mammals. Instead they are provided with an elongated slit in the roof of the mouth.

PANCREAS. This is a large, highly developed gland located between the two horns of the duodenum. It is creamy white in color and is not usually altered during the development of acute infections.

The two known functions of the pancreas are the manufacturing of pancreatic juice, which it empties into the duodenum, and the manufacture of insulin, which is emptied into the blood stream. Failure of this latter function in human subjects gives rise to the condition called **diabetes,** in which the body loses a considerable part of its power to carry on the combustion of sugar. No one, so far as I know, has ever demonstrated the existence of diabetes in birds. But when canaries are taught to do tricks they are subject to considerable nervous shock, and some of the more nervous birds are pretty certain to develop a condition which has many points of similarity to diabetes in man; though I have not investigated the sugar reactions of the blood and urine of such birds—that is something I hope to do in the future.

PARALYSIS. This is the loss of the power of any muscle to expand and contract, usually caused by a failure of the nerve impulses to reach the muscle. It may be either flaccid or spastic; in the former case the muscle is relaxed; in the latter case it is strongly contracted—this condition is sometimes spoken of as tetanic or cataleptic.

There is a paralytic disease of ostriches which appears to be the result of a poison elaborated by bacteria inhabiting the intestines. Young birds are most susceptible. The paralysis begins in the feet and spreads to the wings and neck. The birds may be kept alive for months, but complete recoveries are unknown. There are many points of similarity between this disease and FOWL PARALYSIS.

Paralysis of the wings or feet of chickens, canaries, parrots, sparrows and finches is often the result of hemorrhages pressing on a motor nerve or the motor center in the brain. It is possible that such hemorrhages could result from many causes, but they are most commonly the result of APOPLECTIFORM SEPTICEMIA or FOOD POISONING.

Paralysis of the neck is the principal symptom of FOWL PA-
RALYSIS in canaries. In chickens, the wings and feet are said
to be most frequently involved. Sometimes the optic nerve is said
to be affected.

PAREGORIC. See OPIUM.

PARROT SEPTICEMIA. See PSITTACOSIS.

PARROTS, INDIGESTION IN. Parrots, like other hard-billed
birds, need a supply of suitable gravel for the gizzards. Lacking
this, they are certain to develop a severe indigestion. Proper feeding and plenty of grit of the correct size and kind will often cause
the condition to clear up promptly. Some bird men have recommended the administration of five-drop doses of castor oil, five-
grain doses of bicarbonate of soda or minute doses of nux vomica.

The most common form of indigestion of parrots is that which
attacks young birds during and following importation. Young
parrots are taken out of the nests and raised by hand on a mixture
of cereal and banana chewed up together. When such birds are put
on a seed diet and given drinking water, particularly if the water
has not been boiled, they are almost certain to develop a fatal indigestion which may be attended by symptoms of generalized infection. The primary cause of the trouble in such cases is the
weakened condition of the bird brought about by a sudden change
of diet and the hardships of being shipped over long distances.
When they arrive, young parrots should be placed on a diet of mush
made just stiff enough to be cut when cold. Such a mush can be
made from cornmeal, **Cream of Wheat** and unhulled, cracked rice.
Later they can be given a little banana, and this may be followed
by a little seed, which must be given in very small quantities at
first. No water other than that present in the mush should be
given to newly imported parrots. As they are brought onto a seed
diet, they are gradually introduced to the use of water. For some
time, until they have had a chance to build up their natural resistance to infection, all of their water must be boiled and their cups
should be boiled daily.

Once acclimated, the parrot is one of the hardiest of birds, and
if protected from accidents, preventable diseases and fed just half-
way right, they are very apt to live forever. I have never heard
of anyone who ever knew of a parrot dying of old age. But I have
read of an African gray parrot that was a house pet in one family
for seventy-five years; changed hands, and although for the entire
time it had been thought to be a female, became the father of chicks

when it was placed in a large aviary with some female Cuban parrots. Until acclimated, however, these babies are delicate little creatures, requiring and deserving careful handling and attention. See PSITTACOSIS; APOPLECTIFORM SEPTICEMIA.

PASTEURELLA AVIAN. This is the germ of fowl cholera, **hemorrhagic septicemia of birds.** The organism is a short, plump, non-motile, round-ended rod which, in smears from tissue, takes a bipolar stain. See AVIAN DIPHTHERIA; FOWL CHOLERA; HEMORRHAGIC SEPTICEMIA.

PATELLE. This is the bone of the kneecap—a small, flat, disc-like bone which articulates with the femur and tibia. See SKELETON.

PATHOLOGY. This is the branch of medical science which deals with morbid changes taking place within the body during the development and course of an attack of illness. All material contained in this book under the heading **Morbid anatomy** is pathological data.

PECTORAL MUSCLES. These are the large flight muscles, located in the breast and attached to the sternum, clavicles, and ribs. The superficial or greater pectoral is the muscle which depresses the wing during flight, which furnishes the power of flight. The deep or inferior pectoral, which is much smaller and is located underneath the great pectoral, elevates the wings.

PELVIS. This, as in mammals, is made from the fusion of three bones, the ilium, the ischium and the pubis. It differs from the pelvic arch of mammals in that the horns of the pubis are not joined and in that the highly developed ilium and ischium are combined to form a bony case which almost entirely surrounds the kidneys and affords them a high degree of protection.

PERITONEUM. This is the thin, transparent lining of the abdominal cavity. It covers the abdominal organs and, in birds, forms the walls of the abdominal air sacs. It is formed of a double layer of cells, serous on one side, mucus on the other. Perfectly transparent when in a state of health, the peritoneum may be clouded, opaque, covered with plastic exudate, filled with either fluid or solid exudate, or even partially destroyed during the development and progress of certain diseases. Sometimes the inflammatory changes cause adhesions to form between the peritoneum and the abdominal organs. The exact condition of this membrane should always be observed and noted during the course of a post-mortem examination, for any change found is pretty apt to be of diagnostic importance. Any inflammation of this tissue indicates serious illness and is designated **peritonitis**.

PERITONITIS. This, an inflammation of the peritoneum, is a rather uncommon disease of birds. It usually results from infection gaining entrance to the abdominal cavity through some wound or injury, most often by way of the oviduct, though it may develop as a result of infection of the air sacs, tumefaction of the ovary, a general infection, and there are cases in which no primary lesion can be found and in which no previous general infection has been observed.

Symptoms. In some cases of peritonitis, particularly those resulting from abdominal injuries, the local symptoms appear first, the general symptoms later. There is evidence of great pain and tenderness in the abdominal region. The bird stands high on the perch, legs stiff, wings drooping, head thrust forward to maintain its balance, in some cases; in others, it sits on its heels, using its tail for a brace, its body very erect, its head turned straight back over its back, is suspended from a relaxed and flaccid neck, like an apple on a string. The breathing is very rapid. The abdomen is usually greatly enlarged and reddened; its blood vessels highly congested though there are cases of fatal peritonitis in which there is no enlargement of the abdomen during any stage of the attack. In these cases the abdomen has a shrunken appearance which becomes more pronounced as the illness progresses. The color becomes steadily darker until the whole abdomen has taken on a deep blue-black shade. The general symptoms, fever, thirst, loss of the ability to take food and drink, great weakness, rapid shallow breathing, prostration, coma and death follow in rapid succession. Where peritonitis results from an injury, the area surrounding the injury will take on a blue-black coloration while the rest of the abdomen is very red and greatly distended. This distention of the abdomen is caused by the pressure of fluid filling the peritoneal cavity. This condition may result in death at once from stoppage of the heart, but in cases where that does not happen the fluid is absorbed and the abdomen takes on a shriveled appearance as the blue-black coloration rapidly spreads over its entire area.

In cases where the primary infection is general in character the bird will be found with its feathers puffed out, sleeping in the daytime. At this stage the abdomen may appear to be perfectly normal. It will be noticed, however, that the bird protects the abdomen by leaning back on its heels and tail to sleep. The sick bird makes no effort to eat or drink during the later stages of the illness. Within from six to twenty-four hours from the appearance of the first symptoms the abdomen will start to take on the blue-black color and the shriveled appearance.

There are other cases in which the abdomen is greatly enlarged from the first and continues so through the course of the disease. In these cases there is formation of a heavy, cheesy exudate which fills the abdominal cavity.

Morbid anatomy. There are two general stages to an attack of peritonitis. During the first stage the peritoneal cavity becomes filled with a serous fluid exudate, the pressure of which may become so great as to interfere with breathing and heart action; during the second stage, the effusion is absorbed with the formation of a solid exudate which may take the form of a plastic membrane covering all the abdominal organs and tissues or a cheesy, friable solid which fills the abdominal cavity. The formation of the plastic exudate is associated with the appearance of the blue-black color and great destruction of tissue. The membrane, the organs, the intestines—in fact, all the tissues in contact with the diseased areas become blue-black, shriveled and fused together as a result of this gangrenous process.

In the other class of cases, which undoubtedly involve a different causative agent, in which the exudate is thick, cheesy, yellow or cream colored, and fills the entire cavity, there may be almost complete obliteration of the peritoneum, mesentery and other tissues in contact with the inflammatory process. The interorganic changes, so extensive in the other form of peritonitis are not met with in this form. Those tissues which escape destruction by direct contact remain uninjured.

Etiology. Naturally, we know that peritonitis is caused by germs gaining entrance to the peritoneal cavity, but I regret that I am not in a position to say just what classes of germs are at fault in this respect. These cases do not occur often, and every time one of them has occurred it has caught me unprepared for making a bacteriological study of the condition.

Treatment. Under the heading EGG RUPTURE, I have described what I believe to be the first and most remarkable cure of this condition ever effected. That case occurred almost ten years ago, long before the discovery of sulfanilamide, which has been so useful in the treatment of peritonitis in man, but since that time I have lost just one bird from this condition, and the reason I lost her was an erroneous diagnosis made early in the illness and a pressure of events which caused me to neglect giving her a second examination. There is nothing in the way of treatment to be added to the experience described in connection with that first case of peritonitis resulting from injury and infection of the oviduct.

PERMANGANATES. Sodium, potassium and calcium permanganates are salts of permanganic acid. They come in long, narrow, dark purple crystals which are about the size and shape of niger seed. They are soluble in water with the formation of a deep purple solution which stains organic matter: first, red or purple; later, brown. All of these salts are powerful oxidizing antiseptics. They have the further virtue of forming insoluble compounds with animal tissues, thus promoting the formation of a hard scab over any sore or wound. The potassium salt is very widely used in human as well as veterinary practice; though why it should have preference over the calcium salt, which has one hundred times its germ-killing power, is something that I have never been able to figure out. See GAPE; AVIAN DIPHTHERIA.

For direct application to sores, wounds and scarified tissue the permanganates are used in saturated solution, or they may be applied in the form of pure powder; for injection into the sores, a two per cent solution is strong enough; for internal administration they are used in solutions of from 1:500 to 1:5000.

PHALANGES. These are the bones of your fingers and toes; they are also the bones of a bird's claws and of the tips of his wings. See WING; FEET; SKELETON.

PHENOTHIAZINE. Antithalmintic; dose for a chicken, one to five grains; dose for a canary, 1/50 to 1/10 grain. See TAPEWORMS.

PHOSPHATES. See MINERAL FOOD. Steamed bone meal is the most commonly used source of mineral phosphates for the feeding of poultry. Dibasic sodium orthophosphate is a valuable constituent of effervescent saline preparations.

PIP. This is a condition of the tongue commonly found in diphtheria and infectious bronchitis in poultry. It may be present in any condition where the bird is forced to breathe through its mouth for long periods of time. The tongue becomes dry and cracked and the covering tends to curl and split away from the softer underlying tissue. It is not a direct symptom of any disease, but it is nevertheless a very painful and serious condition. It should be prevented rather than cured, and this can be easily done by following the instructions outlined under the heading GLYCERIN. There is no better method to follow even after the condition has developed.

PLEURISY. This is a rather rare disease of birds. Probably the best method of describing it, and surely the most interesting, will be to give an actual case history. This will serve the additional purpose of illustrating to the reader the blundering process by which truth is often arrived at.*

History. The subject was a three-year-old male canary. When taken sick he was feeding chicks which were fifteen days old. He was in a cage where some draft was possible during sudden changes in the weather. Several other males had developed acute uremia in that cage. The day had been very hot, but thunder storms came up during the night and there was a marked drop in the temperature. Mosquitoes had been bothering the birds a little, too, but they were not plentiful enough to be serious. The bird was found sick the next morning.

At the time the bird was discovered ill his feathers were fluffed out and one eye was closed and watering. For two days the eye was treated with antiseptic solutions. During this time the bird appeared to be blind in the afflicted eye. He had, of course, been placed by himself as soon as discovered and it was then noticed that his breathing was much too fast to be accounted for by the sore eye. He was not eating. His temperature was 110.4 F. There were no droppings, indicating that the kidneys were not functioning.

The case was tentatively diagnosed as acute uremia. Two days later a blood sample was taken from a toe and a plate seeded. He was offered the light treatment but refused to take advantage of it. Diuretics were placed in the drinking water and administered into the crop—there was no earthly reason for putting them in the drinking water, since the bird was neither eating nor drinking. These re-established kidney action. At the time they were first given the bird was sitting on the floor of the cage in a state of coma. As soon as the kidneys began to function the bird showed marked improvement. He was able to make the perches and to eat and drink a little. The rapid breathing and high temperature continued, however. The possibility of his having pneumonia was considered and discarded. He had now lived several days and his temperature was not high enough to indicate pneumonia. By the end of the fourth day the eye was normal.

---

* **Note:** This description of a case of avian pleurisy in a canary is largely a reprint of a copyrighted article, "Dead Birds," which appeared in the November, 1933, issue of the "American Canary and Cage-Bird Life," Chicago, Illinois.

From the third day on the feet were slightly swollen and much redder than usual; by the sixth day he had lost all of his fat and when held in the hand, had a doughy feeling found only in birds that are seriously ill. The breast had become very thin. On the sixth day he was again in coma most of the time but he still aroused himself and drank once in a while. There was some diarrhea and the bird showed evidence of pain.

On the fifth day, forty-eight hours after being seeded, the plate, which had been kept at room temperature, showed colonies of micrococci which were not otherwise identified. Their presence did not throw any light on the condition. All of the symptoms, the complete history convinced me that the bird had first suffered an attack of acute uremia and was now suffering from an acute nephritis. All of my treatment had been directed toward clearing up a kidney infection. I could not bring myself to start treating him for a septicemia when I knew that such treatment would surely aggravate the condition of his kidneys.

On the morning of the seventh day the bird was found in the bottom of the cage in a state of complete coma, sitting on the whole length of his shanks; his tail braced against the floor; his head turned back over his shoulders and hanging down his back. The body was in such an upright position that he would have surely fallen over backwards had it not been for his tail.* He died at noon, and was so well braced that he did not fall over.

Post-mortem. The heart was in systole, somewhat enlarged but otherwise normal. The liver was slightly softened. The spleen seemed to be slightly enlarged and congested, but the change was not marked. The peritoneum was cloudy and slightly thickened, but the change was not sufficient to indicate a serious peritonitis. The digestive organs were normal.

A small inflamed spot was found on the ventral surface of the right kidney. Under a ten-diameter glass it was seen that there was a small bubble of gas in the center of the inflamed area, directly under the capsule, which was not noticeably clouded.

The pleurae were both filled and distended with a thick, dark, bloody, coagulated exudate which escaped into the thoracic cavity when they were opened. The volume of this exudate was equal to the total volume of both lungs. Several small pneumonic spots in the stage of red hepatization were found in both lungs. Under

---

* **Note:** This is the position often taken by birds suffering from peritonitis. The present case is the only instance in which I have seen a bird suffering from another condition assume that exact position.

the glass these were bright red in color, translucent, and had the appearance of small lumps of red jelly—all structure had been destroyed. These spots were very small, however, so, while they were to the type characteristic of sporadic pneumonia, they could not have been the primary cause of death. A bird, because of its extensive system of air sacs, does not die of pneumonia until a very large part of the lung tissue has been destroyed.

Theory. It appears to me that this bird suffered an attack of uremia as a result of his being chilled; that as a result of his lowered resistance, an eye infection which might have been caused by an insect bite, led to a general septicemia which finally settled in the pleurae. I have been able to think of no explanation for the gas bubble in the right kidney when, excepting for this one small area, the organs appeared to be in a healthy condition— something I had not expected to find.

Treatment. This case illustrates better than anything else could the difficulties standing in the way of correct diagnosis when dealing with sporadic illnesses. In the cases of the contagious septicemic diseases, the condition can be positively identified from the bodies of the first few birds to die, and after that may be successfully treated. Had the facts learned at the post-mortem been known during the early stages of the illness, I would have employed an entirely different line of treatment and the bird might have recovered. I would have given him ammoniac, ten drops to the ounce of water or sodium salicylate, ¼ grain to the ounce of drinking water. These treatments would have been given as soon as the kidneys began functioning, for up to that point my treatment had been correct. It was necessary to get the kidneys to functioning before anything else could be accomplished. My error was in not being able to follow the changes taking place from that point onward. Had I recognized those changes, in addition to the internal medications mentioned, I might have given the bird a vapor treatment. This is administered as follows:

The bird is placed in a small cage and the cage is placed on top of a basin containing hot water; a little menthol or oil of eucalyptus is placed on top of the water; and the cage and vessel are covered with two thicknesses of sheeting. A small opening is made in the covering material through which the bird can be watched through the first ten or fifteen minutes of the treatment. If he shows signs of distress (panting, gasping, falling over) he must be given fresh air at once; if he clamps the feathers tight to the body and gasps for air with neck outstretched, it means that the water is too hot. The other symptoms of distress mean that the fumes are too strong. If the bird shows no distress he may be kept under the hood for several hours or longer and small additions of boiling water may be made to the water in the vapor vessel from time to time to maintain its temperature.

This is a very effective method of treating conditions involving the respiratory tract, but it must be handled with care. Birds respond very quickly to vapor treatments, but the response may be unfavorable if the fumes are too strong. Only a small amount of the drug must be placed on top of the water, for owing to the great surface presented by their air tubes and air sacs, birds absorb gases and vapors much more rapidly than do mammals, and retain them. It was this very fact that first led to the domestication of the canary.*

I have discussed this case in some detail because it is the only case of pleurisy to come to my attention and, also, I have never read or heard of any description of the symptoms displayed by birds suffering from this condition.

PNEUMONIA. Most birdmen are under the impression that pneumonia is a rather common condition of birds. This error is undoubtedly the result of their disinclination for making post-mortem examinations. Many of them probably imagine that it takes some special training or special power to be able to recognize a case of pneumonia. Then, too, a very popular little booklet on canaries, over a million copies of which have probably been sold in the last forty years, describes the history and symptoms of acute uremia under the heading pneumonia. I once had a college professor tell me that he was certain a particular bird had pneumonia because it had been chilled and displayed all the symptoms described in connection with that condition. He did not quote the little book referred to above, but that is probably where he got his information concerning pneumonia. He sent me the body of the bird in question. It had died of nephritis. The lungs were in perfect condition.

Actually, while pneumonic lesions are associated with a great

* **Note:** Small birds were first kept and bred by miners for use as gas detectors. They were carried into the mines, and the miners, by watching the birds, could tell by their distress when the air was dangerous. Many types of birds were first used for this purpose, but, when the canary was introduced into Europe, its pleasing song made it a favorite and in a few years it had displaced other species. It was soon discovered that the canary could be trained to sing in the dark and his song influenced by breeding and training. This fact, and the rivalry between the miners over the song of their birds, was responsible for the development of the modern roller canary.

number of septicemic diseases, primary pneumonia in birds is of very rare occurrence.

Etiology. Gallagher,* discussing the etiology of sporadic pneumonia in poultry, states that all cases of pure pneumonia in chickens to come to his attention were due to an organism resembling closely in morphology (appearance under the microscope) and cultural characteristics the pneumococcus of Frankel. I have found such an organism in all cases of bronchial pneumonia associated to with avian diphtheria to come to my attention and associated with many lesions of the respiratory tract, but in all cases of primary sporadic pneumonia to come to my attention, I have found a staphylococcus very smiliar in morphology and cultural characteristics to the **staphylococcus pyogenes albus.**

Symptoms. The bird takes sick suddenly, puffs up like a ball and sleeps most of the time, first on one foot, later on both feet; still later he quits the perch and stands in the corner of the cage, always facing into the corner. He stands well up on his legs, never on his heels. The bird drinks a little and may make attempts to eat during the early stages of the illness but neither eats nor drinks after the first few hours. The breathing is easy but very rapid and shallow. There is never any of the gasping, open-mouthed breathing associated with bronchial pneumonia. After the first day the bird sits in a corner of the cage, his head tucked back into his feathers and makes no effort to return to the perch to eat or drink. Droppings during the early stage of the disease are brown and show little or no urine; there are no droppings during the later stages of the illness. The bird just stands in his corner until he dies.

There are just two points displayed by these symptoms that will differentiate the condition from acute uremia: (1) If there are droppings during the early stages of acute uremia, they will be of normal color, but the urine will be a little more stringy than usual, though in most cases there are no droppings from the start. The uremic bird usually responds to the administration of diuretics. The dry, scanty, reddish-brown droppings of the pneumonic bird are very characteristic, but there are usually not more than two or three passages between the onset of the symptoms and death. The pneumonic bird usually lives from twenty-four to thirty-six hours. I have never known a pneumonic bird to die in less than twenty-four hours; and I have never known a uremic bird, where

---

*Note:** Ward and Gallagher, "Diseases of Domesticated Birds," Macmillan Company, page 163.

PNEUMONIA 305

the suspension of kidney functions was complete, to live twenty-four hours. Should the uremic bird live more than twenty-four hours the case becomes one of nephritis and the bird may linger for a long time.

Morbid anatomy. The liver may be slightly enlarged; the kidneys are about normal in size; though slightly grayish in color, they are not so gray as in acute uremia, however. The principal changes are found in the lungs. There may be from one to four or five spots in either or both lungs; they are reddish-brown in color and vary in size from mere points to spots involving a whole lung. See Figure 70. The spots extend straight through the lung from front to back, are thinner than the surrounding tissue and under a ten-diameter glass have the appearance of translucent gobs of red jelly. All structure appears to have been destroyed and the material of the involved area is much softer than healthy lung tissue. This condition is generally described by the term **red hepatization.** Both lungs are generally involved, but they are never involved to the same extent—one is usually completely hepatized while the other contains only a few small spots and the involvement always retains a distinctly spotted character. In bronchial pneumonia associated with diphtheria, the lungs are usually equally involved, and there is only one spot in each lung located in the center of the organ.

Ward and Gallagher (see note on page 304), describing sporadic pneumonia of chickens, state that the diseased areas are thicker than the surrounding tissue, stand out firmly and that in many cases there are adhesions between the diseased areas and the overlying pleura and pericardium. I have observed lesions similar to those they describe in interstitial and hemorrhagic pneumonia in canaries, but I have never observed them in the type of pneumonia I am here attempting to describe.

Treatment. The great difficulty in treating this condition is the difficulty of arriving at a positive diagnosis early in the illness, or for that matter, of arriving at any kind of a reliable diagnosis during life. The characteristic brown droppings can be depended upon in those cases where they are observed, but there are so few of these that they are apt to escape observation. The most reliable methods would have to be based on blood plates, blood smears or a study of the chest sounds. The former method will detect the presence of bacteria in the blood, but it is too slow to be of any value in outlining a course of treatment, for by the time the plate develops the bird is apt to be dead or so near it that no treatment

Figure 70. PNEUMONIA

A, Sketch giving the general appearance of the lung in sporadic
pneumonia due to a staphylococcus. I am sorry that I have
had no case of this condition
since I have been equipped for
making sections.

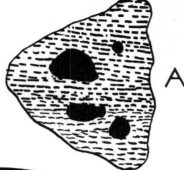

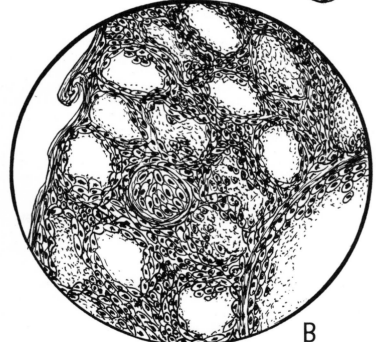

B, Interstitial pneumonia. Sections from the lung of a canary-blackhood
hybrid nine months old. This condition has never been observed in a
canary. It is fairly common in hybrids of the third generation from
parents, both of which are deeply pigmented. This section is from one
of the least diseased areas, chosen because it better illustrated the
development of the interstitial tissue. Notice the infiltration of the walls
between the air cells.

Author's section and drawing.

is of any value. The relations between the cellular composition
of the blood and changes taking place in the lungs of birds have
never been worked out. And suitable instruments for studying the
chest sounds of birds have not yet been invented. And even if
these methods had been worked out, they would not be available
to the average breeder. For several years since writing the above
(this is written in September, 1941), I have been listening to the
chest sounds of all birds examined. These sounds may be purring
—healthy lungs and bronchial tubes—ticking; rasping; bobbling;
or roaring. I have not worked out the meanings of each of these
sounds, but it is possible to locate inflammation in the nostrils,
throat, windpipe, large bronchi, small bronchi and to judge the relative involvement of both lungs. This method offers an infallible
indication as to the presence or absence of disease in the lungs,
however, and thus makes the differentiation of pneumonia and
uremia rather simple.

The examination is performed by holding the bird's back
against the ear and moving the bird around until the location of
each sound can be determined. In health, only a soft purring sound
is heard. There is, of course, always the heart sound, which is like
that of an aeroplane motor.

Some cases of pneumonia have been successfully treated by
administering into the crop ten to fifteen drops of a two to four
per cent solution of STROUD'S SALTS NO. 1. These cases were
diagnosed by the general symptoms and the presence of the brown
droppings. They could not have been uremic cases, since this
treatment is always fatal in such cases. Another prescription
which has given good results is as follows:

Rx To one ounce of I.Q.S. add
   Quinine sulphate ....20 grains
   Tincture of opium........................½ dram
   Caffine .... 1 grain
   Dissolve by warming and then add enough I.Q.S. to
   make up to two ounces.

For administration, this is diluted with warm water in the proportion of 1:100 and administered into the beak in ten-drop doses
twice every twenty-four hours. See SULFANILAMIDE, ETC.

PNEUMONIA, Interstitial. The only case of this kind to come to
my attention occurred in a carmine male hybridized canary (third
generation on father's side, fourth generation on mother's side from
black-hooded siskin; the result of a father-daughter mating).

The bird was turned into flight at the age of two months and remained in good health for about three months. It then began showing slight signs of illness, but for the next two months did not at any time appear ill enough to warrant catching it and caging it alone; at the end of that time it was evident the bird was sick,

Figure 71.   **PNEUMONIA, Hemorrhagic**
A SECTION FROM THE LUNG OF A CANARY SHOWING THE LESIONS OF HEMORRHAGIC PNEUMONIA

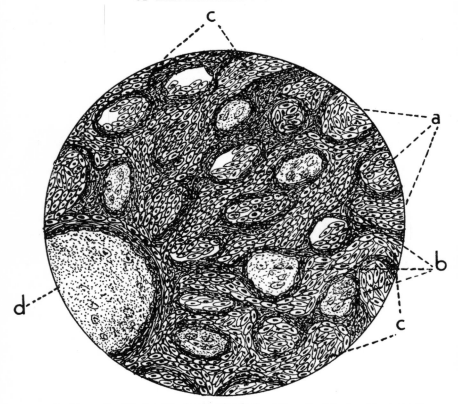

a, Air cells filled with fresh blood; **b,** Air cells filled with granular exudate containing cell debris; **c,** Fresh blood which has escaped into the interstitial tissue; **d,** A plugged bronchus.

however. It was caught and examined. Blood smears showed an unusual number of leucocytes and degenerated blood cells. Epithelial cells and cellular casts were found in the urine. The bird was treated for nephritis for three months. It died at the age of nine months with symptoms of peritonitis. The symptoms during the last three months of life had been persistent but not pronounced diarrhea; subnormal temperature, a number of times its temperature fell so low that it had to be restored by artificial means to keep the bird from dying. On one occasion after bathing, the temperature fell to 92 degrees F. The breathing was very rapid throughout the course of the illness, but on warm days the bird would seem normal in all other respects. It sang up until the last month of its life. B, Figure 70 is a freehand drawing of a section of the lung of this bird and shows advanced interstitial pneumonia.

Post-mortem. Because of the casts and kidney cells found in the urine, I expected to find the kidneys the principal seat of disease. This was not the case, however. The abdominal air sacs were distended with yellowish fluid, but the inflammatory changes in the tissues in contact with this fluid were not extensive. I believe that death resulted from the fact that this fluid prevented the bird from using those air sacs for breathing, since one lung was completely hepatized, and there was very little functioning tissue in the other one. It will be noticed that the only cells present are lymphocytes. Some of the clumps of granular matter looked like they might contain bacteria, but they did not take Loeffler's alkaline-methylene-blue stain, and ox-gall agar tubes seeded from this fluid remained sterile.

The kidneys were normal in size and color. Sections showed the presence of a sub-acute nephritis but the changes were not extensive.

The spleen was normal in size and color, so sections were not made.

The liver was enlarged and congested. Sections showed an excessive number of leucocytes, but the tissue cells stained clearly and their bodies were sharply outlined. No considerable destruction of tissue appeared to have taken place.

The duodenum was distended and slightly inflamed.

One lung, as has already been stated, was about twice as thick as normal and completely hepatized. It was brown in color. The other lung was only slightly thickened, normal in color but examination of sections revealed that at least eighty per cent of the air cells had been obliterated by infiltration of the interstitial tissue. Figure 70 was taken from one of the least diseased areas because it more clearly illustrated the nature of the lesions. In the new drug, sulfothiozol, we now have a treatment that is highly ef-

fective in this whole group of conditions and which may be administered at once, with the onset of the first symptoms and may
be given in conjunction with diurol, so it is no longer necessary
to withhold treatment until a positive diagnosis can be established.
I have given this drug in dose of ⅕ grain into the crop without
fatal effects.   I have recently employed it in the treatment of a

Figure 72. INTERSTITIAL PNEUMONIA

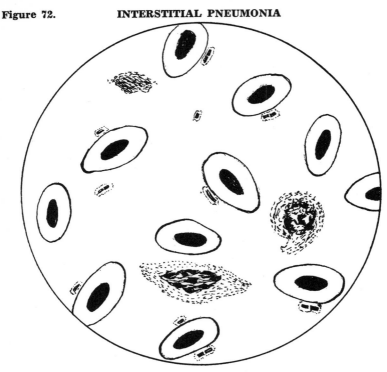

This drawing, which does not do the subject much justice, is from a
smear from the blood of a red-orange canary male suffering from interstitial pneumonia. In order to show all the forms taken by this germ I
have drawn in more organisms than were found in any single field. On a
smear spread this thin not more than one organism per field would be
found. They number about one to each twenty red cells.

Author's preparation and drawing. Drawing made with a magnification of 1,350 ×. November, 1941.

number of cases of interstitial pneumonia in which 1/10 grain
doses were given every two or three days until the symptoms
cleared up.

It is characteristic of interstitial pneumonia that, while a single dose of the drug may cause the symptoms to pass off for a day or two, they have a tendency to return.

Through the perfection of my staining technique—see BLOOD —I have been able to demonstrate in the blood of these birds a pneumococcus that cannot be distinguished from the germ of human pneumonia, and it is now my opinion that these birds were

Figure 73.   PNEUMONIA, HEMORRHAGIC
SECTION FROM THE LUNG OF A CANARY THAT DIED OF HEMOR-
RHAGIC PNEUMONIA OF UNDETERMINED ETIOLOGY

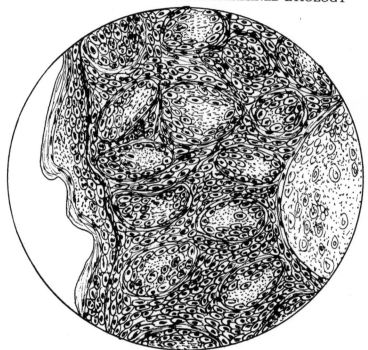

Notice that the cells in the plugged bronchus do not take the stain, which indicates that they were dead and undergoing decomposition at the time the tissue was fixed. Also notice that the interstitial spaces—**interstitial** means between the cells, and it refers to the area between the functioning elements of an organ which is commonly taken up by the supporting connective tissue and lymph spaces, interspersed with capillaries—are filled with blood. In some sections the blood cells are the only thing that can be made out.

Author's section and drawing. Magnification 445 ×.

infected by me while hand feeding them as babies, since every bird to develop the condition had been hand fed some, and most persons carry pneumococci in their mouths and throats. The form taken by the pneumonia is accounted for by the fact that the birds are not very susceptible to the human organism. Figure 72 is from the blood of a bird suffering from interstitial pneumonia. Notice that while we call this germ a coccus (round body) it is actually an incapsulated diplobacterium (rod shaped) having a cylindrical shape and square ends. This is also true of the germs most often associated with human pneumonia.

PNEUMONIA, Hemorrhagic. This condition is often associated with septicemic diseases. I have not observed it as a primary lesion. The air cells and interstitial spaces are filled with blood cells and leucocytes. The small bronchial tubes are plugged with a yellowish granular material in which cells and cell fragments can be seen but which does not stain. Figure 73 is a freehand drawing from a lung section of a bird that died of hemorrhagic pneumonia.

POLYNEURITIS. See AVITAMINOSIS B.

POST-MORTEM EXAMINATIONS. The importance of post-mortem examinations to the diagnosis and treatment of diseases has been emphasized time after time throughout these pages. There is no other method by which one can learn to differentiate one disease from another. It is only by being so familiar with the normal appearances of the organs that any change will stand out like a headlight in a fog, that the breeder can hope to be able to treat his birds intelligently. For you cannot treat a condition until you can recognize it. As I have tried to show both by words and illustrations, each disease has a more or less distinct picture. There are cases where even the most careful methods will lead to failure, but most bird diseases can be recognized by their symptoms and lesions, once the breeder knows what is normal and what is not normal. You do not need any special education; you do not need any special equipment. All you need is two hands and two eyes and the will to use them. If you will take the trouble to carefully pick each bird that dies to pieces and look carefully at each part, look at it as though you intended to draw it from memory (that is not a bad idea, either) you will soon be able to see anything that is not normal. The breeder who will do this will soon find that he is saving a lot of birds which were previously lost.

Years of work, of study, of careful observation; the lives of literally thousands of birds, the disappointments and heartbreaks of hundreds of blasted hopes have gone into these pages; almost every line, every word, is spattered with sweat and blood. For every truth I have outlined to you, I have blundered my way through a hundred errors. I have killed birds when it was almost as hard as killing one's own children. I have had birds die in my hand when their death brought me greater sadness than that I have ever felt over the passing of a member of my own species. And I have dedicated all this to the proposition that fewer birds shall suffer and die because their diseases are not understood. But until the breeder will take the trouble to learn to use his eyes, all of my careful advice is wasted upon him. His medicine chest could contain every prescription I have worked out, but he would never be able to save a bird until he had learned to recognize the circumstance under which each particular line of treatment should be applied. That knowledge can be purchased in but one way. There is but one price. That price is the trouble of making a careful post-mortem examination upon the body of every bird that dies.

Procedure. As shortly after death as possible the body is picked clean and its condition noted. Were the feathers in good condition? Were they oily and elastic, dry and brittle, damp and doughy? Were they louse eaten? Were there any pinfeathers? Are the muscles well filled out? Is there any fat beneath the skin? Are there any sores, bruises or other abnormal marks on the skin? These are the questions the examiner must ask himself and answer before the skin is broken. The skin is then removed—you can tear it right off with your fingernails. Are there any red spots on the skull? Are there any hemorrhagic spots on the fatty tissue? Can you see the abdominal organs clearly through the peritoneum? Are there any dark red or yellow spots in the skeletal muscles? At this point the breast must be removed. You will be able to do a nicer job with a very thin pair of scissors, but you can easily pick it to pieces with your fingernails if necessary. It should be done without disturbing the underlying organs. Look carefully at each organ and notice any off-colored spots or irregularities of contour. Cut or break the bands of connective tissue which hold each organ in place, remove the organ, drop it in a glass of clean water; then pick it up in your hand or on a pin or toothpick and look at it carefully and make a mental note of every line, tone and color; of every spot or other distinguishing mark. Lift up the gizzard and find the spleen underneath it. Take out the intestines in order to see the kidneys. Open the skull, remove the brain and examine the cavities in the bones at the base of the skull. Carefully crush the bones of the spine between your fingernails and remove them from the spinal cord, then note the condition of the cord. Break the big bones and see what is inside of them. Place the intestines in a shallow dish of water and split them from end to end. Wash out the contents and examine the walls closely. Put the washings in a glass dish, add a small drop of bluing, just enough to tint the water, then hold them over a light and study closely. If a drop of bluing or methylene blue solution is added to the washings and worms are present, they will absorb the blue color and be easy to see. Split and study the windpipe, the gullet, the gizzard and the proventriculus in the same manner. If you have a hand lens it will not do any harm to make use of it, but if you haven't, this is perfectly all right. You will be surprised how much you can see with the eyes alone.

I wish the reader to note that I have mentioned no tools whatever as being indispensable. In at least ninety per cent of the post-mortem examinations which have furnished data for this book, nothing but my fingers were used because they were the only tools available. The microscope, the culture tubes, the filter, the reagents and solutions for performing delicate biochemical tests are all very good. They have added much to our understanding of diseases, but it must never be forgotten that more really great discoveries have been made with the unaided eyes and a constructive imagination than with all instruments of research ever invented. When the microscope and culture tube failed Pasteur in his attempt to understand and conquer rabies, he turned his constructive imagination loose on the problem and solved it without their aid and his method has not been improved upon. The finest laboratory equipment money could buy failed to work out a method for the control of FOWL PARALYSIS; though it may be egotistical for me to mention the fact at this place, I solved that problem with a couple of pails of sand and some bird droppings. And I did it at a time when I had never seen a microscope at close range. This preachment may bore some of my readers; they may consider it a waste of space, but if it stimulates just one person to use his eyes and his mind it will have been devoted to a better purpose than any other space in the book.

POTASSIUM CHLORATE. This is the potassium salt of chloric acid. Its chemical formula is $KClO_3$. It is a powerful oxidizing agent and for that reason, is used in the manufacture of matches, fireworks and explosives. It should never be mixed with combustible material, for such mixtures are apt to go off.

When applied to the skin or mucous membranes, potassium chlorate acts as a powerful antiseptic. When taken into the digestive tract it is rapidly absorbed. In the blood it reacts with the hemoglobin, converting it into methemoglobin—a substance which does not combine with oxygen. At the same time it has an injurious effect upon the kidneys, producing a chemical nephritis.

For some little-understood reason, birds are much less susceptible to this poisonous reaction than are mammals. But there are cases on record where this drug has been administered to humans in large doses without producing any symptoms of poisoning. I have administered it to canaries by giving them a 1:1000 solution as drinking water (one-half grain to the ounce) for three months at a time without harming them. It does have a tendency to throw birds into moult, however, and has been used for that purpose. It is a strange and little-understood fact that this drug and a number of other closely related substances, such as peroxide of hydrogen, sodium perborate, the permanganates—all of which produce the same chemical reaction with blood, can, under certain circumstances, produce a reaction in birds and some domesticated animals, and I believe the day will come when it will be produced in man, which destroys the causative agents and toxins of disease in the blood stream almost instantly. The first case of avian diphtheria I ever cured was of the pox variety. I split the lumps and filled the cuts full of powdered permanganate. During half of each day I added one-half grain of potassium chlorate to the ounce of drinking water. During the other half of the day I added one grain of citrocarbonate. The bird was almost at the point of death but within thirty-six hours it was entirely well. The fever was reduced from the very first dose. An hour after she took her first drink of the chlorate solution the bird's temperature was down to 109 F.

POX. This is the form of avian diphtheria in which the principal lesions take the form of wart-like nodules around the beak and head, particularly on the combs and wattles of chickens and the unfeathered areas of the heads of turkeys. In canaries this form of the disease is characterized by large, hard, lumpy swellings developing in the subcutaneous tissues of the head. See AVIAN DIPHTHERIA.

PROLAPSE OF THE OVIDUCT. This is a rare condition in canaries, but it is said to be rather common in high-production poultry, and probably occurs in all species of birds living under artificial conditions. It can result from a rupture of the os-uteri, caused by the passage of an extra large or malformed egg, from injuries re-

ceived in the manual delivery of an egg (see EGG BOUND) or from
breeding exhaustion caused from excess egg production.

The exhausted hen sometimes develops an inflammation of the
oviduct that makes her feel that there is an egg in the oviduct ready
to be laid, when in reality there is none. This causes the hen to
strain and labor in an effort to deliver herself of the nonexistent
egg and in so doing she sometimes forces the oviduct down through
the os-uteri and vent. In rupture cases the injury to the os-uteri
is such that it can no longer hold the oviduct in place.* The organ
slips down into the cloaca and is forced out through the vent.

The protruding tissue attracts the attention of the other birds
which peck at it, sometimes tearing off great chunks of tissue and
so injuring the hen that she has to be destroyed. And because the
protruding tissue worries her, the affected hen will sometimes peck
at it and try to tear it away.

Treatment. Where considerable injury to the tissue has occurred, there is nothing to do but kill the hen. Should the bird be
discovered before the tissue has been greatly injured, however,
she can usually be saved by forcing the prolapsed organ back into
place and injecting into the cloaca a cold solution of common salt,
borax, sodium perborate, peroxide of hydrogen or STROUD'S
SALTS NO. 1. See EGG RUPTURE; EGG, BROKEN; EGG
BOUND.

PROVENTRICULUS. This is the glandular stomach. Its function
is the elaboration and secretion of gastric juices necessary for the
digestion of proteins. It is an expansion of the esophagus, located
just above the gizzard. Unlike the mammalian stomach, it makes
no provision for the retention of food during digestion. The gastric
juices are simply secreted into the food tract and mix with the food
passing through it to the gizzard, where grinding and digestion of
proteins take place simultaneously. See DIGESTIVE TRACT.

PSEUDO LEUKEMIA. It is now generally believed that the condition called **pseudo leukemia** is probably a variety, form or stage
of true leukemia in which the characteristic blood lesions are for
some unknown reason lacking—since the two conditions are often
found associated in the same flock. It is also claimed that an inoculation for leukemia may produce either the regular or pseudo
form of the disease. See LEUKEMIA.

---

* **Note:** Dr. Gustav Eckstein, Department of Physiology, Cincinnati College
of Medicine, has told me of such a case in one of his canary hens. The
bird passed a large double-yolk egg; probably tore the os-uteri; prolapse
developed and she died some days later; no treatment was attempted.

PSITTACOSIS. This is a highly contagious septicemic disease of parrots and other parrot-like birds. It has attracted considerable attention, probably having given rise to more stupid and sensational publicity than any other disease of birds. This is because there is some belief that the disease is transmitted to man. In man the disease is said to take the form of a highly fatal typhoid-pneumonia. It has been studied by Nocard, Palamidessa, Eberth, Wolff and others, and more recently, by Armstrong and McCoy, United States Public Health Service, 1930.

Etiology. Nocard and Palamidessa both isolated from sick parrots an organism of the hog cholera group which they considered to be the causative agent. Armstrong and McCoy demonstrated that the disease could be transmitted to parakeets by inoculation with germ-free filtrates of emulsified visceral organs of birds that had died from the disease.

R. D. Little, who did the pathological work for the investigations by Armstrong and McCoy, reported * the presence in the organs of parrots and parakeets, and in the liver of one laboratory attendant who died during the course of the investigation, of cell inclusions of irregular clumps of very small coccoid or bacillary bodies, varying in size from 0.2 to 0.4 microns and taking a marked bipolar stain.

He found these bodies in the reticulo-endothelial (these are the supporting cells of the liver) cells, the mesothelial cells (these are probably pavement cells derived by the peritonium. My histology does not use the term, but they are derived from the mesoderm), and the mononuclear cells of parrots and in the large mononuclear cells of man. He has suggested that these bodies be designated **Rickettsia psittaci.**

Whether or not the bodies observed by Little are the causative agents of psittacosis is still an unsettled question; but the causative agent has undoubtedly been shown to be something small enough to pass a Berkefeld N filter.

It has long been common knowledge among birdmen that canaries are susceptible to the disease of parrots; that where birds of both species are kept in the same room, a common practice in pet shops, the disease in parrots is certain to spread to the canaries.

During the winters of 1928-29 and 1929-30; I carried out several sets of experiments on canaries which had been exposed to sick parrots before being shipped to me. I noticed that during the early cases the symptoms and lesions corresponded to those observed in

---

* **Note:** U. S. Public Health Service Report, April 11, 1930.

parrots and parakeets, that the birds infected from these first cases developed the bronchial form of avian diphtheria. Still later the pox form of the disease made its appearance. Comparing the results of my experiments with the clinical observations of a number of bird dealers has convinced me that the so-called psittacosis is nothing more or less than a modified pox-virus infection peculiar to parrot-like birds. That I have not had the opportunity of producing the disease in parrots by inoculating them with material from typical cases of pox-virus infection in canaries or other birds is regrettable from a scientific point of view but, from a practical point of view, of little importance. What is important is the fact that I have been able to cure and control all outbreaks of this disease to come to my attention, either in canaries or parrots, by basing my suggestions for treatment upon the assumption that I was dealing with a modified pox-virus infection.*

Symptoms. Psittacosis follows a course very similar to that of avian diphtheria in other birds, excepting that there are no sores. There are fever, fast breathing, thirst and ochre-colored droppings which may turn green or bloody just before death. As the disease progresses the bird becomes greatly emaciated and very weak. It sits in the bottom of the cage, breathing rapidly and paying no attention to its surroundings. When forced to void droppings it often cries out from the pain and whips its tail violently. During the early stages of the illness the sick bird usually eats and drinks, but toward the end refuses both food and water; but in many cases there is an abnormal appetite for soft food, the only kind the bird is able to eat. Often there is a watery discharge from the nostrils and blisters may be found around the vent. In some cases death occurs in a convulsion early in the illness.

Morbid anatomy. There is usually a serous infusion in the pleurae, peritoneum and pericardium. There may be points of coagulation necrosis in the liver, but in many cases, particularly those where death occurs after a short illness, a mulberry liver is

---

* **Note:** When Adams, reasoning from the irregularities in the motion of the planet, Uranus, was able to sit down at his table and calculate the position of the then undiscovered planet Neptune and tell the astronomers: "Point your telescopes at such and such a spot in the heavens at such and such a time and you will see a planet which has never before been observed," the fact that the new planet was found at the spot designated was accepted as ample proof of the soundness of his reasoning. When I, who have had no personal experience with sick parrots, am able to sit down at my table and write: "Do so and so and your bird will recover, and the recovery will take place in such and such a manner," and when my predictions are borne out with as much regularity as the predictions of astronomical calculations are borne out, it appears that my reasoning is sound enough to warrant further investigation.

found. In all cases where the illness has lasted more than a day or two, there will be pneumonic spots in the stage of gray hepatization in both lungs. These lesions are identical with those described in the bronchial form of avian diphtheria in canaries.

Treatment. The following treatment has been used under my direction on a great many parrots suffering with the parrot fever so commonly found among newly imported Amazon parrots and other birds which have been associated with them.* Take away all food and water. Prepare a mush of yellow cornmeal as suggested under the heading PARROTS, INDIGESTION OF. To one ounce of this mush add one-fourth teaspoonful of the best honey and from one to three grains of a mixture of STROUD'S SALTS NO. 1, and STROUD'S EFFERVESCENT BIRD SALTS in equal parts.† If desirable, and if it will make the bird eat the food more readily, a little crushed banana pulp may be added to the mush. The only real difficulty in the application of this treatment is getting the bird to eat the food containing the medicine. Once that is accomplished, he will be well within a very short time. The fever will drop, the breathing become easier and more normal, the diarrhea abate, and then, to all intents and purposes, the bird will be well, though it may take some days for it to regain its flesh and strength. As soon as the symptoms of illness have cleared up the bird can be gradually brought back onto a normal seed diet.

Even in cases where the sick bird is so far gone that he will make no attempt to eat the food of his own volition, he can often be induced to eat it by offering it to him in small bites on a toothpick. Should this fail, add two grains of the mixed treatment to a warm 50:50 dilution of honey and water, and feed that to him a drop at a time from a toothpick or a medicine dropper. Do not try to administer the medicine into the crop by force. The bird that far gone is very apt to die in your hand of heart failure if subjected to any strong excitement. The best plan is to dip the stick in the fluid and then apply it to the edge of the upper mandible, just in front of the corner of the mouth. The drop will run into the mouth and with a little patience the bird can be induced to swallow it. The job can be hastened by using a medicine dropper, applying its tip to the edge of the upper mandible just in front of the corner of the mouth and feeding the solution slowly into

---

* **Note:** If this is not psittacosis, there is a question as to what is.

† **Note:** At the beginning of the treatment the dose should be just as strong as possible. If you can get the bird to accept the food with five grains of the mixture in it, so much the better, though not more than one or two of these large doses are necessary.

the mouth, but care must be taken to see that the bird does not become angry and snap at the glass dropper. Often within half an hour after a dose of the medicine has been administered in this manner, the sick bird will begin to eat the mush. Some of the men who have used this treatment have informed me that they had their birds on a seed diet within forty-eight hours from the time when the first dose of medicine was administered, at which time the birds were almost at the point of death.

Naturally, the same sanitary measures recommended under the heading AVIAN DIPHTHERIA should be put into effect at the first appearance of this or any other disease suspected of being contagious.

Transmission to man. Leichtenstern, in 1899, after summing up and considering all of the evidence available at that time, reached the conclusion that while it was undoubtedly possible for the bacteria involved in outbreaks of psittacosis to become dangerous to man under certain circumstances, the responsibility of the parrot in outbreaks of house epidemics of pneumonia had not been demonstrated—since the disease in man is an atypical typhoid pneumonia and since many outbreaks of this widely prevalent condition could by no stretch of the imagination be traced to an avian source, he considered the relation of parrots and parakeets to certain outbreaks as purely accidental.

Reports of outbreaks of contagious pneumonia in homes into which newly purchased parakeets and parrots, and even canaries, had been introduced, have persisted in spite of all argument. But it is a strange fact that while these outbreaks are always said to follow the taking into the home of some newly purchased bird, bird breeders, bird dealers, bird importers and their families who often handle sick birds by the thousands, ofttimes sleeping in the same room with them and with all windows tightly closed, should be so peculiarly immune to this infection. It is nothing uncommon for men to spend their entire lives in this business, bringing up their children and grandchildren in their shops and aviaries, without their families showing any particular predeliction to disease. On the contrary, they are a healthy, long-lived class of people. I have known several grand old men who were in their eighties when they passed on and I know others who have reached that age and are still going strong, yet they have been associated with birds constantly since early childhood. If you mentioned psittacosis to them they would point to their pink-cheeked grandchildren and laugh you to scorn. It is also very strange how often members of the

families of politicos or politico-medical demagogs are afflicted with
this disease. It is almost as if the germ of psittacosis had a greater
affinity for persons desiring publicity for political reasons than for
birds of the psittacine genera. The law of probability tells us that
such coincidences do not happen unless they are made to happen—
more of this presently.

On the other hand, during the studies of psittacosis conducted
by Armstrong and McCoy in 1930, there were said to have been
eleven cases of what was called psittacosis in the laboratory within
a few weeks of the introduction of the sick birds. And the odd
part of this outbreak is the fact that only one of the persons taken
sick had any contact with the sick birds or even entered the room
where they were kept, while the persons in daily contact with them
were not affected. Nor did any person in contact with these cases
become sick outside of the laboratory—members of their families,
doctors, nurses, etc.

The blood of recovered cases is said to have conferred immunity to the disease and to have proved of considerable therapeutic
value in the treatment of other outbreaks of the disease in man;
but in none of these cases has the diagnosis been established by inoculations.

Aside from the question as to whether or not man is susceptible
to psittacosis, ninety-nine per cent of the so-called human psittacosis
exists only in the stupid ethics of a profession which does not permit its members to employ honest advertising in the selling of
their services, but protects them, by swearing other members of
the profession to secrecy, in the rankest charlatanism.

Some doctor, usually a political doctor rather than a general
practitioner, has or hears of a case of intestinal influenza or typhoid
pneumonia. At once he sees golden opportunity knocking at his
door. If there is a psittacine bird in the neighborhood, he is sitting
on top of the world; he calls the newspapers, the radio stations,
the airports; he has serum flown across the country. There are
pictures and front page stories. Other publicity-seeking politicians
climb on the band wagon and investigations are started; special
restrictive laws are introduced and enacted and the only persons
qualified to express sound opinions on the subject, men who have
specialized in the diseases of birds, are shouted down in the general hullabaloo thus created. And the chances are ten to one that
the patient in the case did not have a thing wrong with him that
a few quinine and opium tablets and a good physic would not cure.

Bird dealers and bird breeders are not, as a rule, rich or influential. They are mostly small businessmen and they are not closely organized, nor do they form a very large proportion of the voting public, and, of course, their birds can't vote. What more ideal victim could be found for the demagog to rail against and, of course, he must have something to make a lot of noise over in order to keep the public from looking too closely at his own person, or doing what would be infinitely worse, ignoring his existence.

The 1930 hubbub about psittacosis was started by Dr. C. H. Ward, Chief of Bureau of Bacteriology of the Maryland State Department of Health. He gave out a statement that he had discovered the germ of psittacosis. At once other politicos began climbing on the band wagon. There was psittacosis everywhere. It just happened that right at that time I was studying the disease in canaries.

I wrote to Dr. Ward and told him that if he had any germ which would cause the symptoms and lesions of psittacosis in a parrot I would be willing to submit to inoculation with that organism or with any material which would cause the disease in a parrot. Of course, the offer was not accepted. Three months later he informed me that pigeons are not susceptible to parrot fever. An honest test is naturally the last thing a demagog ever wants. It is possible to kid the public but no one could laugh off an inoculation test of the kind I suggested.

PUBIS. This is the bone which in mammals forms the ventral or closing segment of the pelvic arch. In birds the two horns of the pubis do not meet and fuse as in mammals. They remain separate throughout life, which makes the passage of large eggs possible. See SKELETON.

PUFFED ABDOMEN. An enlarged abdomen is often a symptom of disease. It may be the result of marked hyperemia or hypertrophy (engorgement with blood or enlargement through tissue cell division) of any of the abdominal organs or the presence of morbid exudates into the abdominal air sacs or the peritoneal cavity. The appearance of the abdomen is one of the most important considerations in the diagnosis of many bird diseases. Inspection of the abdomen holds the same position in bird medicine that taking the pulse holds in human medicine. It is not that a man's pulse will tell the doctor what is wrong with him, but it may tell the doctor a number of things that are not wrong with him. It is the same way with the appearance of a bird's abdomen. We cannot take a bird's pulse but we can usually see his liver and intestines, particularly when there is something wrong with them. If we examine the abdomen and cannot see the liver and intestines, we know at once that there are a number of conditions we do not have to consider in making our diagnosis. See CANARY TYPHOID; AVIAN DIPHTHERIA; APOPLECTIFORM SEPTICEMIA; INFECTIOUS ENTRO-HEPATITIS; B. PARATYPHOSUS B INFECTION; COCCIDIOSIS; LEUKEMIA; PERITONITIS, ETC.

PUFFED FEATHERS. See FEATHERS, FLUFFED.

PULLORUM DISEASE. This is another name for **Bacillary white diarrhea,** but it is more inclusive, since it covers all diseases caused by bacterium pullorum, including the chronic infection of adult hens and the rare outbreaks of pullorum septicemia in adult birds. See BACILLARY WHITE DIARRHEA.

PULSE. See RESPIRATORY SYSTEM.

PYGOSTYLE. This is the expanded, bulbous end of the coccyx. It contains the oil glands and furnishes support for the tail feathers, which radiate from its posterior border.

PYRETHRUM. This is a yellowish brown powder used for killing insects. See CHRYSANTHEMUM FLOWERS.

Q

QUAIL TYPHOID. This condition, also known as **Quail disease, shipping fever, and septic fever of quail, pheasants, and grouse,** is a highly fatal, infectious, septicemic disease of birds of these species which are held in captivity under conditions of great crowding and poor sanitation. The disease usually appears in newly captured birds or birds that are undergoing or have recently undergone the hardships of being shipped from one place to another.

Etiology. According to Morse, who made a study of this disease,* an organism of the colon group is constantly found in the livers of infected birds, though it cannot always be cultivated from the lungs or blood. The organism is pathogenic for mice and guinea pigs. Chickens and pigeons are not susceptible.

The actual cause of the outbreaks is undoubtedly to be found in the lowered resistance of the birds resulting from the hardships of crowding and shipment.

Symptoms. There is nothing characteristic in the symptoms of this disease according to the reports which have come to my attention. The bird takes sick, carries its feathers loosely, loses appetite, has increased thirst, fever, sleeps in the daytime, becomes very weak, and dies generally on the second or third day of the illness. In chronic cases there is great emaciation; this is not true of those cases running an acute course.

Morbid anatomy. The lungs and liver are usually congested, and the latter organ may present necrotic areas varying in size from mere points to single spots involving the greater part of a lobe. A rather consistent lesion is the presence of numerous minute spots of suppurative necrosis (small abscesses or pus-filled pimples) in the inner wall of the intestines. Some of these ulcers, which may be as large as the head of a pin, may perforate the intestinal walls. At other times they may be mere points; and there are cases in which only reddened areas of intestinal mucosa are observed.

Prevention. The logical methods of preventing this disease are: to keep the birds in clean quarters; to refrain from crowding them as much as possible; to make shipments with only a few birds in each box; to store them with only a few birds in each coop; to see that the coops and shipping boxes are so constructed as to

---

* **Note:** Circular 109, Bureau of Animal Industry, 1907.

prevent the droppings from contaminating the food and water; and by placing one teaspoonful of STROUD'S EFFERVESCENT BIRD SALTS in each quart of drinking water, or, lacking it, to use one of the effervescent salines put up for human use. But do not forget that medicine must never be given in metal drinkers.

Treatment. Having had no experience in the treatment of this disease, I can only reason from my years of experience in treating similar conditions in other species of birds. I would expect the birds to respond to the use of one teaspoonful of STROUD'S EFFERVESCENT BIRD SALTS in each quart of drinking water. Should this fail, I would then try STROUD'S SPECIAL PRESCRIPTION in the same dosage. That failing, I would give them STROUD'S SALTS NO. 1. This failing, I would administer salol into the crops three times per day in 1/10 to 1 grain doses. I am pretty certain that one of these three lines of treatment would clear up the condition, however.

QUASSIA. This is the wood and bark of the **Bitterwood** trees, **Picrasma excelas** and **Quassia amara**—two distinct but closely related species of trees native to the West Indies.

The first contains two bitter principles; the latter, the true quassia, contains four. Their extracts are employed as tonics, for the removal of intestinal worms, and in the manufacture of fly poison. An infusion of quassia is said to be of great value for the extermination of lice and mites. See NAPHTHALENE.

Quassia comes on the market as chips of wood or bark, as an alcoholic extract, a fluid extract and an alcoholic tincture. I have not tested the tonic qualities of this substance, but the correct dose for birds would be one drop of the alcoholic tincture to the ounce of drinking water.

QUININE. This is the principal alkaloid contained in cinchona bark. Although the pure alkaloid is not used in medicine to any considerable extent, it forms a large number of salts holding important places in both human and animal medicine. The sulphate is the salt most commonly used in human medicine, and in various combinations with opium, caffeine, belladonna, strychnine and cathartics—it provides us with some of our most valuable prescriptions.

Quinine acts as an antiseptic, antipyretic and tonic. Because it is extremely poisonous to ameba, it is a specific for malaria and amebic dysentery. Because it opens the pores and expands the smaller blood vessels, it makes the removal of heat from the body

much more rapid. It also stimulates the excretion of waste product through the skin and takes a load off the heart, which gives it
the power to overcome fatigue in a really remarkable manner.

The only specific disease of birds upon which I have tested
this salt is diphtheria, and in that case it did not prove of value.
It is of value in the treatment of pneumonic conditions, however.
See PNEUMONIA. The two most valuable bird tonics known con-
tain quinine. They are: IRON AND QUININE CITRATE and
I.Q.S.—Elixir of Iron, Quinine and Strychnine phosphates.*

---

* Note: The action of quinine in expanding the capillaries and how this
relieves the strain on the heart in attacks of disease is well illustrated by
an incident which had nothing to do with illness: I was once placed in a
position where, to avoid embarrassment, I had to accept a challenge to
play handball against a man whom I knew could normally beat me any
day in the week. I had been playing sociable games with him for six
months and had never beaten him. It was not that he played a better
game; he had better wind. He played a fast game. I could outplay him
as long as I could last, but I could not last long at the pace he set. The
challenge was made; bets placed. I could not afford to lose. Two hours
before the game I took three tablets which contained 15 grains of quinine,
¾ grain of opium and small amounts of caffeine, belladonna and strychnine.
The quinine opened my pores and steadied my heart action. The opium
slowed down my reflexes just enough to give me perfect control. The
open pores permitted me to sweat out the poisons of fatigue as fast as
they were formed. The result was that I ran rings around the man; beat
him by such a one-sided score and did it with such a little show of effort,
that he was always convinced that I had been stringing him along for
six months just to hook him. I was perfectly willing to let him keep on
thinking that, since it would keep others from trying to rope me into a
money game. I did not let him see me the next day, however, for such
abuse must be paid for. Of course, I had known that and what to expect
in the way of reaction.

RACHITIS (Rickets). This is a disease of the skeleton resulting from insufficient lime and phosphates for the growing bone structures. It may develop as the result of an insufficiency of these elements in the diet, but is usually caused by the inability of the individual to metabolize the minerals which are in the diet. This results from an inadequate supply of Vitamin D or direct sunlight. See VITAMIN D.

The condition is indicated in old birds by inappetence, inability of the male to fertilize eggs, inability of the female to produce firm-shelled, hatchable eggs. In young birds the condition is indicated by a tough, dry, horny or leathery condition of the bones; an overgrowth of the long bones of the legs and the upper beak, which makes the baby bird look like a cross between a young crane and an eaglet; an inability to maintain normal growth or to grow a full coat of feathers; a darkening of the body; emaciation; weakness and death.

Treatment. Both prevention and treatment of this condition consists of correcting the diet or environment. The birds should have plenty of mineral food constantly before them and either an opportunity for daily exposure to direct sunlight or an adequate supply of the sunshine vitamin in the diet.

This condition is discussed much more fully under the heading VITAMIN D.

RAPE SEED. Rape is a plant somewhat similar to kale and mustard, and it exists in several varieties, some of which are raised for hog and cattle forage. There are other varieties which are raised for oil, and two that are grown exclusively for bird food. The seeds of the varieties which are raised for forage and oil are large (the size of number eight shot), usually black in color, and have a bitter, burning taste resembling mustard. Though these seeds are unfit for bird food, many dealers substitute them for the more expensive seeds grown especially for birds. Some disreputable dealer may even substitute mustard, cabbage and turnip seeds for rape. The two varieties of bird rape are German Summer Rape and Rubsen.

The seeds of the small red German summer rape are about twice the size of maw seeds. They should be round and full bodied, uniform in size, a uniform reddish-brown in color and have a rather pleasant taste. Some writers describe the taste of good rape as similar to that of the English walnut—though this, I think is a little bit too farfetched. The taste should be rather pleasant, however, and not more than one seed in twenty should bite the tongue.

Rubsen is slightly larger than the German Summer Rape, is darker, more purplish in cast and has an even milder taste. Neither of these seeds should ever have a wrinkled surface, which would mean that the seed was either green and immature when harvested or very old and had lost all of its oil. In either case it would be of very low feeding quality.

When fresh rape seed is placed between two pieces of white paper and rolled with a bottle or rolling pin, each seed should flatten out into a paper-thin disc and remain intact until disturbed; it should leave a distinctly oily spot on the paper. If the seed is crushed to powder and does not leave oily spots on the paper, it is stale and unfit for bird food.

RED BLOOD CORPUSCLES. See BLOOD.

RED CANARY. In the year 1914, Bruno Martin, Loetzen, Germany, let a bright, humane idea step in and question a well-established fact, or what everyone else thought was a fact. A breeder friend of his had raised a large number of canary-finch hybrids. The males had been sold and the females were to be killed, since they were mules and of no commercial value. Martin did not like to think of such nice birds being destroyed, and he could not convince himself that they would prove entirely infertile, regardless of what all the books said; so he asked his friend to give him the flight full of females—about forty in all.

He took these birds home, placed them in a large flight and gave them good treatment. When the breeding season came around, male canaries were placed in the flight, and the birds were given nests and nesting material. They mated and went to work. All of the hens laid eggs, but from the forty hens only one egg was fertile. The bird was raised and turned out to be a female. For the first four years only one bird was raised each year, and it was nine years before Mr. Martin had fully fertile birds of both sexes. He did, however, succeed in establishing a strain of copper-red canaries.

In 1928, Mr. Martin wrote a series of articles on color-breeding canaries in which he recounted his experience with the red hybrids. Martin's article was translated and republished in the United

States by A. H. Hasseler, who was then owner and editor of "American Cage Birds," a trade journal devoted to canary breeding.

There was great interest among American canary breeders, and a number of them attempted to arrange for importations of these red birds. This failing, there was a demand for information concerning which red finch had been used in their production, since Martin's identification of the bird as "Kapuzen Zeisgi" (red hooded) had been a little vague.

In 1931, William C. Dustin published an article in which he stated that the bird used in Martin's experiments was the South American Black-hooded Siskin, **Spinus Cuculatus;** that he had secured some of these birds and experimented with them and learned that though the females were almost wholly infertile the males were about fifty per cent fertile and in three years he had been successful in producing good bronze rollers.

From that time on the quest for the red canary has gone on in a thousand aviaries and breeding rooms. Good naturally colored orange birds have been produced, but the quest for a pure red still goes on. The work has been hampered by the fact that we are treading new ground. Mendal taught us how to calculate the inheritance of unit characteristics when dealing with strains within a species, but here we are dealing with the first instance of the crossing of two distinct species possessing many distinct characteristics, and there have been no precedents for our guidance. To illustrate:

Most of us had the idea the use of deep yellow canaries would be of advantage—reasoning that the color of the canary would reinforce the color of the finch. It was not until 1936 that I guessed, and later demonstrated, that there was a link between the inheritance of red pigment and buff feathers. The laws are not yet fully worked out, but they operate about as follows so far as red pigmentation is concerned.

Each male hybrid inherits from the male finch a pigmentation which is about half the intensity of that of the finch. The male hybrid can pass this pigmentation on to about half of his offspring, and they in turn can pass it along to about half of their offspring without any further loss of intensity. Thus, a bird of the sixth generation will be 1/32 blackhood, but if he is pigmented at all, his pigmentation will be about half that of the blackhood, which indicates that the blackhood's pigmentation is the result of two factors which cannot be further subdivided. It must not be assumed from this that all of these birds show the same intensity of pigmentation in their feathers, however, for there are many other factors which influence the actual color of the feathers. My breeding results further indicate that only buff birds show pigmented feathers. The males with black skins and black underfeathers are copper colored as are the males of the first cross; the males with white skins are orange or apricot in color. Buff females inheriting the one factor for pigmentation, may be copper colored, pale creamy buff or grayish white in color. **Yellow** males (the word is here used as the antonym of buff. See BALDNESS) inheriting the pigmentation may pass it on to their offspring but do not show pigment in their feathers. Whether or not a **yellow** bird receiving a factor for pigmentation from both parents would have pigmented feathers, I do not know. I am here discussing the inheritance of pigment, as it occurs when normal canary hens are mated to pigmented males. So far as I know, the yellow female does not inherit the pigment factor, and up to the fourth generation, these yellow hens are all infertile, though buff females of the third generation are partly fertile.

The above reduced to the following law:

A single factor for red pigmentation is dominant in buff males, recessive in **yellow** males, dominant or **recessive** * in buff females, lost in **yellow** females. There is an unrelated sex factor inherited from the finch which tends to suppress the development of pigmentation in females. Canaries do not have this factor, so that females of the third and later generations may or may not have it, depending upon whether they inherit their female factor from the canary or the finch.

While the distinctions **yellow** and **buff, pigmented** and **nonpigmented** are broad enough to include all possible occurrences, since, in fact, they are all inclusive, they give but a faint idea of the complexities of this subject or the color combinations possible. It must be remembered that in the normal canary we have three pigments, six color factors and six other factors for the manifestation of the colors inherited, and three possible factors for the loss of color factors; in the finch we have all of these factors but the last three—the colors of the finch have not been segregated as have those of the canary—and in addition a factor which is responsible for the suppression of bright colors in the females. It is easily seen that the combinations are limitless. To unscramble all

---

* **Note:** I have set the word **recessive** in bold face type in connection with buff females, for although these birds inherit the factor for pigmentation and may pass it on to their young, though they are not pigmented themselves, they are not true mendalian recessives.

of these factors and work out the inheritance of all possible color combinations will take years of research and a book much larger than this one will be required to explain the results.

To date, birds have been produced in carmine, pink, orange, apricot, orange-brown, copper-red, grayish white, silver-gray, gray-green, moss-green, brownish green, lemon-yellow, orange-yellow, mahogany and bronze.

This line of experimentation has already thrown light upon one of nature's mysteries and may throw light upon others. For generations it has been known that certain red-pigmented birds

Figure 74.   **RED MITES**

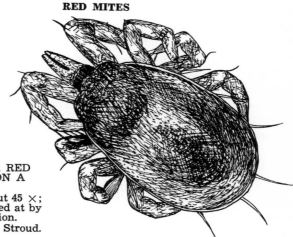

DRAWING OF A RED MITE FOUND ON A CANARY
Magnification about 45 ×; measurements arrived at by microscopic projection.
Drawn by Robert Stroud.

kept in captivity lost the red pigment from their feathers. In 1935, I observed this to be true of the finch-bred birds moulted indoors. Those carried into the sunshine every day developed a good color. Investigation has revealed that the pigment as manufactured by the skin cells and deposited in the feathers is not red but yellow; it is soluble and photoactive. If not acted upon by ultra-violet light it is soon lost, but when it is exposed to direct sunlight it turns from yellow to red and becomes fixed in the feathers. I believe that I was the first to work out the relationship between red color and direct sunlight.

RED MITES. This is a small tick-like creature which lives by sucking blood from the birds during the night. It does not as a rule remain upon the birds in the daytime. The individuals are about 1/75 to 1/100 of an inch long. Figure 74 is a microscopic drawing of a red mite found on a canary.

These pests can do great harm where they are permitted to multiply unmolested. They will invade the nests, suck blood from the hen until they either drive her from the nest or lower her vitality to such an extent that she is no longer fit for breeding. And they will literally bleed the babies white—leaving them as bloodless as if their throats had been cut. But they can do these things only because the breeder permits them.

Control. The control of mites and all the other bloodsuckers—blue bugs, bedbugs, etc., is no great problem if attacked in a systematic manner. The first problem is the common one of cleanliness. Make it a practice to wash all equipment at frequent intervals, using a strong, hot solution of lye soap. Remove and burn all litter and spray all cracks or other places where mites might breed, with a good commercial spray which may be reinforced by adding two ounces of naphthalene and two ounces of castor oil to each quart. The best way to demite chicken houses is to spray them once each week with a power sprayer, using a mixture of eights parts of kerosene, one part engine oil and one part crude carbolic acid. The bird room should afford no breeding places for mites. This can be assured by filling all cracks with putty, giving the room two coats of flat paint and then a top coat of hard zinc enamel. Unpainted quarters can be frequently whitewashed, using a power sprayer to make sure that all cracks and crevices are filled and sealed. It is the practice of continued cleanliness rather than drastic delousing measures which should be relied upon. See FEATHER LICE; MITES, ETC.*

RESPIRATORY FREQUENCIES. These, of course, vary with the species and somewhat with the age of the individual. Young birds breathe faster than adults, and, like humans, birds breathe faster when they are frightened, excited or after exertion of any kind.

---

* **Note:** There is now on the market a vapor method of destroying all manner of insects without harming either the birds or the food. The initial expenditure is greater than with the more common method of exterminating insects, but the results fully warrant it, since in the long run there is a considerable saving. The outfit, which costs about $25.00 for the electric vaporizer and a gallon of the special insecticide is guaranteed to destroy all insects in five thousand cubic feet of air space in thirty minutes and at a cost of about 60c. There is no labor involved, since all one has to do is close the doors and windows and plug the vaporizer into a light socket. The method has been recently tested out by a large number of bird breeders and they all contend that it is the ideal solution of the lice and mite problem. Even seed stored in the bird room is freed of any worms that may happen to be present. The job of exterminating is so thoroughly done that one application every four to six weeks is all that is required.

The average respiratory frequencies of healthy adult birds at rest, expressed in times per minute, are:

Black-hooded siskin 98
Canary-Bh S hybrids...........................92 to 96
Canary 86
Sparrow 80
Chicken 20
Turkey 14
Pigeon 26
Duck 22
Goose 16

During the progress of many diseases the breathing becomes very rapid. In the bronchial form of avian diphtheria I have on many occasions counted respiratory frequencies between two and three hundred per minute; in sporadic pneumonia and peritonitis the breathing is even more rapid, while in the later stages of the toxic * form of diphtheria and in the last stages of aspergillosis the breathing is much slower than normal—in the first case the rate may drop to forty and in the latter cases to five or six per minute.

RESPIRATORY SYSTEM. See AIR SACS; LUNGS.

RESPIRATORY DISEASES. See ASPERGILLOSIS; INFEC-TIOUS BRONCHITIS; AVIAN DIPHTHERIA; GAPE; PNEUMO-NIA. There are respiratory symptoms and lesions in a great many diseases, particularly the bacterial septicemias, such as **B. para-typhosus B infections, Canary necrosis, Fowl cholera,** etc. Hemorrhages into the air sacs and the air cavities in the bones are common lesions of apoplectiform septicemia and food poisoning, but in these conditions there are no respiratory symptoms.

RHEUMATISM. A true rheumatism, similar to that to which man is so susceptible, is probably unknown in birds. Rheumatic symptoms may be associated with chronic nephritis and the chronic cases of bacterial septicemias.

RIBS. Birds have five full ribs and two short ribs on each side. Each full rib of one of the larger birds consists of two parts: the superior rib, which articulates with or is fused to a spinal verte-bra, sweeps out in a graceful curve to the point on the side of the

---

* **Note:** I have used the word **toxic** in this paragraph to refer to certain chronic cases of avian diphtheria in which there are no diphtheric lesions, either external or internal. In these cases the birds may live for several months but finally succumb to a general toxemia and exhaustion. Such birds can be identified as diphtheric only by the fact that all birds asso-ciated with them develop the typical forms of the disease.

body where it meets and articulates with the inferior rib; the inferior rib articulates with the superior rib by means of a cartilaginous attachment (it could hardly be called a joint) and then runs forward in an almost straight line to its point of attachment just back of the anterior edge of the sternum.

These inferior ribs are attached to the sternum in a close-packed group and radiate from the attachment point like the leaves of a fan. In small birds, like canaries, sparrows and finches, there are no divisions between the superior and inferior ribs. Each rib sweeps out in a long graceful curve which is almost "U" shaped, and reaches from the spine to the sternum without a break, since the flexibility of the bones of these little birds makes a joint unnecessary. Unlike mammals, birds have two short ribs located at the apex of the thoracic cavity. Each rib, excepting the first and last, is provided with a posteriorly extending process which overlaps the adjacent rib and helps bind them all into a compact, strong, yet flexible unit.

RICKETS. See RACHITIS; VITAMIN D.

REPRODUCTIVE ORGANS. See GENERATIVE SYSTEM; EGG STRUCTURE AND FORMATION.

REPRODUCTIVE VITAMIN. See VITAMIN E; WHEAT GERM OIL.

ROUNDWORMS. There are a great many varieties of roundworms to be found in the digestive tracts of various species of birds. Those found in poultry and water fowls vary in length from two to four inches; those found in pigeons are from one and one-half to two inches long; those found in canaries and sparrows are from one-quarter to three-quarters of an inch long.

All species of birds are susceptible to roundworm infestation, but because canaries spend most of their lives caged alone or in small groups, never coming in contact with contaminated ground, they are seldom infested with intestinal worms. The same applies to the other species of pet birds.

In poultry and pigeons intestinal worms cause considerable damage. They sometimes accumulate in such great numbers that they block the intestines; again, they sometimes perforate the intestinal wall and make their way into the peritoneal and thoracic cavities.

Diagnosis. Birds that are heavily infested with roundworms become unthrifty, emaciated and extremely susceptible to bacterial infections. The only certain methods of diagnosis are the finding of the worms in the birds' droppings and their discovery at post-mortem examinations. Post-mortem diagnosis of this condition is of value in handling poultry, since where one bird of a flock is heavily infected the rest are pretty sure to be in a similar condition; but is of no value in the case of caged birds since here there is little opportunity for the worms to pass from one bird to another.

To locate the worms in the droppings, the dropping is broken up with a little water in a watch glass or Petri dish and examined in a strong light. The small thread-like worms of the smaller species of birds can be more easily located by adding a trace of methylene blue solution to the emulsified dropping.

Treatment. This is a subject upon which I am unable to give advice. In all of my experience with pet birds I have found just one case of worm infestation. The bird was an English sparrow, one of the first birds I ever owned. Acting on advice found in a Government bulletin on the care of canaries, I gave him three drops of castor oil and a little santonin. The treatment killed him. Another bird was given the same dose of santonin without the oil. It was not made ill; therefore I blamed the oil for the death.

I have had reports from others of good results attending the use of cascara and creosote. See CASCARA and NAPHTHA-LENE. The dose of the cascara prescription was ten drops to the ounce of drinking water and it was kept before the bird for three days. The dose of naphthalene was one-tenth of a grain administered into the crop and followed several hours later with about five drops of olive oil—a single dose being used. These doses are, of course, for birds the size of a canary. For larger birds, larger doses would have to be employed.

One of the methods highly recommended for the removal of intestinal worms from poultry consists of feeding the birds a soft mash containing one pound of tobacco stems for each one hundred adult birds. The finely chopped stems are placed in water and simmered for several hours; then the stems and the water they have been simmered in are mixed with the required amount of ground food and given to the chickens, which should have been previously fasted for twenty-four hours. The amount of mash given should be about half of what the birds normally consume at a single feeding. Three hours later they are given another feeding which, this time, contains ten ounces of Epsom salts for each one hundred birds. See TAPEWORMS.

ROUP. SEE AVIAN DIPHTHERIA.

RUMP GLAND. See OIL GLAND.

RUPTURE OF THE OVIDUCT. See PROLAPSE OF THE OVI-
DUCT; EGG RUPTURE.

SALICYLIC ACID AND SALICYLATES. Salicylic acid, which is a natural constituent of many vegetable products, such as **ammoniac, oil of wintergreen, oil of sweetbirch,** is a crystalline powder made by the action of sodium hydroxide and carbonic acid on carbolic acid. It enters into a great many chemical combinations to produce artificial products, some of which are widely used in medicine and are of considerable value; for instance, aspirin (Acetylsalicylic acid) and salol (Phenyl salicylate).

Salicylic acid and the salicylates are antiseptics, antirheumatics, antipyretics, analgesics (drugs which stop pain) and diuretics, and they appear to have some specific action on inflammations involving the serous surfaces, especially those of the joints. In human medicine they are used: externally, for the treatment of wounds, skin diseases, inflamed surfaces; internally, for the treatment of rheumatism, pleurisy, scarlet fever, influenza, pericarditis, headache and neuralgia.

Salicylates have been recommended for the treatment of colds, inflammation of the bowels and respiratory tract. See SODIUM SALICYLATE and AMMONIAC, which are most commonly used in the treatment of respiratory conditions, and SALOL, which is employed chiefly as an intestinal antiseptic. The dose for an adult chicken is said to be from five to fifteen grains administered into the crop. The dose for a canary is from one-quarter to one-half grain of sodium salicylate to the ounce of drinking water and one-twentieth to one-tenth grain of salol into the crop.

SALIMONELLOSIS, AVIAN. See B. PARATYPHOSUS B INFECTION.

SALOL. This is a combination of carbolic and salicylic acids and it combines the action of both. It comes as an almost tasteless, insoluble white powder. It is decomposed in the intestines by the action of the steapsin of the pancreatic juice into carbolic and salicylic acids. The salicylic acid is absorbed and produces the characteristic effects of other salicylates; the carbolic acid acts as an antiseptic in the intestines, exercising an inhibitory influence upon the growth and development of bacteria and other parasites. Because it is insoluble in water, salol is usually employed in bird medicine in a 1:20 sugar dilution, which may be dusted on bread or other soft food or made into pills and administered into the crop. The dose for a canary is from one-twentieth to one-tenth of a grain every twenty-four hours.

SALT. Some persons have the erroneous idea that salt should never be given to birds, that it is a deadly poison to them. The truth is that salt is as necessary for birds as for mammals and performs necessary functions in their physical economy. Birds differ from mammals in one important respect in regards to salt, however, their machinery is not designed for getting rid of a large excess. A uniform amount of salt in the blood is as important to birds as it is to you.* When the salt content of the blood becomes too low, as often happens in man and animals during very hot weather, a condition called **heat exhaustion** develops. This condition, and it is a highly fatal one, results from the fact that the blood cells can function only in a plasma of fixed and normal saline content. When the proportion of salt falls below what it should be, the red blood cells absorb water, swell and burst. They are not able to perform their function of carrying oxygen under these conditions and without the necessary oxygen the subject dies. On the other hand, when there is too much salt in the blood, the cells give up water, become smaller in size and shriveled in appearance, and the protoplasm of the cell body (the cytoplasm) becomes collected into granules which arrange themselves around the periphery of the cell. Such red blood cells are spoken of as being **crenated**. Under the dark-field microscope they appear as rings composed of many burning points of light. These cells, too, have lost their power to carry on their normal function; but this condition is not serious to man and most animals, and for a very simple reason; any time the salt concentration of the blood becomes too great the subject, be he man or animal, becomes very thirsty, drinks a lot of water, dilutes the blood and then his kidneys throw off the excess water and the excess salt with it. Thus no great harm is done, since the crenated cells return to normal just as soon as their plasma has its normal proportion of salt restored. Birds do not have this power of getting rid of excess salt so quickly and con-

---

* **Note:** It is interesting to note here that the proportion of salt in the blood is just about half the proportion present in sea water. It is estimated that between one and two billion years ago, which is also estimated to be about the time terrestrial creatures made their first appearance upon earth, the proportion of salt in the sea was identical with the proportion of salt in blood. It is argued that while the proportion of salt in sea water has been constantly increasing, the composition of the blood has remained constant. If that is true, the most fragile thing in existence has remained constant in the face of forces which have not only changed all living things but have changed all living conditions and the forms of life itself thousands of times and have even swept away great continents.

veniently. Their kidneys are constructed for handling urine in a thick, pasty state, not for handling large quantities of fluid urine. For this reason, when a bird gets too much salt it is very apt to die.

The birds seem to know this, for birds that are not starved for salt will never overeat of foods containing it. The bird that has been starved for salt may overeat of such foods and dies as a result, however. The solution of this problem is not found in depriving your birds of the salt they need, but in keeping before them at all times a mineral-food mixture containing sufficient salt to satisfy their requirements.

Gallagher and Edwards * have tested the toxicity of sodium chloride on poultry and have found that the lethal dose for a medium-sized chicken is 150 grains; they found 75 grains of salt introduced directly into the crop produced no noticeable symptoms of illness. Now let us figure a little.

If a bird weighing three pounds can withstand 75 grains of salt, a man weighing 150 pounds should be able to withstand 3750 grains, about one-half pound. Now if you took one-half pound of salt at a single dose you might survive but I don't think you would ever look the same. I am pretty certain that you would not carry it without showing symptoms of illness, and I most certainly do not advise you to try the experiment on yourself.

It is evident from this material that salt is probably less poisonous to birds than it is to you. It should show you how idiotic it is to deprive your birds of all salt just because you have heard of some bird dying because he was starved for salt and overate of the first food he got hold of containing it. I do not know whether a man starved for salt would overeat of it and kill himself, but I do know that he would certainly kill anyone else or commit any other crime to obtain the supply his system craved.

I once had a pet sparrow which was very fond of salted peanuts. I used to crush them up for him and keep a dish of them before him at all times. He would never overeat of them. Another sparrow, one that had been deprived of salt, was turned into my room. He tasted the salted peanuts and refused to stop eating them until the dish was empty. The next morning he was dead. I have kept mineral food containing from two to four per cent of sodium chloride before my birds constantly for years. They do not die of salt poisoning.

---

* **Note:** Edwards, Journal of Comparative Pathology and Therapeutics, Volume 31, 1918; Gallagher, Journal of the American Veterinary Association, Volume 7, 1919.

SANGUINARIUM BACTERIUM. This is the causative agent of
FOWL TYPHOID.

SANTONIN. This comes as a yellow, crystalline powder, and is
used as an anthelmintic (a drug which expels intestinal worms).
The dose for a chicken is said to be from five to fifteen grains administered into the crop.

I have not used this drug on canaries. I employed it once on a
sparrow with fatal results, though I do not think that this drug
caused the death. I at once gave the same size dose to a normal,
healthy sparrow without ill effects. The dose used was one-fifth of
a grain introduced directly into the crop. The minimum therapeutic dose for a bird about the size of a canary, would be about
one-twentieth of a grain.

SCALY-LEG. If your bird's feet look unsightly, always appear to
be dirty, have large scales of extraordinary thickness, it is just possible that he is suffering from **scaly-leg.** This condition is caused by
infestation with a very small mite which bores under the scales of
the feet and lives by eating the connective tissue. This mite has two
long, hair-like processes protruding posteriorly. Ignoring the length
of these processes, the mite is about 1/200 of an inch long, which is
a little too small to be seen by the unaided eyes. They are easily
visible with a ten diameter hand lens. The excrement of these mites
accumulates under the scales as a fine, white powder.

The condition is spread by unclean perches, but it spreads through
the flock very slowly. Some birds appear to be entirely immune.

Treatment. This is one condition for which there is absolutely
no excuse. Of all the bird pests the scaly-leg mite is the easiest to
destroy. To cure the condition it is only necessary to anoint the
bird's feet with a little olive oil. The first application will soften
the scales; at the second, which should be given about three days
later, the old scales may be removed and this will let the oil come
in contact with the mites and kill them. It is as simple as that.

Of course, the perches must be cleaned. If the bird keeper will
make it a habit to wash his perches at regular intervals and will
clean up the feet of all new birds before permitting them to mix
with his flock, he will never be bothered by this condition and his
birds will be saved much annoyance.

SCAPULA. This is the shoulder blade. In birds it is a long, saber-
like bone which extends straight down the back from the shoulder
to the fifth or sixth rib.

SEED TESTING. Hemp seed is tested by crushing five or six ounces, placing it in a closed jar over night and, in the morning, smelling the enclosed air. If the odor is suggestive of English walnuts the seed is first rate; if the odor is that of stale butter the seed is unfit for bird food.

Canary seed is tested for freshness in the same manner, excepting that the uncrushed seed is used. If the odor resembles that of mouldy bread the seed is unfit for bird food.

Another test for canary seed is to double up your fist and thrust it down into the bag. If the fist goes down into the seed easily, it means the seed is sun-cured; if the fist goes down into the seed only with great difficulty, it means that the seed has been kiln-dried and is of inferior quality.

Rape seed is tested by chewing half a teaspoonful of it until all the seeds are broken. Good rape does not bite the tongue. One hot seed in twenty means that the seed is of good average quality.

Both rape and hemp should be tested for oil. See RAPE SEED.

There are numerous unscrupulous dealers who mix wild mustard and other harmful seeds with their rape. The best test for contaminated seed is to plant a half-teaspoonful of it. You may be surprised at what comes up. I once grew twenty-three species of plants from a single teaspoonful of what was supposed to be pure rape seed. But I have planted other samples which did not average one off-species plant per thousand.

All seeds may be tested for dust by letting them fall through several feet of air, pouring from one container to another.

SEPTIC ENTERITIS OF CROSS BILLS. This is a bacterial septicemia of cross bills, canaries and finches in general. It is rather uncommon in America, though it is said to be of common occurrence in Europe. Whether or not birds other than finches are susceptible is not known.

Symptoms. The disease appears to follow a periodic course similar to malaria in man. There are periods of depression and illness followed by periods of apparently perfect health. There is probably a periodic fluctuation of temperature, since during the periods of illness there is loss of appetite and increased thirst. The bird dies within from ten to twelve days.

Morbid anatomy. This disease stands out from all others because the breast muscles appear yellow, as if cooked. The heart and kidneys may be yellow, too. The liver and spleen are consistently congested and enlarged.

Etiology. Pure cultures of a slender, active-motile, Gram-negative, non-liquefying, non-coagulating, gas-forming rod, which varies in length from two to two and one-half microns and in width from six-tenths to one micron can be obtained from the heart blood and organs of infected birds.

Treatment. Having had no experience with this disease, I am in no position to recommend treatment. It is possible that the same lines of treatment which have proven effective in other septicemic diseases might be efficacious in this one, too. See AVIAN DIPHTHERIA; FOWL CHOLERA; CANARY TYPHOID; B. PARATYPHOSUS B INFECTION. Should other things fail I would try quinine and anthroquinone violet. Sulfanilamide might be worth trying, too. The dosages of these three drugs would be about the same and should start at about four milligrams per bird per day and be increased gradually while the bird's reactions were studied. See SULFANILAMIDE.*

SEPTIC FEVER OF CANARIES. In America the name **Septic fever** as applied to a disease of canaries and finches, always refers to an outbreak of Avian diphtheria; in English and European bird literature, however, this name usually refers to the disease that has been described in this book under the heading CANARY NECROSIS.

SEPTIC FEVER OF PARROTS. See PSITTACOSIS.

SEPTICEMIA OF DUCKS. A number of cholera-like septicemias of ducks and geese have been reported. The descriptions of these diseases and of the organisms isolated from the various outbreaks differ somewhat, one from another, but from what I have been able to learn of them, they are in the vast majority of cases outbreaks of hemorrhagic septicemia. They are amendable to the same lines of treatment that are effective in hemorrhagic septicemia in other species of birds. It is my experience that species have little to do with the treatment of this disease. I have treated it in about two dozen species of birds and one mammal and have found that while the methods of administration and the dosages must be varied to meet the requirements of various species, the action of the treatment is about the same in all of them. The whole problem is to get the correct amounts of the drugs into the patients, be they finches or flamingoes, eagles or ostriches. See HEMORRHAGIC SEPTICEMIA; FOWL CHOLERA; AVIAN DIPHTHERIA.

---

* **Note:** This disease was studied by Tarakowski in 1899. It is described in Ward and Gallagher's "Diseases of Domesticated Birds," Macmillan Company, 1926.

SEX BREEDING. Some years ago Bernarr McFadden published an article in "Physical Culture Magazine," in which he outlined the theory that the female child was always the result of early impregnation; that the male child was always the result of late impregnation. He contended that, should a woman become pregnant during the first seven days following menstruation, the child was certain to be a female; should she become pregnant during the next five days, the child might be either male or female; should she become pregnant more than twelve days after menstruation, the child was certain to be a male. He asked his feminine readers to record their careless moments and inform him of the results.

Two years later he published another article in which he discussed the results reported in more than one thousand letters he claimed to have received from his feminine readers. The evidence offered was overwhelmingly in support of the theory. Whether this evidence actually existed or was worth the paper it was written on is something I am not prepared to pass an opinion on.

Notwithstanding that this theory appears to be in conflict with our present views regarding the inheritance of sex, as based upon the presence of sex chromosomes in the reproductive cells of male mammals and female birds, I made up my mind to put it to a test. It has now been twelve years since I started keeping sex records based upon this theory, and all of the facts at my disposal seem to indicate that it is the expression of a biological law.

It has long been known to canary breeders that the early hatches of the season predominated in male chicks, and that the chicks of the later hatches were predominantly female. Since birds are usually mated sometime after the females are ready and since the males and females are constantly together from that time until the end of the season, it is seen that the first nest would in most cases be the result of a delayed mating, while the second and third clutch of eggs would be fertilized as soon as the hen was ready. So these constantly observed fluctuations in the production of males and females are explained by this theory.

The bird breeders have had a theory of their own to account for this difference in the proportion of males and females in the early and late hatches. They have been of the opinion that the vigor of the female was the controlling factor in the development of male or female chicks—that the rested hen, full of vigor, had a tendency to produce males; that the exhausted hen had a tendency to produce females.

Experimentation. I have never made any pretenses of being a pure scientist. First, last and all the time, I am a practical bird breeder. Birds, being my only source of income, have always been my first consideration. So it will be understood that I have had no particular interest in establishing which of these theories is true; my whole interest has been in producing baby birds of the desired sexes. These facts should be borne in mind while considering the conditions of the following experiments. Had I been less breeder and more scientist, I would have arranged the conditions of my experiments in such a manner as to exclude the operation of one of these theories while I was testing the other one. I did not do that; I arranged my tests in such a manner as to take advantage of any merit there might be in either.

When the young of the first clutch have left the nest, it is the habit of the canary hen to lay a second clutch of eggs and start sitting on them while the male finishes the weaning of the birds from the first clutch. Now, since at this time the presence of the cock in the cage with the hen is a necessity—he must be there to take over the care of the babies if they are not to be neglected—it is impossible to keep him from fertilizing the second clutch of eggs as soon as the hen comes into heat. Should he refuse, as he sometimes does toward the end of the season, she would jump on his neck and try to knock his eyes out. These little ladies do not like to be neglected.

In testing these theories I permitted the hens to lay their second clutches of eggs in the normal manner, but as soon as those eggs were laid they were taken from the hen laying them and set under other hens. The test hen was taken from the breeding cage and turned into a large flight room where she would get plenty of direct sunlight and flying exercise, and, of course, the very best of food. The old man was left to wean the chicks.

Long before the chicks were weaned the hen was ready to build a third nest, but she was held back for another week. She was then put back with the same cock, and she would often be so much overdue that she would build and lay within forty-eight hours after being returned to the breeding cage. This third clutch of eggs the hen was permitted to hatch out, but when she laid her fourth clutch, when this second nest of babies was about twenty days old, the eggs were again taken from her and she was again turned into the flight for two weeks' rest, while, as before, the cock weaned the chicks.

It will be seen that each test hen was permitted to lay five clutches of eggs. Three clutches, the eggs she was permitted to set on, were all the result of delayed impregnation. The other two clutches, which were taken from her, were the result of early impregnation. These two sets of chicks were kept separate by marking the eggs and young babies with ink and then banding the older babies with different colored leg bands.

I found that the eggs from the late matings ran a little better than ninety per cent males; that the eggs laid as soon as the hen came into heat produced a little better than forty per cent males. By combining these results, I found that I was able to get from seventy to seventy-five per cent males for the entire season; also, I was able to boost the production of my hens from ten to twelve birds per season up to from fifteen to eighteen birds per season, and at the same time have them close the season in a less exhausted condition than they would have been from raising three nests in a row with no rest.

I do not say which, if either, theory is correct; but I do say that by following the method just outlined, it is possible to get half again as many chicks from the same number of pairs and to boost the percentage of males from a little over fifty per cent on the average to almost seventy-five per cent.

I have used this method for eight out of the last twelve years, but because there is a little scientist hidden somewhere in my make-up, I could not resist the temptation to try the reverse method during the other four seasons, though the practical side of my nature kept telling me I was a damn fool for doing it. I paired the birds before any of the hens were in breeding condition and then let them come into condition in the breeding cages, and I bred them straight through without a break. My average production for three of these years was forty-two per cent males. In one year the results could hardly be accepted as valuable, however, since due to some mouldy food, four hundred out of four hundred and fifty of the chicks hatched were lost from aspergillosis. A five per cent error should be allowed in all of these figures since the variation in mortality among the chicks from year to year could easily have influenced the results to that extent. When the nest mortality is high, the production of males will also be higher, since the females, being weaker, are more apt to get starved or trampled in the nest. The male's greater vigor enables him to put up a better fight for food and the attention of the parents. Once the babies leave the nests, however, the influence of mortality swings in the other direction. Many of the finest and strongest males are often lost as a result of their strength. Often, the first time one of these fine big babies is taken up in the hand he will jerk his wings with such force as to break them, or he may get his head or a foot caught in something and injure himself so badly during his struggling that he has to be killed, while a hen in the same situation would take things more quietly until she were found and released.

SHADOW CELLS. See BLOOD.

SHIVERING. A bird shivers when he is cold, the same as you do. A sick bird may shiver when the temperature is subnormal or during a rising fever. I once knew of a case where two birds were badly chilled when they were ten days old. They had suffered prolonged chilling. This hardship so affected their development that they could not grow full coats of feathers. They shivered constantly even on the hottest days. I killed one of these birds and should have killed them both but let a person talk me into giving him the other one, since it was a male and a good singer. This bird lived for more than five years that I know of and shivered constantly through the whole time.

SILICON. This metallic element has such great affinity for oxygen that it does not occur free in nature. Its most abundant compound is silica of which quartz, glass sand and agate are familiar examples. It is present in straw and in the outer coatings of some seed, particularly the brown coating of canary seeds. Silicon enters into animal and bird economy in very small quantities and is found principally in hair and feathers. See FEATHERS; BALDNESS.

SIMPLE DIARRHEA. See BISMUTH.

SILVER NITRATE. This is the silver salt of nitric acid. It comes as white crystals which darken when exposed to the light. Because it is very caustic, it is fused into sticks and used for the destruction of tissue—burning off warts, pimples, etc. See LUMPS—and for cauterizing wounds and foci of infection located on the skin and accessible mucous membranes. In this connection it is sometimes employed in the treatment of diphtheric skin lesion. See AVIAN DIPHTHERIA.

Silver nitrate is also a powerful antiseptic. It can be used on the skin in solutions up to five per cent. Two per cent solutions are used in treating the eyes. Some states have laws requiring that the eyes of every newborn infant shall be washed with a two per cent solution of silver nitrate, as a preventative for gonorrheal conjunctivitis, a condition which usually results in blindness. It is unfortunate that such laws are not universal. Several breeders have told me of good results following the treatment of diphtheric sores around the eyes and vent with silver nitrate solutions. From five to ten per cent of alcohol added to any solution of silver nitrate will greatly increase its effectiveness as an antiseptic.

SILVER PROTEIN PREPARATIONS. There are a number of these such as **protargin, argyn, lunosol, argyrol,** etc., and they come in various strengths. The only one that I have used on birds is the ten per cent solution of argyrol. This solution is strong enough to be effective and still is not irritating to the tissue. It is very valuable in the treatment of nasal infections. See ANTISEPTICS FOR THE EYES.

Figure 75.

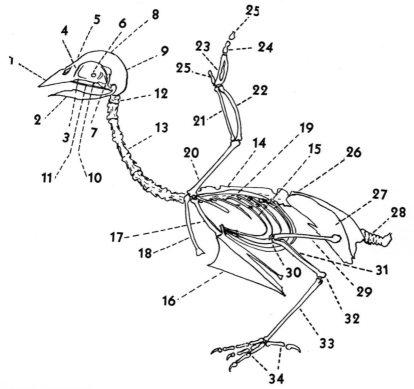

SINUS INFECTION. See ASTHMA; NASAL CAVITY; AVIAN DIPHTHERIA.

SKELETON. Figure 75 shows the Skeleton of a canary and the following list describes the principal bones:

HEAD:

(1) **Incisive.** This is upper bill. It is supported by the super-maxillary, nasal, frontal and lacrymal bones.

(2) **Mandible.** This is the lower bill. It is supported by the submaxillary (jaw) bones.

(3) **Temporals.** These bones are located at the sides of the face, just back of the eyes.

(4) **Lacrymals.** These bones are located just in front of the eyes. Together with the frontal they support the front of the face.

(5) **Frontal.** This bone extends from just above the bill to the crown of the head and takes up most of the space between the eyes.

(6) **Orbital.** This is the bony structure of the eye socket. The orbitals of birds are very large in proportion to the visible areas of their eyes.

(7) **Quadrate.** This is a bone process located at the angle of the jaw and containing the jaw socket. In birds it is set well back on the side of the head.

(8) **Parietal.** This bone forms the crown of the head. It is fused with the frontal, lacrymals, temporals in front with the mastoidals back of the ears, and with the occipital at the back of the head.

(9) **Occipital.** This bone forms the back of the skull.

(10) **Sphenoids.** These bones, there are four or more of them, form the floor of the cranium, extending from the back of the head to a point a little above the termination of the hard palate. They are formed of a number of thin plates, and it is difficult to say which of these should be considered independent bones and which parts of the same bones.

(11) **Quadrajugals.** These are long narrow strips of bone connecting the malar bones (supermaxillae) with the quadrate regions, adding strength to the supporting structure of the upper bill.

There are a great many other divisions of the bones of the head, particularly of those forming the structures surrounding the eyes and ears and supporting the beak, but these are all small bones of interest only to anatomists. Many of the divisions exist only as a basis for academic argument.

A knowledge of these structures beyond what can be obtained by dissecting a few heads is of no importance to a discussion of bird diseases.

NECK:

(12) **Atlas.** This is the first of the cervical vertebrae. It is the bone which supports the skull.

(13) **Cervical vertebrae.** The bones of the neck column. The number of cervical vertebrae vary in different species of birds, and different investigators often ascribe different numbers to the same species, as a result of lack of unanimity among anatomists concerning the point where the cervical vertebrae end and the thoracic vertebrae begin. Considering the vertebra supporting the first short rib as belonging to the thorax, a canary has eight cervical vertebrae.

THORAX:

(14) **Thoracic vertebrae.** These are seven in number and they support the ribs. The first thoracic vertebra may be free, and the last may be free or fused to the lumbar vertebrae, but the rest are usually fused together by the consolidation of their processes.

(15) **Ribs.** These are seven in number—five complete ribs and two short ribs.

(16) **Sternum.** This is the breast bone. In birds it has a high development, made necessary by the requirements of the large flight muscles for attachment space.

(17) **Coracoids.** These bones are missing from the shoulder girdles of man and animals. In birds they are very important, since they perform the function of the clavicles in man, and as we shall presently see, birds' clavicles have been modified to fulfill functions non-existent in mammals. The coracoid articulates with the sternum at one end and with the scapula at the other—their attachment being at a point just back of the shoulder socket.

(18) **Clavicles.** These are your collarbone. In birds these bones are fused at their anterior junction to form the "wishbone." They are no longer attached directly to the head of the sternum, as in mammals, but their junction point is bound to it by a short, powerful tendon. The function of the clavicles in birds is to act as a powerful spring to take up

the momentum of the wings. The flight impulses of the wings are so powerful that the bones would snap if it were not for the cushioning effect of this spring. In a previous section, SEX BREEDING, I have mentioned the fact that a fine young canary male frequently snaps a wing bone when he gets scared, excited, caught in something or is picked up unexpectedly.

(19) **Scapulae.** These are the shoulder blades. In birds they are long, saber-like bones extending down the back from the shoulders to the sixth or seventh rib.

WING:

(20) **Humerus.** This is the first bone of the wing. It corresponds to the bone of your upper arm.

(21) **Radius.** This is the small, outside bone of your forearm and the corresponding bone of a bird's wing.

(22) **Ulna.** This is the large inside bone of the forearm and of the wing. In birds it is much heavier than the radius and is curved; so that while the two bones are joined at both ends, there is considerable space between their centers.

(23) **Carpi.** These are the small bones of the wrist. In birds they are two small bones located between the ends of the radius and ulna respectively and the metacarpus.

(24) **Metacarpus.** These are the bones of the back of your hand. In birds they are fused into a single flat bone having an oblong opening running lengthwise, left by the last metacarpus being fused to the others only at its ends.

(25) **Phalanges.** These are the bones of your fingers. In the wings they fuse into one rather heavy bone which corresponds to the last joints of your finger and a light bone corresponding to the rest of the finger. The heavy phalange which corresponds to the outer side of your little finger carries the primary flight feathers. The metacarpus, which corresponds to the back edge of your hand, carries the secondary flight feathers. There is a rudimentary thumb, but the feather it carries is purely decorative.

HIPS:

(26) **Lumbar and sacral vertebrae.** These bones are fused to add their bit to that massive structure usually called the **ilium,** the pelvic arch.

(27) **Ilium, Ischium, Pubis.** These three bones are fused to make up the rest of the pelvic arch, which has been more thoroughly discussed under the heading PELVIC ARCH.

TAIL:

(28) **Coccygeal vertebrae.** There are seven coccygeal vertebrae. The last one, which supports the tail, is flattened on both sides and curved at the end. It is called the **Pygostyle.**

LEG:

(29) **Femu.** This is the upper bone of the leg.

(30) **Patella.** This is the kneecap.

(31) **Fibula.** This is the small shin bone in birds—it does not reach to the ankle.

(32) **Tibia.** This is the large bone of the foreleg.

(33) **Metatarsus.** This is the first bone of the foot. It is the familiar scaly shank but it really corresponds to that group of bones which form the arch of your foot. If you should ever dissolve the flesh off of a bird's leg and foot by immersing them in a solution of sodium hypochlorite, you would discover that birds have a heel as distinct as yours but it is located at the top of the scaly shank.

(34) **Phalanges.** These are the bones of the fingers and toes. In birds they form the tips of the wings and the claws.

SKIN. The feathered areas of a bird's skin are considerably thicker than the unfeathered areas and are provided with muscles for elevating and depressing the feathers; there are no sweat glands and the only oil glands are a few small ones located in the ears and the large glands located in the pygostyle. The skin as well as the rest of the body of a small bird is rather porous, however. Mineral oil administered into the crop in food will penetrate the body tissues and escape through the skin to foul the feathers. From what tests I have made, though I have not run controlled tests on well birds, I am convinced that mineral oil is distinctly harmful.

The most common skin lesions are those of diphtheria and of the mould infections such as favus. See FUNGOID SKIN.

SKULL. A bird's skull is formed of two thin layers of bone separated by a web-like structure containing many air cavities. The principal lesions involving the bone structure of the skull are those resulting from exudates into the suborbital and mastoid sinuses and hemorrhages into the air cavities. The suborbital sinus may become involved as the result of any infection of the nasal passages, but the only cases of mastoiditis to come to my attention were the aftermath of diphtheria. Hemorrhages into the air spaces are common lesions of apoplectiform septicemia and food poisoning, though they sometimes occur as the result of head injuries caused by striking unseen objects in flight. The heavy varieties of canaries, Yorkshires, Norwiches, Coppies, often suffer fatal head injuries from bumps received during flight, though rollers and the other light varieties seldom injure themselves in this manner.

The principal bones of the skull have been enumerated and their locations pointed out under the heading SKELETON. See AVIAN DIPHTHERIA; APOPLECTIFORM SEPTICEMIA; NASAL CAVITY.

SLEEPING SICKNESS. So far as I know, this disease has never been observed in America. It has been studied in Germany, where it exists as a natural disease of poultry, by Dammann and Manegold and later by Greve. It is not known to attack pet birds. The disease runs a rather chronic course; its most pronounced symptom being a marked desire to sleep in the daytime.* Sometimes the conjunctiva of one eye becomes reddened and swollen. There is usually diarrhea.

This disease is caused by a streptococcus which is distinguished from the streptococcus of apoplectiform septicemia by the fact that it is encapsulated while that of apoplectiform septicemia is not. There are many points of resemblance between sleeping sickness of fowls and gastro-enteritic form of apoplectiform septicemia.

SLIPPED CLAW. This condition is the result of a nest injury.† It is a dislocation of the back claw, which usually occurs when there are but one or two chicks in the nest. The hen, in her efforts to keep the chicks warm, covers them too closely. In moving around the baby gets one of its back claws slipped forward, between the front toes and, because of the weight of the hen, is unable to raise up and get the claw back into the correct position. The chick is growing very fast and it takes only a short time for the claw to grow into the abnormal position and for the baby to lose the power of moving it.

---

* **Note:** I would not consider sleeping in the daytime a very characteristic symptom, since it is a common symptom of many bird diseases.

† **Note:** Dr. Herbert Sanborn has informed me that he has observed cases of slipped claw in the blackbirds which had been taken from the nest shortly after hatching and raised by hand. It was his opinion that the condition resulted from a deficiency of vitamin D in the diet. When the affected birds were given cod-liver oil they recovered the control of their back claws. I have never seen a canary recover from this condition without the intervention of local, mechanical treatment.

By the time the baby is ready to leave the nest all voluntary control over the affected claw has been lost. Naturally, the affected bird is unable to grasp the perches. See Figure 76.

Treatment. The treatment for slipped claw is very simple. All that is required is to catch the bird and bind the affected claw back against the shank with a small piece of adhesive tape and let it remain in that position for several weeks. Sometimes the claw can

Figure 76. **SLIPPED CLAW**

Freehand sketches by the author illustrating slipped claw and the method of treatment.

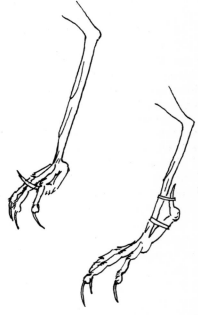

be bent back against the shank and held in place with an open celluloid leg band. Care must be taken not to bind the leg so tightly that the circulation will be cut off, for then the foot will be lost. There are some cases of long standing in which the claw cannot be bent back against the shank without breaking it. In such cases the claw is bent back as far as possible and bound in that position for a week or two; it is then rebandaged, taking it back a little more. This is continued until the claw has been held back against the shank for about two weeks. If the claw slips forward again when the tape is taken off, it is bandaged back for a couple of weeks more. Some of these cases are very persistent, but they can all be cured with a little patience. I have cured cases which were of two years' standing at the time the first treatments were given.

SODIUM SALICYLATE. This is the sodium salt of salicylic acid. See SALICYLIC ACID AND SALICYLATES. It is employed in human medicine as an antiseptic for the intestinal and urogenital tracts and the serous surfaces, particularly those of the pleurae and joints. It is a specific for acute articular rheumatism (inflammatory rheumatism). It is also employed in the treatment of colds and headaches.

Sodium salicylate is of value in bird medicine for the treatment of colds and other inflammations of the respiratory tract. The dose for a pet bird is from ¼ to ½ grain to the ounce of drinking water. It should never be administered for more than four consecutive days at one time; and it should always be discontinued at the first signs of salicylate poisoning, which are: loss of appetite, dullness of hearing; dimness of vision; shortness of breath; diarrhea—sometimes there is rapid, irregular, deep breathing, followed by collapse, coma and death.

The treatment of salicylic poisoning in birds consists of placing the bird in a warm place and administering stimulants. Three drops of I.Q.S. may be added to the ounce of drinking water. A cropful of strong, lukewarm coffee may be administered with a medicine dropper.

SODIUM FLUORIDE. This is one of the natural constituents of bone, but it is not used in food or medicine, excepting as it occurs as a natural constituent of foods. It comes on the market as a heavy white powder, which, when dry, is only slightly irritating to the skin, though when it is moist or in strong solution, sodium fluoride is very caustic. It is one of the best insecticides known and it is extremely effective against bird lice. See FEATHER LICE.

This powder is poisonous and should never be used in the nests. Should sodium fluoride be taken by a person by mistake, it should be followed by a large quantity of egg white and a teaspoonful of Epsom salts dissolved in a glass of warm water, which will convert the sodium fluoride into the insoluble magnesium salt. In using this powder around birds, care should be taken to see that it does not get into the food and water. A 1:4 dilution of sodium fluoride with white flour is much more effective as an insect powder than the pure chemical; it is lighter and more apt to be carried into the insect's respiratory mechanism.

SOFT MOULT. French moult. This is a condition in which birds continue to moult and grow feathers until they become exhausted and die, usually from some minor infection to which their lowered resistance and weakened condition has made them susceptible.

Etiology. Soft moult is usually caused by keeping a bird in a place that is too warm. Continuous feeding of bread and milk will sometimes cause soft moult. The feeding of lettuce is said to predispose to its development. And, it may follow over-dosing with potassium chlorate.* This drug is sometimes used in medicines for the cure of baldness and for that reason such foods and medicines should be avoided.

Treatment. The best treatment for soft moult is to place the ailing birds in a large, cool flight room and feed them on a diet containing good quality seeds and plenty of green food. A very little egg food that is not too rich will help build up their strength. An iron tonic, either I.Q.S. or IRON AND QUININE CITRATE may be used, but no tonic can correct the effects of an overheated room if the temperature is not corrected.

SOFT SHELL EGGS. See VITAMIN D; EGG STRUCTURE AND FORMATION; MINERAL FOOD.

SONG RESTORERS. There are many foods on the market advertised as song restorers, concerning which one point should always be borne in mind: any healthy, happy, tight-feathered, mature, male canary will sing without inducement. It is his natural way of working off his surplus energy. To keep a bird healthy and happy it is necessary to see that his diet contains small amounts of certain foods which will supply certain elements that may be missing from his standard diet. There are many mixtures on the market built around this idea. Some of these contain from twenty to thirty species of garden and weed seeds together with a little dried egg yolk and finely chopped dried fruit. The theory is that the bird's natural cravings will cause him to pick out and eat the foods that will supply the elements lacking from his regular diet. This is a fairly sound theory, and a good song restorer or **tonic-seed** mixture will do much to keep a bird in health and song. The bird's natural cravings do tell him things about his condition that his owner can never know. It must be remembered, however, that these mixtures are not a general diet, but a supplement to it. A child may like and need candy, cake and ice cream; war conditions have shown us that persons deprived of these things will do absolutely anything to obtain them, sell their bodies or commit murder with equal readiness, but, candy, cake and ice cream would be a

* **Note:** What I have said here should not be misunderstood. Potassium chlorate is a valuable drug, but when you use drugs you should know what you are doing. For that reason all prepared food suspected of containing drugs should always be avoided.

very poor substitute for beef and potatoes as a regular diet. Most of the good tonic seed mixture can be given to hens making eggs and to moulting birds in unlimited quantities, and where this is the general practice, the birds are not apt to overeat. At other times, however, each bird should receive not more than one eggdrawer (these are little cups which hold about ¼ of a teaspoonful and slip between the wires of the cage) of tonic seed per day.

Not all manufacturers are satisfied to trust to the bird's natural craving for the success of their products. Some are tempted to add stimulating drugs to their song restorers—drugs which may make an ailing bird sing for a day or two but wind up by poisoning him and ruining his health beyond repair. If your bird is sick, learn what is wrong with him and treat his illness in exactly the same manner as your doctor would treat yours. Use drugs, naturally, but know what you are about when you are doing it. A sick bird does not sing but there is no special food that is a general cure-all. It would be as stupid to expect such results as it would be to believe all that the human food faddists claim for their particular eating systems.

When a bird is well, you might try to keep him that way by supplying him with a reasonable amount of good tonic seed, but do not expect such preparations to perform miracles—it can't happen.

Formula for a Song Restorer or Tonic Seed Mixture:

Niger seed .... 5 parts
Maw seed .... 3 parts
Whole groat oats.......................... 2 parts
Mixed red millet.......................... 2 parts
Flax .... 2 parts
Sesame .... 2 parts
Gold of pleasure seed..................... 1 part
Dandelion seed .... 1 part
White lettuce seed........................ 1 part
Wild weed seeds * .... 3 parts

---

* **Note:** At the large seed houses, the bulk seeds which are received from all parts of the world, are run through recleaning machinery to remove all dirt and foreign seeds. Among the materials removed from the cultivated bird seeds are dozens of varieties of weed seeds. These are again recleaned to remove the dust and dirt and then sold as **wild weed seeds** or **wild bird-seed.** Now there is a good chance that some of the seeds contained in such a mixture are going to be poisonous, and though I have seen samples of wild weed seeds that could be fed to birds with day-old chicks without harming those chicks, this is not the general rule. Other samples have killed every chick, but the old birds receiving small quantities of these mixtures seem to be greatly benefited. It will be noticed, however, that they soon learn to pick out certain of the seeds and discard the others. In view of these facts, tonic-seed mixtures containing wild weed seeds should not be given to birds having babies under ten days old.

And, if to this mixture you will add five parts of finely chopped figs and raisins and five parts of egg-yolk powder, you will have as fine a tonic seed mixture as you could get anywhere.

The figs and raisins should be run through the fine plate of a food chopper and the egg yolk and a little ground bread, if necessary, should be rubbed into the chopped fruit until it is no longer sticky.

SOOR. See OIDIUM ALBICANS.

SPINAL CORD. See NERVOUS SYSTEM.

SPIROCHETES. These are thread-like, corkscrew-shaped organisms. Some species are motile by means of flagella located at one end; others are motile by means of a peculiar corkscrew motion. They are observed to best advantage in fresh preparations under the dark field microscope.

Spirochetes are generally classified as protozoa,* though some investigators have classified them with the bacteria. Some species of spirochetes have been cultivated by the use of a special media and technique.

Spirochetes are responsible for morbid lesions in man, animals and birds. Syphilis, relapsing fever and Vincent's angina (a common disease of the gums) are examples of human spirochetosis.

In addition to the pathogenic spirochetes, there are hundreds of harmless varieties, one of which is a normal inhabitant of the human mouth. Other harmless varieties are found in water and on the skin and mucous membranes of man and animals. Those forms which are blood parasites, the hematozoa,† are often transmitted by biting insects which act as secondary hosts for the parasites. In some cases the parasites pass from one generation of ticks to the next by means of the egg of the parent tick and can still cause disease in susceptible animals after a number of such passages. Thus, the bite of the great-granddaughter of an infested tick can cause disease in a susceptible animal.

SPIROCHETOSIS. Avian spirochetosis is a highly fatal, acute septicemic disease of birds characterized by ruffled feathers, som-

---

* **Note:** The classification **protozoan** includes all of the single-cell animals; the **bacteria** are single-cell vegetable organisms. As a general rule, bacteria can be cultivated with ease; protozoa, on the other hand, are artificially cultivated with great difficulty or not at all.

† **Note:** A **hematozoon** is a **protozoon** invader of the blood stream.

nolence, high fever, and diarrhea. It is caused by a spirochete which is transmitted by the bite of the fowl ticks, **Argus miniatis, Argus persicus.***

Geese, ducks, chickens, guinea fowls, turtle doves, pigeons, sparrows, canaries and finches are known to be susceptible to spirochetic septicemia, though there is some doubt as to whether causative organisms and transmitting insects are the same in all cases. All species of birds are probably susceptible.

The carrier. The fowl ticks, **Argus miniatis, Argus persicus,** are sometimes called **blue bugs** and range from southwestern Arkansas through southern and western Texas, southern New Mexico, southern Arizona, southern and western California, to a point slightly north of San Francisco. Climatic conditions in other parts of the United States do not seem to be suitable for this pest, though ticks imported with birds may sometimes find conditions favorable to them for a short time and may cause transitory outbreaks of spirochetosis.

The habits of the fowl tick resemble closely those of the red mite and our domestic bedbug. It lives in cracks and crevices during the day, depositing its egg there; it comes out at night to feed on the blood of roosting birds.

The destruction of fowl ticks is not so simple. Adult ticks have been known to live for two and one-half years without food; they display a very high resistance to ordinary disinfectants and insecticides. One of the methods suggested for their control is the construction of all metal poultry houses of galvanized sheet steel over frames of iron pipe set in concrete. This construction makes the extermination of ticks very simple. The poultryman turns his birds out in the morning, covers the floor of the house with a little litter, throws a gallon or two of gasoline over the litter and touches a match to it. By evening, the house is cool enough for the chickens to be returned to it. Fair results are said to be obtainable by spraying the houses at frequent intervals with a power sprayer; using, first, a mixture of carbolineum, crude oil and kerosene in

---

* **Note:** Some writers mention **Argus miniatis** and others mention **Argus persicus** as the carrier of **Sp. gallinarum** or **Sp. avian**—whichever we care to call the spirochete responsible for this disease, depending on whether we consider it strictly a chicken disease or a disease of birds in general— but whether or not these are two distinct species of ticks or two names for a single species is not clear. The entomologists I have consulted have been able to throw no light on the subject.

equal parts; then, after several days, respraying with a thick white-wash which will fill all cracks.

The fowl tick is known to attack chickens, turkeys, geese, pigeons, sparrows, ostriches and canaries.

Whether or not spirochetosis is spread by insects other than the fowl tick, does not appear to be definitely known, though there is some reason for suspecting nest bugs and bedbugs. The latter is the carrier of **relapsing fever**, which is the human counterpart of **Avian spirochetosis.**

Etiology. The cause of avian spirochetosis has been variously designated **Spirocheta gallinatum, Spirocheta anserinum, Treponema anserina,** etc., etc. I think, however, that until such time as they are definitely shown to be distinct species, the designation **Sp. avian** is much preferable.*

The organism in question is a slender, thread-like, spiral shaped, active motile body of an average length of nine to ten microns and a maximum length of about eighteen to twenty microns. The average width is about 0.5 micron. It forms from three to four nodes and is sharply pointed at the ends.

The life history of this spirochete has been worked out by Hindle,† who has shown that multiplication takes place by two methods. First, the free-swimming parasite in the blood plasma grows until it has attained a length of eighteen to twenty microns; then one end bends back upon itself and coils around the body until it is even with the other end, until the organism takes on the appearance of a thread twisted upon itself and then cut off so that both ends are equal distance from the point of flexure. The ends are slightly uncoiled as the ends of the twisted thread would be. Then the organism begins to uncoil, while at the same time division begins to take place at the point of flexure. By the time the uncoiling is complete the division is usually complete, though sometimes the daughter parasites remain attached to each other for some time after the uncoiling has been completed. At a certain stage in the attack the spirochetes break up into small coccoid bodies about one-half micron in diameter. These bodies are not known or thought to undergo further development in the affected bird.

Second, when a spirochete is taken into the body of a feeding

---

* **Note:** In the classification of spirochetes and other organisms, too—for that matter—the terms **gallinarum, anserinum, muris,** etc., mean simply: "pertaining to chickens"—"pertaining to geese"—"pertaining to mice." spirochete found in the blood of a parrot would be called **Sp. psittacum,** found in the blood of a canary it would be designated **Sp. canarias.** The designation **avian** simply means "pertaining to birds."
† **Note:** Hindle, Parasitology, Volume IV, 1911, p. 463.

tick, it makes its way through the intestinal wall and invades the
cells of such organs as the gonads, salivary gland and other organs.
Some of the spirochetes remain in the intestines of the tick.   After

Figure 77.   **SPIROCHETOSIS**

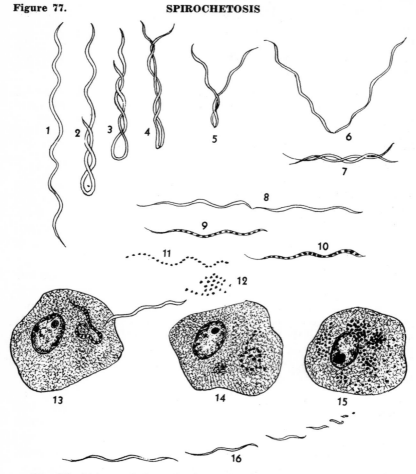

The life history of the spirochete of avian tick fever as worked out
by Hindle.
Figures **1** to **8,** inclusive, illustrate the method of division in the blood
of the infected bird.
Figures **9** to **12,** inclusive, illustrate coccoid division in the blood, which
takes place rarely.
Figures **13** to **15,** inclusive, illustrate coccoid division in the invaded
cell of the infected tick.
Figure **16** shows the growth of a coccoid body into a mature spirochete.
(After Hindle.)

invading a cell of the tick the spirochete breaks up into coccoid bodies which continue to divide by fission (simple division). Some of the coccoid bodies are passed out in the excrement of the tick, and though it was formerly thought that coccoid bodies were introduced into the blood of the bird directly by the bite of the tick, it is now believed that infection takes place by the contamination of the bite wound with tick excrement. In some cases spirochetes have been observed to invade the blood cells of birds and there undergo coccoid division, but this is not usual. Figure 77 illustrates the life history of the spirochete as it was worked out by Hindle.

Sp. avian has been cultivated by Noguchi in a special media consisting of a piece of fresh rabbit kidney or fowl muscle, which has been aseptically removed from the body and placed in a sterile tube with ascitic fluid. The ascitic fluid is poured into the tube on top of the fresh tissue to a depth of about ten centimeters. Then a few drops of blood aseptically drawn from an affected fowl and mixed with an equal amount of sterile physiological salt solution, to which has been added 1.5 per cent of sodium citrate are dropped into the tube. The culture is then sealed with a half-inch cap of sterile mineral oil.

The organism has been cultivated on this media for thirteen generations without loss of virulence; although under some conditions of cultivation, it has been known to lose its virulence. Inoculation with an avirulent (no longer able to produce disease) strain is said to confer resistance against infection by a virulent strain.

The disease may be experimentally produced by means of an infected tick, by placing infective material on scarified skin, or even on the unscarified skin or by placing infective material in the food or drinking water, which suggests that under favorable circumstances, spirochetosis may possibly become epizootic without the intervention of a secondary host.

Symptoms. Like most septicemic diseases, spirochetosis occurs in three forms, peracute, acute, and chronic. In the peracute form birds which were apparently well in the evening are found dead the next morning. In the acute form there are the general symptoms of illness: dullness, ruffled feathers, a tendency to sleep in the daytime, high fever and diarrhea. The attack has a distinct crisis, at which time the spirochetes disappear from the blood and the temperature drops to normal, much as it does in relapsing fever and malaria in man. During the course of the disease there is a large destruction of red blood cells and an increase in the number of polymorphonuclear leucocytes; but as soon as the spirochetes disappear from the blood there is a decrease in the number of polymorphonuclear leucocytes and an increase in the number of mononuclear leucocytes. The bird often dies in convulsions on the fourth or fifth day of the illness.

The chronic form of the disease often makes its appearance towards the end of the outbreak, though there are outbreaks which are chronic from the onset. In this form of the disease there are marked paralytic symptoms. The head may be twisted back as in fowl paralysis, or the wings and legs may be affected; the claws become useless. The bird may lose the ability to hold the ankle joints straight, and thus appears to be knock-kneed or bowlegged. There is great emaciation. Death may occur from the tenth to the fifteenth day.

Morbid anatomy. When the disease has run an acute course, the liver and the spleen are always congested and enlarged; the spleen to two or three times normal size. The liver is often yellow in color, as a result of fatty degeneration, and may contain necrotic spots. Other tissues are usually pale because of the pronounced anemia, though in some cases there are congested areas or small hemorrhagic spots in the intestines.

Spirochetes can be found in the blood only during the febrile stage which means, while there is an active fever.

Treatment. According to Huaer, and also Araggao, Salvarsan * in doses of from 0.005 gram to 0.05 gram per kilo of body weight, injected intramuscularly, acts as an absolute specific for this condition even when administered on the fourth or fifth day of the illness when the bird is in a state of coma and almost at the point of death, it is said to bring about the most remarkable and immediate recovery. Salvarsan also confers upon the birds treated a high degree of immunity which lasts for a considerable period. Dose for a 28-gram canary would be 0.14 milligram.

SPLEEN. If after opening the abdomen the investigator will cut away the connective tissue which holds the left side of the gizzard and duodenum in place and lift them up, he will see a small, red, sausage-shaped, gland-like organ lying between the left lower mar-

---

* **Note:** Salvarsan is a poison. The fatal dose for a chicken has been found to be 0.3 gram (5 grains) per kilo of body weight. The maximum therapeutic dose tolerated is 0.15 gram per kilo of body weight, or about half of the lethal dose, which in turn, is about three times the largest dose used in the treatment of the disease.

Figure 78.   SPLEEN

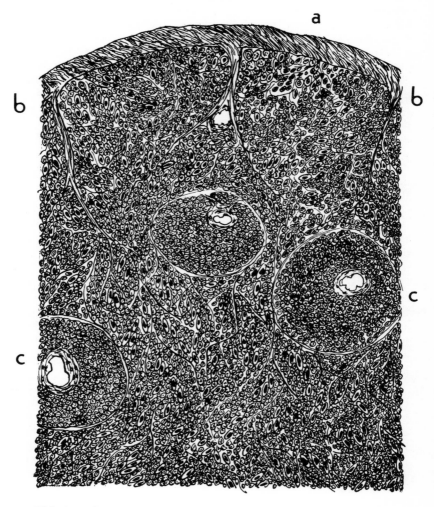

This is a freehand drawing from the spleen of a sparrow that died of FOWL CHOLERA. The organ was somewhat enlarged and congested.

a, Muscular capsule.

b, b, Trabeculae.

c, c, Malpighian bodies.

Magnification about 445 ×.

Tissue fixed in mercury-iron solution and stained in toto in hematoxylin and eosin.

Section and drawing by Robert Stroud.

gin of the liver and the coiled intestines and attached to the dorsal side of the duodenum. This is the spleen. In an adult canary in a state of health, this organ is about three-thirty-seconds of an inch thick and about three-eighths of an inch long. See "C," Figure 1.

The functions of the spleen and the lymphatic tissues in general are the filtering of blood and the destruction of foreign bodies contained therein, such as bacteria, bits of protein, and degenerated blood cells; the formation of blood cells, particularly those of the lymphocyte series, but in disease and cases involving rapid blood destruction, this tissue seems to be able to take over part of the load placed on the red marrow of the bones and assist in the formation of red cells for the blood; and there is some evidence for believing that the spleen also elaborates hormones acting on the bone marrow and exercising a restraining influence upon the formation of cells for the blood.

The cells in the centers of the small compartments into which this tissue is divided are those concerned with the production of new cells. Those closely packed cells—not very well shown on this drawing—hugging the trabeculae—Figure 78—are circulating cells of the lymphatic system.

The supporting structure of the spleen is formed of what is called reticulo-endothelial tissue, the cells of which are believed to be the most powerful phagcytes (cells that destroy germs and other foreign proteins in the blood by ingesting and digesting them, in plain language, eating them) in the body.

The exact part played in these functions by the malpighian bodies seem to be still in doubt.*

The lesions found in the spleens of canaries which have died of canary necrosis, tuberculosis, apoplectiform septicemia and B. paratyphosus B infection are so characteristic that it is almost possible to base a diagnosis on the examination of this one organ; but it is also the seat of marked lesion in a great many other conditions caused both by infections and poisons. These changes may vary from slight hyperemic enlargement to complete necrotic destruction of its medullary tissue.

SPLINTS. See BROKEN BONES.

SPORADIC PNEUMONIA. See PNEUMONIA.

STAPHYLOCOCCUS PYOGENES ALBUS AND AUREUS. This is one of the common pus germs. The elements are small cocci

---

* **Note:** See Hill's "Manual of Histology," Fourth Edition, 1937, page 150, and Osgood's "Atlas of Hematology," 1937, page 152.

which vary in diameter from 0.4 to 1.2 microns (the average diameter is about 0.8 micron) and grows in grape-like clusters by dividing in two plans. It is the cause of **pyemia** in man, **sporadic pneumonia** in canaries, **osteo arthritis** in ducks and geese and has been found in a great many lesions in man, animals and birds, one of which is a paralytic disease of ostriches in which, although another organism is considered the etiological factor, the staphylococcus pyogenes aureus is consistently found in the sub-mucous tissue of the duodenum. Figure 79 shows the general appearance of this organism under the microscope. For a complete description see any work on pathogenic bacteria.*

Figure 79. STAPHYLOCOCCUS. PYOGENES AUREUS

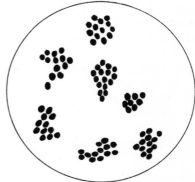

FREEHAND SKETCH ILLUSTRATING SOME OF THE FORMS COMMONLY TAKEN BY CLUMPS OF STAPHYLOCOCCI

Drawn by Robert Stroud.

STERILITY. This is the inability to reproduce. Hens that have been improperly cared for, that have been overworked, may lose the power to produce hatchable eggs. Males that are out of condition for any reason, that are moulting, that have been fed on certain harmful foods, such as mustard seed, may lose the power to fertilize eggs. See CLEAR EGGS; GENERATIVE SYSTEM.

STERNUM. See SKELETON.

STOMACH. See DIGESTIVE TRACT.

STOMACH DISORDERS. See DIGESTIVE DISORDERS; PARROTS, INDIGESTION IN.

STREPTOCOCCI. The organisms of this classification grow in long chains. See Figure 3. They are small spherical or oval bodies varying in diameter from 0.5 to 2.5 microns. The chains may contain from three or four to a hundred or more units. In some species of oval units the chains are formed on the short axis of the ele-

---

* **Note:** Sulfathiazol and sulfadiazine should be tried in all diseases caused by this germ. Dose as of sulfanilamide.

ments; in other species they are formed on the long axis. Unstained, fresh preparations of these organisms look like strings or skeins of pearls. Stained, they look like colored beads.

STROUD'S SPECIFIC. Many times in this book I have mentioned STROUD'S SPECIFIC, STROUD'S SALTS NO. 1, STROUD'S EFFERVESCENT BIRD SALTS, and STROUD'S SPECIAL PRESCRIPTION, and you have probably thought that these preparations were some deep and magical secret. That is not the case, however. They are magical in that the results they produce in certain types of diseases are most astounding, and the more so when the simplicity of the preparations is considered.

STROUD'S SPECIFIC consists of STROUD'S EFFERVESCENT BIRD SALTS and STROUD'S SALTS NO. 1, packed separately. It was so called because used together these two preparations act as an absolute specific for avian diphtheria and a number of other diseases of a septicemic nature.

STROUD'S EFFERVESCENT BIRD SALTS consists of:

Citric acid	2 parts
Tartaric acid	2 parts
Dibasic ortho sodium phosphate	2 parts
Sodium sulphate	2 parts
Sodium bicarbonate	8 parts

Only pure, dehydrated drugs are used. The citric acid is mixed with the bicarbonate and the result dried slowly in a warmer, since the mixture becomes moist as the result of chemical action. The resulting product is crushed and mixed with the other ingredients and the mixture stored in tight containers.

STROUD'S SALTS NO. 1. This was formerly called STROUD'S AVIAN ANTISEPTIC. It consists of nothing more than the very best grade of sodium perborate. Any sample assaying less than ten per cent available oxygen is discarded, and by paying a special premium for this drug I used to attempt to secure lots assaying from 11.5 to 12 per cent available oxygen. During the five or six years this product was on the market I was able to cure hundreds of thousands of sick birds of dozens of different species with it.

STROUD'S SPECIAL PRESCRIPTION is nothing more than a mixture of these two products in equal proportions. It was found that in some conditions they worked best that way, but, as the mixture did not keep well, it was only mixed in small lots to fill special orders; hence, the name.

STRYCHNINE. This is an alkaloid present in **nux vomica.** A bitter tonic, a motor stimulant, a dangerous poison, strychnine is a valuable constituent of a number of very useful prescriptions.

Experiments on the poisonous effects of strychnine on birds have been conducted by Gallagher and by Schneider. Gallagher worked with chickens; Schneider worked with geese, ducks, chickens and pigeons.

Gallagher found that 2 grains of strychnine was fatal to a three-pound fowl but not fatal to a five-pound fowl.* The drug was administered in gelatin capsules per os and by injection.

Schneider's results were given in terms of milligrams per kilo of body weight. He found the therapeutic doses administered subcutaneously to be:

Geese 0.4; Ducks 0.5 to 0.6; Chickens 1.0; Pigeons 0.5 to 0.75. The lethal dose, subcutaneously:

Geese 1.0 to 2; Ducks 1.0 to 1.1; Chickens 3.0 to 5.0; Pigeons 1 to 1.5.

The therapeutic dose per os:†

Geese 0.6; Ducks 1.5 to 2.0; Chickens 2.0 to 3.0; Pigeons 6.0. The lethal dose per os:

Geese 2.5; Ducks 3.0 to 4.5; Chickens 30.0; Pigeons 8.5 to 11.0.

I have found that one minim of I.Q.S. tonic, containing 0.0275 per cent of strychnine, administered to a canary per os, is almost instantly fatal, and that three minims of this preparation to the ounce of drinking water for one week will usually cause pronounced symptoms of strychnine poisoning—violent colonic convulsions lasting from four to ten seconds whenever the bird is disturbed—continuous nervous twitchings. Calculating from this data we find that the lethal dose for a canary is something less than 1/4000 of a grain and that the maximum therapeutic dose is from 1/8000 to to 1/10000 of a grain every twenty-four hours. See I.Q.S.; NUX VOMICA.

SUBORBITAL SINUSES. These are small cavities located on the sides of the head, anteriorly and ventrally to the forward margins of the sphenoid bones, between the nasal cavity, with which they communicate and the orbital region. The floor of the suborbital cavity is below the floor of the nasal cavity; the communication is by means of a short, curved tube which dips sharply downward from the floor of the nasal cavity. This arrangement affords very poor natural drainage. See NASAL CAVITIES.

---

* **Note:** Two grains is just about the fatal dose for a hundred and fifty-pound man, which shows that chickens are only about 1/30 as susceptible to this drug as we are.

† **Note: Per os** means by way of the mouth.

SULFANILAMIDE. Para-aminobenzene-sulfonamide, which for convenience has been shortened to **sulfanilamide,** was discovered by a German chemical worker, named Gelmo, something over thirty years ago. The therapeutic properties of this substance remained undiscovered until 1932, when two other chemical workers combined it with a naphthalene compound and obtained a red dyestuff. Under the name **prontosyl,** this dye was placed on the market as a patent medicine for use in gonorrhea. Soon it was discovered that it had wonderful curative powers in a wide range of diseases resulting from micrococci infections, particularly those of the most deadly strains of streptococci.

At first, investigators were puzzled to explain the fact that while the drug killed the germs inside of the body, it would not kill them in the test tube. And in this respect, it is worthy of noting in this place, that had these dye workers been living in the United States their product would have been driven from the market by the Pure Food and Drug Administration. Fortunately, they were living in Germany before the advent of Hitler. Their preparation was not driven from the market and it was soon discovered that the germ-killing power of the drug was due to the fact that it was decomposed in the human body and the para-aminobenzene-sulfonamide set free, and that it was this substance which destroyed the germs of disease.

This drug has been used in no less than fourteen highly fatal diseases of man with wonderful results. So far as I know, it has never been used in the treatment of the diseases of birds, but there is no reason for believing that it would not give the same results in bird diseases. It should be of particular value in any of the bacterial septicemias. The only micrococcus disease of man for which it has proved of little value is pneumonia, which is due to thirty-two different varieties of encapsulated diplococci.

It appears that sulfanilamide is ineffective against these organisms because it has no power to penetrate their capsule.

I have recently tested this drug and one of its derivatives, sulfathiazol, on a number of chronic conditions affecting canaries and I have found that sulfanilamide will cure Fowl Paralysis in a single application. The dose for a 28-gram canary is 1/10 grain into the crop. A second dose of this same size given to a 24-gram canary 24 hours after the first dose caused death; though a second 1/10 grain dose given to a 30-gram canary 24 hours after it had received the first dose did not cause death.

It appears that repeat doses are unadvisable, and, if given, should never be larger than ½ the initial or preceding dose.

SULFAPYRIDINE. This is a sulfanilamide derivative which combines the germ-killing power of the latter drug with a unique power to penetrate the capsule of pneumococci. It is an even more effective drug than sulfanilamide, and its use is indicated in all of the infectious diseases of birds. In human medicines it has been found effective against several of the virus diseases as well as against the bacterial infections. The dose for a bird would be about the same as the dose of sulfanilamide. In human subjects in conditions not involving pus this drug is less toxic than sulfanilamide, but in conditions involving pus it enters into chemical combination with the pus and the resulting compound is plenty toxic, and I don't mean maybe. A short time ago I had lobar pneumonia and was badly poisoned by an overdose of this drug. I have not used it on birds. Dose as of sulfanilamide.

SULFATHIAZOL. This is a still more recent derivative of sulfanilamide and is said to be both less toxic and more effective than either sulfanilamide or sulfapyridine. It is claimed that sulfathiazol is as effective as sulfanilamide against gonococci and more effective than sulfapyridine against pneumococci infection, while it is also effective against staphylococci infections. I have used it on canaries suffering with cold; mild attacks of bronchitis, associated with noisy breathing; and on several birds affected with chronic bowel and liver conditions that had resisted all other forms of treatment, with very good results. The dose should be 1/10 grain the first day; 1/15 grain the second day; 1/20 grain the third day. The drug is introduced into the crop in pill form. A saline in the drinking water lessens the danger of poisoning, which is not as great with this drug as with the other two. Three days' treatment should be sufficient for curing any infection against which the drug is effective.

SUET. This is the hard fat of cattle and sheep, and all birds that eat animal food of any kind are very fond of it. Where canaries and finches are wintered in a cold flight room, a chunk or two of suet, nailed in places where they can be conveniently pecked at, is a valuable addition to the diet.

SUISEPTICUM BACTERIUM. This is a member of the **Pasteurella** or **hemorrhagic septicemia** group of organisms. It is the cause of swine plague and is to all intents and purposes identical with the organism of fowl cholera.

SULPHUR AS FOOD, MEDICINE, OINTMENT. Sulphur is a nonmetallic element occurring free in nature as **brimstone**. It enters into a large number of inorganic and organic compounds and is one of the elements essential to life and health. It is found in such animal products as albumens and caseins—blood, milk, eggs, muscle, skin, hair and feathers. Because of this fact, many breeders are under the impression that free sulphur added to the diet will benefit their birds; that it will act as a tonic and improve the nutrition; that it will promote the growth of feathers. I think that this is an erroneous opinion. Only a very small proportion of the sulphur consumed can be absorbed and metabolized, and I am not certain that the part which is used does the body any particular good.

When sulphur is consumed, that part which is absorbed appears to act as a mild tonic and alterative. Many persons can remember when it used to be a habit to feed molasses and sulphur to children every spring. The medical profession has exposed and exploded that fad and millions of children are thankful. We now feed them canned spinach and cod-liver oil and the spinach probably does them just about as much good and harm as the sulphur—certainly no more good. The spinach would be of value if eaten fresh and raw, however, and the kids would not find it so hard to take.

The part of the sulphur which is unabsorbed is probably of more value than the part which is absorbed, for in passing through the intestines, it acts as a mild laxative, antiseptic and vermicide. Free sulphur is not a poisonous substance but the benefits derived from its use in bird medicine are not great. Birds living on a balanced diet containing the correct amounts of animal, vegetable and mineral foods for their particular needs will have no need for free sulphur either as food or medicine.

From five to ten per cent of flowers of sulphur is sometimes mixed with lard, cocoa butter or vaseline and employed as an ointment for the treatment of skin lesions and the destruction of skin parasites. I have found such ointments of little value in the treatment of any condition met with in canaries. Where a real ointment is needed, I prefer two per cent yellow oxide of mercury in cocoa butter. Lard and cocoa butter are preferable to vaseline as a base for bird ointment, since the latter will often blister the skin of small birds.

SWEATING HENS. This is a condition of canary hens, and probably the hens of other species that nest-raise their young, resulting from a digestive disorder of the baby birds which causes the nest to become damp and foul and the feathers on the hen's breast to become matted as though she had been sweating. Hens do not sweat, however. Therefore, the name is a misnomer.

This condition is fully discussed under the heading NESTLING DIARRHEA. Also see ASPERGILLOSIS; DIGESTIVE DISORDERS.

SYRINX. This is the voice box, the true larynx, the seat of voice and song in birds. It is a cartilaginous, box-like structure located at the lower end of the trachea.

SYMPTOMS. If the reader who has gotten this far does not know what a symptom is, there is little hope for him. A symptom of a disease is any abnormality of conduct, structure or function, or any other fact which can be observed during the course of an illness and which may be caused by the illness or throw light upon its nature. From the point of view of persons interested in the treatment of diseases, symptoms are of value and importance where they assist in differentiating one disease from another. The description of the symptoms of any particular disease should contain a description of the bird's actions, habits of eating, drinking, sleeping, color and texture of the droppings, condition of the body (whether in good flesh or emaciated), appearance of the abdomen, the respiratory rate, the body temperature, a description of any lesions appearing upon the surface of the body and any other fact which might be of value in distinguishing that particular illness from all others. See DIAGNOSIS.

SYRUP OF BUCKTHORN. Buckthorn is the dried root of a plant, **Rhamnus Frangula,** native to Southern Europe, Southern Asiatic Russia and Northern Africa. The bark when freshly gathered is an emetic (a drug that causes vomiting) but after being stored for one year it loses this property and becomes valuable as a mild laxative, tonic and diuretic. Syrup of buckthorn contains extract of buckthorn, licorice and syrup. Its action is very similar to that of cascara. As a tonic for birds it may be administered in doses of one drop to the ounce of drinking water; as a laxative, it may be given in doses up to five drops to the ounce of drinking water.

TAPEWORMS. Although they have not been thoroughly investigated, tapeworms probably infest all species of birds living in an environment favorable to the completion of their involved life cycles. How many different species of avian tapeworms there are is still an open question. Ransom found nine species in chickens and turkeys. Pheasants, ducks, geese, pigeons and a large number of wild birds have been found infested. Canaries are probably susceptible to tapeworm infestation, but the opportunity for the completion of the life cycle of the worm is broken by the routine of cage life.

Life history. From time to time the feces of infested birds contain ripe, egg-filled worm segments. For the carrying out of the life cycle of the worms, it is necessary for one of these eggs to be eaten by some creature which acts as a secondary host for that particular species of worm. The egg hatches in the body of the secondary host; the worm makes its way to some organ and there becomes encysted. When the infested secondary host is eaten by a susceptible bird, the cyst is digested and the infant worm set free. The worm then attaches itself to the mucous membrane of the intestine and the life cycle is completed. It is easily seen that the chances of such an involved life cycle being completed cannot under ordinary circumstances be much more than about one in a million. That tapeworms survive in spite of this adverse percentage is because they produce millions upon millions of eggs.

What creatures serve as secondary hosts for the various species of tapeworms is still undetermined. We know that the housefly is the secondary host for one species; the earthworm is suspected of being host to some of the worms infesting poultry; the secondary host of some of the worms infesting water fowls is probably to be found among the snails and crustacea upon which these birds so often feed.

Symptoms. In heavy tapeworm infestating, the symptoms are identical with those of chronic digestive disorders. There is diarrhea. At first the droppings are clear and watery; later they are mixed with brown or brownish-yellow mucus, due to the hemorrhages caused by the worms. The most diagnostic symptom, outside of the presence of worm segments in the droppings, is the fact that droppings sometimes contain gas bubbles. There is abnormal appetite, increasing thirst and progressive emaciation.

Morbid anatomy. The carcass is anemic and greatly emaciated. When the intestines are cut open the worms can be seen clinging to the intestinal walls. In some cases there are nodule-like ulcerations at the point of attachment which can be seen from the serous surface of the intestines. The worms can be more readily observed by opening the intestines under water.

Treatment. Because their heads are buried in the mucous membrane, tapeworms are very resistant to the action of vermicides and vermifuges (drugs that kill worms and drugs that expel worms). Many drugs have been recommended for their destruction and removal. Of the lot, tobacco and turpentine stand high in the opinions of poultrymen, though I cannot personally vouch for either their effectiveness or safety. These treatments appear to me to be rather drastic; it may be, however, that only drastic treatments can afford any hope of effectiveness. The method of administering tobacco to chickens has been discussed under the heading ROUNDWORMS. That for the administration of turpentine is as follows:

The chickens are fasted for a day; then in the evening they are given a feeding of mash containing one teaspoonful of Epsom salts per bird. The next morning each bird is given about a teaspoonful of turpentine. This substance is so offensive that it is almost a waste of time to attempt to administer it per os. The quickest and simplest method of administering turpentine is to inject it directly into the crop with a small, sharp hypodermic needle. If this is impossible or impractical, it may be introduced into the crop with a large-sized medicine dropper fitted with a piece of small, stiff rubber tubing long enough to reach the crop through the mouth. Another method is to dilute the turpentine with one to two parts of olive oil and then feed it to the birds slowly from a medicine dropper. It is said to usually be possible to get chickens to swallow turpentine in this manner. Four hours after the administration of the turpentine, the birds are given another feeding of mash containing Epsom salts.

Sodium hydroxide has been used and highly recommended as a taeniafuge * for poultry. One ounce of the hydroxide is added to each gallon of cracked grain necessary for a single feeding of cooked mash; enough water is added to cover the mixture which is then stirred and placed in a closed water bath and cooked for several hours. After being fasted all day, the birds are permitted to eat this mash before going to roost. They are given another

_____
* **Note:** A **taeniafuge** is a drug that expels tapeworms.

meal of it the next morning. There is now on the market a new synthetic drug called PHENOTHIAZINE, which is said to be more powerful and less toxic than any antithalmintic we have had up until this time, and certain published experiments seem to indicate that it is highly effective against both tapeworms and roundworms, especially in poultry. I have not used this drug myself, but the reports indicate that it should be worth trying. The dose for a chicken is from one to five grains into the crop. The dose for a canary is from 1/50 to one 1/10 grain into the crop.

TARAXACUM. This is the juice of dandelion roots preserved in alcohol. It is a bitter tonic and is considered of value for bringing run-down birds into condition. Where possible, however, it is preferable to feed the birds all the fresh dandelions they will eat.

TARTARIC ACID. This is the acid of grapes, pears and some other fruits. It is found on the market in the forms of colorless crystals and white powder. Tartaric acid is a laxative and diuretic and it acts on the bowels by causing large quantities of fluid to be thrown off by their mucous glands. It is nonpoisonous but in large doses has a tendency to be extremely irritating to the stomach. This tendency is counteracted by combining tartaric acid with sodium bicarbonate to form effervescent mixtures. The well-known **Seidletz powders** of a generation ago consisted of two little paper packages of white powder. One of the powders was sodium bicarbonate; the other was tartaric acid; they were dissolved separately and the solutions were mixed and taken while still forming. Today, we mix the dry powders, but the principles and effects are still the same. There are many excellent and justly popular effervescent saline preparations on the market and most of them are superior in every respect to the cathartic drugs. Taken in large doses, the action is almost immediate, yet it is not drastic. In small doses, one teaspoonful to the quart of drinking water, these preparations are invaluable for removing the poisons of waste and disease from the system because they keep both the bowels and the kidneys working at top capacity. I consider certain of these preparations among the most valuable prescriptions known to bird medicine. They act as absolute specific for certain highly contagious and hitherto incurable septicemias of birds, and are of great value in the treatment of many other conditions. This book is little more than a testimonial to their effectiveness, for had I not discovered their effectiveness, I would never have made the studies which make this writing possible.

TEMPERATURE. The body temperatures of birds are considerably higher than those of mammals. They are so high, in fact, during fevers they often pass beyond the range of an ordinary clinical thermometer. The reason I have not been able to give exact temperatures in my description of many diseases, is because they were too high for my thermometer to register. The normal temperatures of some of our domesticated birds are as follows:

	Min.	Max.
Black-hooded siskin	108.5	109
Bh S-Canary hybrid	108	109
Canary	106	107.5
Chicken	104.9	107.6
Turkey	104	106.7
Pheasant	105.8	111.2
Pigeon	105.8	109.4
Duck	105.8	109.4
Goose	104	105.8

During the course of some diseases the temperature may reach a height of 113 degrees F., plus. And I do not know how big that **plus** may be. There are cases where it drops as low as 96 just before death.

THRUSH. This is a mould infection of the mouth, throat and crop caused by a pathogenic fungus, OIDIUM ALBACANS, under which heading the condition is discussed.

THYMOL. This is a phenol found in the volatile oil of. **thymus vulgaris,** a plant growing in Southern Europe. It comes on the market as colorless crystals and white powder and has the thyme-like odor. It is an antiseptic, antipyretic and anthelmintic. It is used in human medicine as a specific for hookworms and for the treatment of gout, rheumatism, typhus fever, influenza and gastric fermentation. It is used externally as an antiseptic for the skin and mucous membranes, for the treatment of wounds and in surgery and dentistry. For external use it is employed in a one per cent aqueous-alcoholic solution containing twenty-five per cent of alcohol.

This drug has been recommended for the destruction of intestinal worms in birds. The dose for a chicken is ten grains every hour until thirty grains have been given. Several hours later this is followed by a laxative.

THYROID. This is a gland located on the right side of the neck. Its functions have to do with the control of growth and the basal metabolism,* and the development of intellect. The thyroid can carry on its necessary activity only when a sufficient amount of iodides are available in the food or water. When they are not present a condition called **Goiter** develops. See IODIDES; OBESITY.

THYROID. (This is sometimes called **Thyroid extract,** though it is not an extract.) It is a dry, brown powder obtained from the thyroids of cattle and sheep. It is sometimes used to increase the basal metabolism and bring about the reduction of fat. See OBESITY.

TIBIA. This is a bone of the leg. See SKELETON.

TICKS. See SPIROCHETOSIS.

TOBACCO. See ROUNDWORMS.

TOES. Most of our domesticated birds have four toes—three in front and one behind. Exceptions are the ostrich which has but two toes, both pointing frontwards, and the psittacine birds which have two toes in front and two behind. See FEET; BREEDING CONDITION; BROKEN BONES; SCALY-LEG; MOSQUITOES.

TONICS. Tonics are drugs which improve the appetite and the general nutrition of the body. See CASCARA; I.Q.S.; CITRATE OF IRON AND QUININE; SONG RESTORERS.

TONIC SEED. These are seed mixtures made from a large number of weed and garden seeds which are thought to have a tonic action upon birds by supplying them with elements lacking from the ordinary diet. I have given the formula for an excellent tonic seed mixture under the heading SONG RESTORERS.

TRACHEA. This is the windpipe. See RESPIRATORY SYSTEM.

TUBERCULOSIS. This is a common disease of man, animals and birds, characterized by emaciation, anemia and the formation of characteristic nodules in various parts of the body. The disease runs a chronic course. The older members of the flock are most frequently affected. Guinea fowls, peafowls, turkeys, ducks, geese, swans, parrots, pigeons, canaries, pheasants, sparrows and many species of wild birds kept in zoological gardens have been found affected. It is a common disease of chickens that have been fed on creamery-skimmed milk. I found the lesions of this disease in

---

* **Note: Basal metabolism** is the rate at which the body burns up sugar and fat for the production of heat, energy and carbon dioxide. It is measured by measuring the amount of carbon dioxide exhaled by the lungs in a given time, during which the patient remains at rest.

the bodies of a blackbird and an African finch which had been sent to me for examination. These birds had died from other causes.

Etiology. The cause of tuberculosis in birds is an avian strain of **B. tuberculosis.** This avian variety differs in several respects from the mammalian organism. The individual cells are much broader than those from human tuberculosis. The avian strain is

Figure 80.   **TUBERCULOSIS**

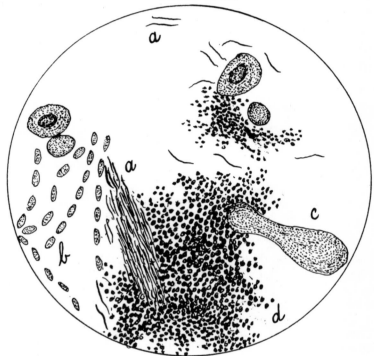

a, a, Tuberculosis bacteria, in the original preparation these were stained red. All else was stained blue. Staining by Gabbett's method.
b, Streptococci.
c, Cells.
d, Mucus debris.
    Bureau of Animal Industry.

much more readily cultivated on artificial media seeded directly from tissue, and the colonies are distinctly different. The human strain grows in a uniform layer on the surface of the media while the avian strain produces a number of distinct colonies which do not coalesce. Figures 80 and 81 illustrate the most striking difference between the two strains. Figure 82 shows cultures of avian tubercular bacteria.

Birds have been found affected with human tuberculosis, and both animals and man have been found affected with avian tuberculosis, yet in both cases the isolated organisms have retained their distinctive characteristics. Hogs on the same premises have been found infected by both strains, and in some cases it has been possible to trace each strain to its source. All of these facts seem to indicate that there is no relationship between avian and mammalian tuberculosis; but the simple fact that flocks of chickens fed on creamery-skimmed milk show an extremely high tuberculosis

Figure 81.   **TUBERCULOSIS**

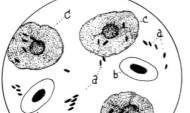

THE BACILLUS OF AVIAN TUBER-
CULOSIS FROM THE LIVER OF A
BIRD
(Bureau of Animal Industry)

a, a, Bacilli. Notice that the organisms are shorter and plumper than those of the human variety.

b, b, Blood cells.

c, c, c, Tissue cells.

Magnification about 1,000 ×.

Freehand copy by Robert Stroud.

incidence indicates that there must be a relationship. Dawson (page 351, Annual Report of the Bureau of Animal Industry, 1898) suggested the possibility of the observed differences between the mammalian and avian strains of tuberculosis being the result of environmental adaptations. The differences in pathogenicity of tubercle bacteria of human and avian origin are certainly no greater than the difference between the **street virus** and **fixed virus** of rabies. And in the case of rabies, we know that the difference in the two strains is the result of adaptations. (This is a good argument, that's why I use it so often; it is easier than trying to think up another.)

Symptoms. There is nothing characteristic enough about the symptoms of avian tuberculosis to make a positive diagnosis during life possible, excepting in those cases where there are external lesions. During the early stages of the disease the birds appear to be well, though they may seem a little less thrifty than some of their mates. Later they become anemic, emaciated and very weak. They have a disinclination to move, and walk with an unsteady gait.

Involvement of the skin and joints is not uncommon, and in these cases the disease is easily recognized. The tubercles form hard, horny growths upon the skin and either hard, horny or soft cheesy swellings on the joints.

Among strictly domesticated birds, recoveries from tubercu-

Figure 82. **TUBERCULOSIS**
AGAR CULTURE OF AVIAN TUBERCULOSIS

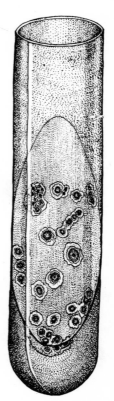

BACTERIA
Human tubercular bacteria do not grow well on agar. It forms a mould-like growth on the surface of liquid media containing glycerin or blood serum.

Drawn by Robert Stroud.

losis are probably very rare, but I have observed a number of spontaneous recoveries among free-flying pigeons affected with skin lesions.

For many years I have daily thrown the waste food from my canaries to the wild birds. Sparrows, pigeons, turtle doves, blackbirds, bluejays and starlings have visited this feeding ground. Often the same group of pigeons have fed there daily for years at a time. Naturally, these birds became as well known to me as members of my own flock and some of them became a lot tamer than my canaries. I have seen these birds develop skin and joint lesions as large as hickory nuts. I have killed some of them and verified my diagnosis by examination of the liver and spleen. But, others I have permitted to live and I have seen the lesions disappear within from six to nine months. During the attack the birds became very thin and weak and spent most of their time sleeping in the

Figure 83.   **TUBERCULOSIS**

SKIN LESION OF TUBERCULOSIS ON A PIGEON

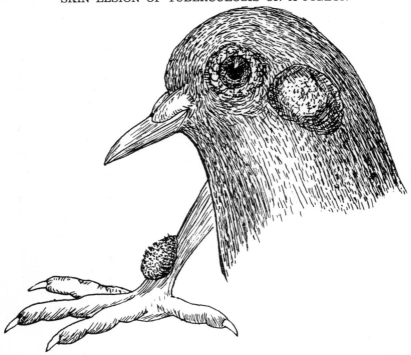

The tubercular skin nodules appear as large, gray, horny, wart-like growths.

Drawn from memory by Robert Stroud.

sun, but as soon as the skin lesions disappeared they put on weight and became to all appearance normal, healthy birds. Figure 83 is a free-hand drawing of the head and foot of one of these birds. The bird in question lived for about three years after the lesion had disappeared.

Morbid anatomy. The carcass is very light; the breast muscles almost gone; the lymphatic glands may be greatly enlarged and contain a caseous (cheesy) material that often has a gritty feeling when it is rubbed between the fingers or between two microscopic slides. Almost any part of the body may be involved. Parrots and pigeons frequently develop skin lesions; involvement of the joints is not uncommon in chickens. Their feet often become enlarged with the development of lumps containing caseous of fluid exudates. In practically all cases of avian tuberculosis, round, hard, yellow lumps are found in the spleen and liver and usually in the walls of the intestines. Usually there are a great many nodules in these organs. The larger ones will be found to contain a cheesy material in which there are gritty particles.

In all cases of chronic disease where the characteristic lesions of tuberculosis are found in both liver and spleen a diagnosis of tuberculosis is justified, but where nodules in the liver and intestines are associated with a healthy spleen, the investigator should be slow to pronounce the case that of tuberculosis. Nodules in the intestines may be the result of tapeworm infestation; abscesses in the liver may be mistaken for tubercles.

Tuberculin test. Tuberculine is prepared from the ground bodies of the tubercle bacteria. It was first developed by Koch in 1890 and has long been used for the detection of tuberculosis in man and animals. That intended for use on birds must be made from the avian strain of organisms. Chickens are tested with from 1/30 to 1/20 of a cubic centimeter of a fifty per cent solution of avian tuberculine injected into the thick skin of the wattle. A very fine needle is used so as to injure the tissue as little as possible. The injection should be made into the skin, not into the underlying tissues. To accomplish this, the needle should be inserted at an acute angle. In reacting cases the wattle is said to sometimes swell to two or three times normal size, sometimes only slightly. The test, as checked by post-mortem examinations, is said to be about ninety per cent accurate.

Transmission and prevention. Tuberculosis is transmitted from bird to bird in the flock by means of dropping-contaminated food and water. It is most effectively prevented by culling out all unthrifty birds, keeping the various age groups separate and maintaining as high a standard of sanitation as possible. Because such measures are standard practice in all well organized poultry plants and bird rooms, tuberculosis is no problem in such plants. It is on the small farm, where the various age groups are permitted to mix freely among themselves and with the other farm animals, and in zoos, where birds of all ages and species are associated in large, crowded flights which are not thoroughly cleaned from one year's end to the other, that tuberculosis often becomes a serious problem. Among zoological birds it is said to account for thirty per cent of the total mortality.

Treatment. There is no treatment for avian tuberculosis. As has been pointed out, free-flying birds may sometimes recover. I have read of no recoveries among confined birds, however.

Tuberculosis has resisted all attempts at the development of a specific therapy. We have developed methods by which the disease can sometimes be arrested or controlled in human subjects, if it is taken during the early stages, but to date, no drug, either of chemical or biological origin, has proved of any great value, notwithstanding that the clue to the cause of this high resistance of the tuberculosis bacilli was pointed out by Schweinitz and Dorset, 43 years ago.*

They found that the dry organisms contained no less than 37 per cent of crude fat; that a small amount of this fat was the glyceride of a volatile fatty acid, but that by far the largest part of it was the glycerides of palmitic acid and a heavy acid, probably arachidic, with a melting point higher than the boiling point of water.

It takes no great stretch of the imagination to understand that when more than ⅓ of the weight of the dried organism is composed of heavy fat, that organism is apt to be pretty well protected against the action of water-soluble reagents, though the corollary of this proposition seems to have escaped the attention of the medical profession, which is not surprising when we consider that more than ninety per cent of the great medical discoveries made during the last 75 years have been made by men who were not doctors.

These facts suggest, however, that the therapeutic properties of Du Pont's Anthroquinone Violet (see ASPERGILLOSIS) should be as effective against the tuberculosis bacillus as they are against the aspergillus fungus, which is another organism that owes its great resistance to therapeutic agents to the presence of a high fat content. This is one agent against which fats or gums can offer no protection, since it passes through such substances with the greatest of ease. This may be demonstrated by placing a little of the dry

---

* **Note:** Journal of American Chemical Society for May, 1896.

dye on a toothbrush handle, a pair of rubber gloves or the varnished top of your desk.

Wherever a flock of birds is known to be suffering with tuberculosis, all sick or ailing birds should be placed on the anthroquinone treatment as suggested for acute generalized aspergillosis. The dosage should be about one one-thousandth part of the body weight of the bird per day. It should not be necessary to apply the treatment for more than three weeks, since this drug, once absorbed, remains in the body for some months.

I also wish to suggest that should this work fall into the hands of a competent investigator, he test the effect of this drug on inoculated rabbits, and that in reporting his results, he remembers the source of this suggestion.

TUMORS. See CANCER; LEUKEMIA.

ULNA. This is the large bone of the forearm and the second division of the wing. See SKELETON.

UREMIA. Acute uremia is a condition resulting from the complete suppression of the functions of the kidneys. The urinary products remain in the blood stream, where they exercise a poisonous reaction upon the body tissues, particularly nerve tissues. It is a rather common symptom of acute Bright's disease in man, and the condition I am about to describe might really be better named had I chosen to call it Acute Bright's disease of birds or Acute avian **nephritis.** I have avoided these names because the condition, at least at its inception, is not associated with inflammatory changes in the interstitial or medullary tissues of the kidneys. I have chosen the designation **Uremia** because it is my belief that in the beginning the condition is always purely functional and mechanical; that if injuries to the kidneys occur, they are always of a secondary nature; and that the entire phenomenon — depression, coma and death, is the result of uremic poisoning.

This condition is often confused with sporadic pneumonia by those who do not make a habit of performing post-mortem examinations. Many breeders, and others who should know better, having read that pneumonia is a highly fatal disease of birds, that the illness develops following exposure and is of short duration, jump to the conclusion that every bird to die under such circumstances is a victim of pneumonia. This attitude on the part of bird breeders and poultrymen can be overlooked; but what is hard to understand and overlook is the fact that not one of the books I have read on bird or poultry diseases, not one out of the hundreds of bulletins from state and governmental experimental stations, not one of the literally thousands of articles I have read in poultry and canary journals, has made any mention of this condition. It is hard to believe that the hundreds of trained investigators engaged in the study of poultry could have overlooked such a common condition. Since both poultrymen and aviculturists have written to me about many deaths which could have resulted from no other cause, I can hardly believe that anyone associated with birds in any way for any length of time could have failed to come in contact with it.

Etiology. While the primary cause of the symptoms of uremia is the retention of waste products in the body, the real underlying cause is found in the conditions responsible for that retention. One of these is the structure of the bird's kidneys, which is designed to handle urine in a thick, pasty state, which is possible only because of the bird's high body temperature.

In every case of uremia to come to my attention, there has been a distinct history of chilling, of the bird sleeping in a draft or of a bird bathing in the open air during very cold weather, getting so wet that it could not fly to dry itself.

We know that such conditions of exposure are responsible for the greater part of nephritis in man. Why this is so, we do not know. In the case of birds, however, it is my opinion, and I shall presently offer pathological evidence in support of it, that lowering of the bird's body temperature caused the almost solid urine to crystallize in the small uriniferous tubes, thereby plugging them.

It is my belief that a fall in body temperature causes the formation of these large crystals; that their points penetrate the wall of the small tubes; that the resulting congestion causes an increase in the pressure exerted by the surrounding tissue upon the tubes which results in the plugging becoming complete. Thus the functioning of the kidneys is suspended and uremic poisoning follows in short order.

Symptoms. There are two distinct forms of acute uremia. In the first form a bird that has been in perfect health is left in a draft, or, there may have been a sudden change in the weather which caused a draft of cold air to play upon the bird during the night while he was sleeping. A short time later he is discovered puffed up like a ball. He eats or drinks little, if at all. He shivers, seems cold and wants to sleep all the time. He will tuck his head back over his wing and go to sleep while you are talking to him. He becomes weaker by the minute, which is evident from the fact that when discovered the bird will usually be standing on one foot, is soon standing on both feet, and a little later has found it impossible to cling to the perch and has sought a corner of the cage where he finds it very difficult to keep from falling over. He does not sit on his heels and tail, however. He soon goes into a state of coma from which he can be only partially aroused.

As the illness progresses toward a fatal termination, the breathing becomes more rapid and shallow, but at no time is there ever any gasping or open-mouthed breathing. There is no struggle of any kind. There are no droppings. The bird just sits quietly in his corner until he falls over, dead. Death may occur within from two to twenty-four hours of the onset of the attack. This form of the disease occurs almost exclusively in birds that are chilled during sleep.

In the second form of this condition, the bird may fly into a stream of cold air coming through a crack or a partly opened window; a bird may take a bath in the open air and get his feathers so wet he cannot fly to dry himself and thus stands in the cold air shivering until his owner notices him and takes him into the house. In either case the bird suffers from muscular cramps which appear to extend to the involuntary muscles of the kidneys. In any case, there is immediate and complete suspension of kidney functioning. I have seen canaries fly through a small shaft of cold air and fall to the floor as if they had been shot. Regardless of how the chilling occurs, the bird falls to the floor and lies there jerking. There may be a cataleptic contraction of the muscles of one side of the body which lasts for a few moments and is followed by a rhythmic jerking of all the muscles of the affected side. The beak opens, the eye blinks, the wing jerks down against the side, the foot jerks upward. The period of this jerking may be from ten to ninety per minute, but it is fairly uniform throughout the violent period of the illness. There is no kidney action, no droppings. Without treatment, the bird will die within from two to six hours. If kidney action can be re-established, the frequency of the jerking will become slower until it finally ceases, though this may take from two to forty-eight hours from the time the first droppings appear.

Morbid anatomy. There may be a few punctiform hemorrhages in the brain and in some cases there is a slight effusion into the peritoneum and pericardium. The principal changes are in the kidneys, however.

In the first form of the disease the kidneys have a gray granular appearance. There is not, as a rule, much, if any, enlargement. Under a ten diameter hand lens the grayness can be resolved into a series of alternating, white and purple, curved lines. The white lines are the plugged tubes; the purple lines are the highly congested medullary tissues.

If the whole pelvis is fixed to the stage of a microscope and the kidney studied **in situ** in a thin, strong beam of light directed down upon it at an angle of about thirty degrees, it is possible to see the tubes and their contents. By using a 44 x, high-working-distance objective and a 5 x eyepiece, it was possible to see the spear-shaped crystals with their points thrust through the walls of the tubes. By using a 10 x objective and a 15 x eyepiece, it was possible to get better light and wider view, though the image was not so good, and it could then be seen that above these points where the concretions of crystals plugged the tubes, the tubes were distended and varicosed—this was not noticed in cases where the bird died within two or three hours of the onset of the attack. E, Figure 84 gives a rough idea of the type of crystals found in the kidney tubes.

Figure 84.

UREMIA

SOME OF THE CRYSTALLINE FORMS FOUND IN BIRD URINE

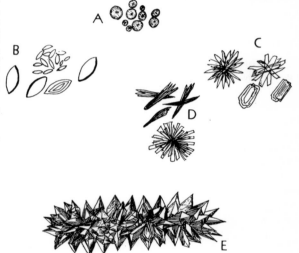

A, Globules of normal bird urine. It is in this form that solids are usually present in bird urine. Crystals are not found until the urine has been exposed to the air or diluted.

B, Normal crystals of uric acid.

C, These forms are also composed of uric acid, but they occur less frequently than those shown at **B.**

D, These crystals are calcium phosphate. They appear rapidly as the globules disintegrate.

E, These concretions probably uric acid, urates, and phosphates. They are formed on the microscopic slide when fresh bird urine is treated first with one-tenth normal sodium hydroxide and then with dilute hydrochloric acid. They are also found in the uriniferous tubes of birds that have died of acute uremia as a result of sleeping in a draft. Magnification about 600 ×.

Drawn by Robert Stroud.

In the spasmodic form of the disease, this plugging of the kidney tube was not observed.

Differential diagnosis. The symptoms of the spasmodic form of the disease cannot be mistaken. (See LEAD POISONING.) The only condition even remotely resembling it is cinchopin poisoning, which probably brings about a similar physiological condition. In any case, the two conditions are amendable to the same lines of treatment. Too, the breeder knows whether or not he has been administering cinchopin.

It is impossible to distinguish between the somnolent form of acute uremia and the early stages of sporadic pneumonia excepting by the droppings, and there are usually none in either case. The pneumonic bird does try to eat and drink a little at first and there may be a few droppings of a brown color. The uremic bird does not make any attempt to eat or drink, and if there are any droppings early in the attack, they will be of normal color. There are at least fifty cases of acute uremia in canaries for every case of sporadic pneumonia, so the safest course is to treat all such cases for uremia. This was true when written. I have now found that chest sounds give a reliable differentiation of these two conditions. See PNEUMONIA.

Treatment. If treated in time, all cases of acute uremia can be cured. The bird must be put in a warm place at once. I have found it a good plan to hang a 40-watt electric light inside the hospital cage and cover the cage with a cloth. Many birds will recover within a few hours without any other treatment. They should always be watched to see that they do not become over-heated, which would do more harm than good. Birds suffering from the somnolent form of the disease will usually snuggle up alongside of the light and go to sleep. If the light is hung so that they can get under it, they will lie down and spread their feathers and allow the light and heat to beat down upon their backs, over their kidneys. Sometimes this light treatment will start the kidneys functioning in a very short time, and birds apparently at the point of death may be eating and singing within an hour.

These observations led me to arrange a box and a 100-watt light in my cold flight room, so that the birds could either snuggle against the light or crawl directly under it and sun themselves by it whenever they wished. There was an immediate and marked reduction in the number of uremic cases occurring in the room.

Birds suffering from the spasmodic form of the disease are unable to get under the light or do anything else for themselves. They are utterly helpless. I have found it advisable to wrap them in handkerchiefs and place them in a warm, but not too warm, place; since the handkerchief retains most of the body heat, less external heat is necessary.

To all birds suffering with the symptoms of acute uremia, the following prescription should be administered in the manner presently to be described:

DIUROL

F. E. Triticum	16 minims
F. E. Hydrangae	16 minims
F. E. Hyoscyamus	2 minims
F. E. Sabal	16 minims
F. E. Dichi	16 minims
F. E. Buchu	16 minims
Potassium Carbonate	8 grains
Lithium Carbonate	4 grains
Glycerine	1 ounce

50% alcohol to make 4 ounces.

For use on canaries or other small birds suffering from uremia, one part of this preparation is mixed with three parts of warm water, and ten drops to one c.c. of the mixture is introduced into the crop with a blunt-tipped medicine dropper.* The dose should be repeated every hour or two until the bird's kidneys start to functioning; then thirty drops of the undiluted preparation can be added to each ounce of drinking water for a day. Once the bird's kidneys start to functioning he will be able to eat and drink.

There are a few mild cases of uremia in which complete suppression of kidney functioning does not occur. In such cases, diurol may be given in the drinking water from the first, the dose being varied from ten to thirty drops to the ounce of water, depending on the severity of the attack.

When the symptoms of the uremic attack are spasmodic and the attack is discovered at once, the bird will always respond to the treatment just described, and the recovery, even though it takes thirty to forty hours to bring it about, will always be complete. There will be no aftereffects. There is no danger of the bird developing chronic nephritis following recovery.

Most of the somnolent cases respond to this treatment, but in these cases the illness is not so apt to be discovered at its onset. Then, too, uncertainty of the diagnosis may cause delay in the application of the treatment, while all the time those big crystals are ripping the linings out of the kidney tubes. As a result, about fifty per cent of the birds affected with the somnolent form of acute uremia do not completely recover; they develop chronic nephritis as an aftereffect. Even some of these may regain a fair degree of good health for a while, but they are pretty certain to die of nephritis within two years.

---

* **Note:** It is a waste of effort to attempt to induce a bird suffering from an attack of uremia to eat or drink. The only way of getting the medicine into them is by introducing it into the crop.

Theory concerning the development of the uremic attack. I have noticed that cases of uremia developing during the breeding season are confined to males. From a single cage, hung facing a doorway, I lost two or three males every season for about four years. The cases always occurred during hot weather, and the attack always followed a sudden change in the weather occurring at night. Normally, no draft reached this cage for it was six feet from the door, but a sudden thunderstorm occurring at night would set up a circulation of air in the building of sufficient force to blow into this cage; and when that occurred I was pretty certain to find a very sick male in that cage next morning. Outside nest boxes were used, so that the hen, especially when she was standing over some well-grown chicks, was much more exposed to the draft than was the male sleeping in the back of the cage. None of these hens were affected. Their bodies received as much or more draft than the bodies of the males could have received, but their feet, down in the nest or among the babies, were protected.

Reasoning from this fact and from my studies of the uric acid crystals in the plugged tubes, I have come to believe that air blowing on a bird's feet during sleep caused a slow drop in body temperature, and that as the temperature falls the uric acid in the urine has a tendency to form larger and larger crystals, until a point is finally reached at which the concretions become so large that their points dig into the walls of the tubes. It must be remembered in this connection that the chilling which takes place during sleep, sudden as it may appear to be, is always more or less gradual. Its causes are of a nature which would be harmless to the waking bird—if they were violent enough to cause the bird * to awaken, quit his perch and seek the floor of the cage, he would probably escape unharmed. We sometimes have storms of that nature in Kansas, and the birds come through them in good condition; it is the gentle, insidious draft playing on that unprotected foot which seems to be at the root of the whole trouble. And it is worth noting at this point, that while scientific investigators seem to have overlooked this condition entirely and practical breeders have been laboring under a misapprehension concerning its pathology, the latter have had sense enough to associate cause with effect and universally adopt the practice of covering the cages of their pet birds at night.

---

* **Note:** I would be a fool if I did not realize that this theory may be all wrong. It is possible that the draft sucks the blanket of warm air from among the bird's feathers, but in that case I cannot account for the hen's escape.

The phenomenon of the spasmodic form of acute uremia is something entirely different, so different, in fact, that the two conditions probably should have been discussed separately. Why a sudden and severe chill should cause violent muscular contractions and cramps seems to have escaped explanation—many swimmers who have experienced such attacks while in the water have not been lucky enough to escape with their lives, however, but it is such a condition we seem to be dealing with in spasmodic uremia. There are no changes in the kidney structure. It appears to me that cramping extends to the involuntary muscles of the kidneys and the uremic poisoning which follows, in some manner, tends to prevent these contracted muscles from relaxing. This conclusion is partly supported by several cases which were discovered at the moment of attack. The birds were taken in the hand and held with their backs up against a 100-watt lamp until they started to pant. I had these birds flying in less than an hour. But in other cases where a short but unavoidable delay had taken place between the onset of the attack and the application of heat, the application of strong heat to the back proved ineffective; they responded to the diurol treatment, however.*

URETERS. These are the small tubes that carry the urine from the kidneys to the cloaca. If the kidneys are in a state of health, the courses of the ureters over the ventral surfaces of the kidneys can be easily traced, since the white urine they contain causes them to stand out against the dark background of kidney tissue.

URINARY SYSTEM. See KIDNEYS.

UROPYGIUM. This is the correct name for the oil or rump gland, naturally, no one uses it. See OIL GLAND.

UROTROPINE (Hexamethylenamine). This is a complex chemical product having the formula $(CH_2)_6N_4$. It comes in white crystals soluble in water and has the unique property of breaking down

---

* **Note:** Much of this discussion of acute uremia is a rewrite of a copyrighted article which appeared in the October, 1933, issue of the "American Canary and Cage-Bird Life," Chicago, Illinois. At that time, however, I had given very little study to the spasmodic form of uremia, nor had I developed an effective drug-treatment for the condition.

* **Note:** Dr. Herbert Sanborn has informed me that he has had good results in the treatment of the somnolent form of uremia with pills containing red pepper and cod-liver oil. The birds were moved to warm quarters and the pills forced down their throats. He was under the impression that the condition was a pneumonia. Some of the bodies he had sent to me with the explanation that the birds had died with what he thought to be a pneumonic attack, first turned my attention to the study of the kidney diseases of birds; for all but one of these presumably pneumonic cases had healthy lungs. The lesions were those of uremia and nephritis.

in the presence of organic material in an acid solution and forming formaldehyde. When urotropine is administered to humans having an acid urine, it breaks down in the kidneys and the formaldehyde formed acts as a powerful antiseptic. Since the reaction takes place only in the presence of an acid, it is customary in human medicine to administer urotropine in conjunction with sodium acid phosphate or sodium benzoate, which causes the urine to have an acid reaction. Bird urine is always strongly acid, so it is not necessary to administer any drug to put it in that condition.

Urotropine is the most effective and reliable kidney antiseptic known to human medicine, but my experience with it in the treatment of nephritis in birds has not been happy. The great difficulty has been in arriving at the correct dosage. Very small doses have produced no noticeable effects over short periods, and increased doses have caused fatal hemorrhages from the kidneys. Under the heading NEPHRITIS, I have outlined an experimental method of using this drug on birds. The method outlined is far from satisfactory but it is the best I have to offer until such time as my own experiments shall definitely establish the exact dosages of this drug to be employed. This was written before the discovery of sulfa drugs. These conditions can now be treated with SULFA-THIAZOL.

UTERUS. See OVIDUCT; GENERATIVE SYSTEM; EGG STRUCTURE AND FORMATION.

V

VEINS. See CIRCULATORY SYSTEM.

VENT GLEET. In the literature of poultry diseases, **Vent gleet** is mentioned as a specific disease of unknown etiology. Whether or not this view is correct, I do not know. I do know that in every case where a poultryman has written to me about vent gleet in his flock, I have instructed him to treat the condition exactly as he would an outbreak of diphtheria; I have informed him that in my opinion the lesions of vent gleet were the result of a more or less chronic diphtheric infection. I advised that the entire flock be given STROUD'S SALTS NO. 1, in their food and STROUD'S EFFERVESCENT BIRD SALTS in their water in the proportion of one teaspoonful to the quart. I suggested that the sick birds should be isolated and the vent lesions treated with a saturated solution of STROUD'S SALTS NO. 1. In every case wherein I have subsequently heard from a person to whom this advice had been given, I have been informed that the condition had cleared up within the three weeks' period of treatment suggested.

Symptoms. It is contended that this is an infectious venereal disease of fowl, spread only by coition. There is inflammation of the cloaca and vent. At first the discharge is watery; later it is purulent (pertaining to pus) and foul smelling. The passage of droppings causes the bird considerable pain. Its irritation is apt to cause the affected bird to peck at the inflamed tissue, and its mates are apt to join in and do such a thorough job of it that the affected bird has to be destroyed.

Prevention. It is recommended that all roosters be removed from the flock, all affected roosters destroyed, all affected hens either isolated or destroyed. See DIPHTHERIA.

VENT, INFLAMED. See AVIAN DIPHTHERIA; NEPHRITIS; BACILLARY WHITE DIARRHEA; VENT GLEET.

VENTRICULUS BULBOSUS. You probably would not guess it, but this is the official name of the gizzard.

VISCERA. This is the sum total of the internal organs as heart, liver, lungs, spleen, intestines, gizzard, kidneys, etc.

VISCERAL GOUT. Avian gout takes two forms, the **articular** and the **visceral**. In articular gout uric acid and urates are deposited in the joints and their vicinity, causing swellings which sometimes rupture and discharge. In visceral gout the retained uric acid and urates are deposited on the serous surfaces of the abdominal and thoracic cavities as white powder and crystals. In all other respects the two conditions are identical. See GOUT; VITAMIN A.

VITAMINS. Vitamins are rare chemical compounds present in living matter in minute quantities and exerting a vital influence upon certain of the life processes. They are formed in nature under circumstances which were until recently little understood.

In the last few years our knowledge of the vitamins has advanced by leaps and bounds. We have learned how some of them are produced in nature; we have succeeded in synthesizing some of them, and in one or two cases the chemists have been able to make closely related products which are even more potent than the natural vitamins; we know that each of these substances exerts its influence upon one specific set of functions and that when the living creature is deprived of that particular vitamin, those functions fail; but concerning the action of these substances in the living body, we know practically nothing.

The views presented in this section are as complete and up to date as I have been able to make them, but with our knowledge of this subject advancing so rapidly, they are very apt to be out of date before they are in print.

Vitamins are designated by letter, A, B, C, etcetera, by names relating to their particular functions, such as **antiscrobutic, antirachitic** (which means **stops scurvy; stops rickets), nervous, reproductive,** etc., or by words indicating their mode of production or occurrence in nature, as the **sunshine** vitamin. Recently some of the artificially produced vitamins have been given names relating to their chemical composition or have been assigned trade names by the laboratories engaged in their manufacture such as **irradiated ergosterol, thiamin,** etc.

Some of the morbid conditions resulting from vitamin deficiency were known for generations before the existence of vitamins was suspected, and, hence, have special names like Rickets, Scurvy, Beriberi. It is now becoming the general practice to group all of these conditions under the generic term **avitaminosis** (meaning disease due to lack of vitamins) and differentiate them one from the other by the letters by which their respective vitamins are designated. That is the plan I shall follow as far as possible in the succeeding sections.

VITAMIN A. Until recently it was thought that this vitamin was produced in growing plants. We now know that the yellow coloring matters of most plants and fruits, carotenes and cryptoxanthin, are converted by the liver into Vitamin A, which is one of the higher alcohols. It usually occurs in animal tissue as an ester (a salt produced by two organic compounds) of a fatty acid. It is colorless and fat soluble.

The food sources of Vitamin A are the parts of plants retaining a green or yellow color, animal fat, liver, fish-liver oils, cream, and egg yolk. The vitamin is destroyed by the action of light and oxygen, though it resists drying and ordinary cooking. The chief source of Vitamin A in the diet of our birds is fresh green food, though rape seed may retain some of this substance.

Avitaminosis A. This condition always develops when there is an insufficiency of Vitamin A producing substances in the diet. It has been found that chickens fed on a diet containing little or no Vitamin A producing substances always develop a condition resembling roup and which, for that reason, is called nutritional roup. It has been found that such a diet will cause the death of old birds within from six to eight months and young birds within three months.

Symptoms. As stated above, the symptoms of avitaminosis A are very similar to roup. There is a watery discharge from the eyes and nostrils. Sometimes there is the formation of exudates in the lachrymal duct and the suborbital and nasal sinuses, which may become plugged. This is accompanied by asthmatic breathing. In the ordinary course of events bacteria invade these lesions, gain entrance to the blood and set up a septicemia that causes death.

There is a retention of uric acid and urates in the body with resulting symptoms of gout, which may be either articular or visceral in form.*

Other conditions resulting from varying degrees of deficiency are retarded growth; diarrhea; intestinal disorders; poor vision, particularly night blindness; loss of weight; weakness; and sterility, but the first and most pronounced of these symptoms in birds is always asthmatic breathing that does not respond to the ordinary treatments. Death always results if the deficiency is continued over

---

* **Note:** It is very likely that there is a direct relationship between the need for Vitamin A and the amount of amo acids (proteins are broken up into amo acids for absorption) absorbed. It is known that there is a relationship between the presence of Vitamin A in the body and the ability of the individual to use proteins for body-building purposes. And I am convinced from my own experiments that green food is the best possible insurance against gout.

a sufficient period of time, though some old birds have enough of the vitamin stored in their bodies to carry them over many months.*

Morbid anatomy. Uric acid in the blood may be increased from forty to fifty times the normal amount. There are apt to be deposits of uric acid and urates on the serous surfaces of the visceral membranes. The inside of the esophagus will be found covered with pimple-like nodules. The general anatomical picture corresponds to that of visceral gout. In fact, the symptoms and lesions of gout associated with a nasal discharge and asthmatic breathing give a perfect picture of advitaminosis A.

Treatment. I have not treated this condition in poultry, nor has it developed in my own canaries. At different times, though, many birds suffering with it have been sent to me for study and treatment. I have given them cinchopen for the elimination of the uric acid and turned them into my large flight room where they have the best of living conditions. Naturally, along with the rest of my birds, they had all the green food they could eat every day, and their supply of direct sunlight was limited only by weather conditions and their own desires. If they wished, they could sit in the sun all day long. About seventy per cent of the treated birds recovered and came to enjoy reasonably good health, but not one of them ever achieved the vigorous health enjoyed by birds which had never been deprived of this important vitamin.

VITAMIN B. This substance is sometimes referred to as the **nerve** vitamin, since its absence from the diet is always followed by certain nervous symptoms. It is found in the outer covers of all grain and seeds, though some seeds are much richer in it than others. It has been recently synthesized, and studies of the synthetic products have shown that what we have considered a single vitamin actually consists of at least two and probably three or four distinct substances, each having its distinct function. So what was formerly referred to as Vitamin B is now referred to as the B complex and is known to contain **thiamin**, B_1; riboflavin, B_2; nicotinic acid, B_3, and there are at least three other substances associated in this complex about which very little is known.

These substances occur in the outer covering of grain and seeds, usually in close association, though some seeds and grains are richer in one member of the complex than in others. For

* **Note:** For most of my material concerning recent vitamin research I am indebted to J. George Claffey of HEGER PRODUCTS, St. Paul, Minn., who has supplied me with a number of valuable papers that would have otherwise been unavailable to me.

instance, yellow corn is rich in thiamin and deficient in nicotinic acid. Fresh yeast and liver are said to contain the complete complex.

The B vitamins are soluble in water and are not destroyed by moderate cooking, but they are apt to be leached out of the food and thrown down the drain. I once read of an interesting case occurring in India. There was a monastery and a convent located in the same locality. During one of their periodic famines both the monks and the nuns were reduced to a diet of dried fish and polished rice. The nuns were cleanly in the preparation of their food; they washed their rice before cooking it, and they all died. The monks, who were extremely filthy in their housekeeping, boiled their rice as it came from the bags, dirt and all. They did not die. There had been enough Vitamin B in the dust from the polishing machine adhering to the outside of the rice grains to save their lives. People who boil their grains and vegetables with the skins on and then use the water for making soup do not suffer from lack of this vitamin complex.

Thiamin. This substance is now made synthetically and comes on the market as the hydrochloride of thiamin. It is a preventive of beriberi and has the following positive effects: Promotes growth; stimulates appetite; aids digestion and the metabolism of carbohydrates and fats.

Yellow corn and kaffir are probably the best sources of this substance in poultry food. Rape seed contains it in greater quantities than any other item in the canary's diet.

Riboflavin. This substance is now made synthetically. It improves growth, promotes general health, prolongs active life span, and is essential to the functioning of nerve and other tissue cells.

Animal proteins, whole seeds, grains, and yeast are the best sources of riboflavin.

Nicotinic acid. This substance is made synthetically and is found in nature in grain; seeds; lean meats, particularly liver; yeast; and egg yolk. It promotes health and growth and is essential to the proper functioning of the gastrointestinal tract and skin. Its lack causes the disease known as pellagra.

Avitaminosis B. This condition, also called **beriberi** and **polyneuritis,** is a common cause of death in man. This is especially true in those countries where the poorer classes are forced to live on a diet of polished rice and dried fish. Typical cases of this condition are so rare in America that not one doctor in twenty would recognize the condition if he saw it, but don't conclude from this we do not suffer from lack of this vitamin. It is my opinion that much of our craving for drink, for narcotic drugs and even for swing music is a nervous affliction traceable directly to our overrefined diet of steam-cooked and processed food; that about ninety per cent of our digestive disorders are the direct result of the habit of the American cook and American housewife of pouring the first water in which anything is cooked down the drain. It is little wonder that we are the greatest consumers of digestive, headache and sedative pills that the world has ever known; that constipation is our normal state; that aspirin and bicarbonate of soda are household necessities.

Very little of this vitamin can be stored in the body, so the symptoms of disease follow quickly when the foods containing it are removed from the diet. A twenty-day-old canary fed on a diet containing bread, apple pulp, dried egg yolk, polished rice, cod-liver oil and cuttlebone, that is, on a diet containing everything a bird needs with the one exception of Vitamin B, will develop polyneuritis within from two to four days; it will die within from four to ten days. This is not a common disease of birds, since most birds are fed on uncooked seeds and grains, but it causes the death of many hand-fed canaries.

Symptoms. The symptoms of avitaminosis B in birds are identical with those of beriberi in man. It was the reading of a description of the disease in man which first enabled me to recognize it in young canaries. The symptoms are: digestive disorders; loss of weight; loss of appetite—at first the appetite is increased. The bird is hungry all the time but has no stomach for the food offered—constipation, followed by a thin, bright yellow diarrhea; nervous twitchings; loss of control of the limbs; continuous colonic convulsions which continue until death. The course of the disease in young canaries is from three days to one week. Of course, where there is a deficiency, rather than a total absence of the vitamin from the diet, the symptoms and course of the illness will be influenced by the amount of the vitamin actually present.

For several days before the convulsions make their appearance, it will have been noticed that the baby is off its feed. It sits with its feathers ruffled, crying for food, but refuses to swallow the food offered. The yellow, dribbling diarrhea may run down onto the abdomen from the vent. For a time the bird shivers, as if cold, and then it goes into a violent convulsion which is distinguished from the convulsion of apoplectiform septicemia by the fact that there is no period of wild aimless flight, and from the convulsions of strychnine poisoning by the fact that the disturbance is less violent at first and more continuous. The first attack may be of short duration; it is quickly followed by one that lasts until death.

In apoplectiform septicemia and food poisoning, the bird is undoubtedly unconscious, but the flight, wild as it is, is always on an even keel, showing that there is nothing wrong with the nerve centers which coordinate the flight impulses. In avitaminosis

Figure 85   **VITAMIN B**
CANARY IN THE LAST STAGES OF BERIBERI

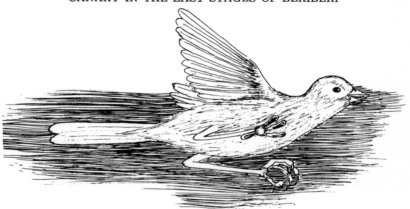

Drawn from memory by Robert Stroud. I am afraid that this drawing falls far short of perfection in almost every particular, but maybe it will help some breeder to recognize the condition I have tried to illustrate. The bird lies on its side; its feet either drawn up or grasping futilely at the air, and its free wing fluttering constantly. The beak may be either closed or open. The feathers around the vent are usually somewhat matted from the diarrhea which preceded the convulsions.

B all muscular coordination is lost, but the bird is fully conscious at all times. The head may be drawn back, or it may be thrust forward, the neck limp. The bird usually lies on one side with the free wing fluttering continuously. The spasms become weaker and weaker as the bird becomes exhausted. Finally it dies. Figure 85 shows a baby canary in the last stages of polyneuritis.

Treatment. A single cropful of food rich in Vitamin B will make the affected bird a new creature, almost instantly. The best source of Vitamin B for baby canaries is ground rape seed; the best source for poultry is cracked yellow corn. The rape seed is prepared by placing a handful of rape between two pieces of paper;

rolling it with a roller or rolling pin until the seeds are crushed; blowing off most of the hulls; and mixing what is left with an equal amount of ground bread. A little of this mixture is chewed until it is the consistency of thick mush; it is then fed to the baby by force. The struggling bird is taken up in the hand; its beak forced open; some of the food placed in the mouth with a match stick; and then, with the blunt end of the stick, the food is forced down into the crop. I have often seen young canaries that had lain in convulsions from five to ten hours able to return to the perch after a single feeding of rape seed. After two or three such feedings, they are able to open their mouths and swallow the food without assistance. The digestive symptoms are the first to appear and the last to disappear. As little as ten per cent of ground rape in the food will keep a hand-fed baby from developing this condition.

VITAMIN C. This substance is called the **antiscrobutic** vitamin, since its presence in the human diet prevents a disease known as **scurvy,** and characterized by a disorganization of the blood, from developing. Scurvy is the oldest disease known to man. Evidence of it has been found in skeletons considered to be more than one hundred thousand years old.

Recently this vitamin has been shown to be ascrobutic acid and its chemistry has been worked out and the substance made synthetically. The vitamin is destroyed by ordinary cooking or drying, but it is now known that the destruction takes place as a result of oxidization, particularly in the presence of alkalis. Food may be cooked in an atmosphere of steam or in vacuum without the destruction of their Vitamin C content.

Birds have the power of manufacturing Vitamin C for themselves.

VITAMIN D. This is the sunshine vitamin. It is produced by the action of ultraviolet light upon certain chemical compounds which are widely distributed in the tissues of both animals and plants ergosterol, 7-Dehydrocholesterol, and a number of other sterols (fatty compounds present in tissue), when these substances are acted upon by ultraviolet light. In that respect, it is closely related to Vitamin A. Both are fat-soluble vitamins and they are usually found closely associated in nature. It is produced wherever ultraviolet light shines on the necessary compounds or upon tissues containing them, and it can be produced in dead tissues as readily as in living tissues. Visible light takes no part in its production, however. In the temperate latitudes, the amount of ultraviolet light which can fall on the body of a bird in ten minutes' exposure to the noonday sun, will manufacture enough Vitamin D to last the bird for one day.

Vitamin D is manufactured in man whenever his skin is exposed to any light which will tan it. The light of the open electric arc, the mercury-vapor arc, or any other light rich in radiation of wave lengths beyond the visible range. It has been recently manufactured and is now available commercially and sold under the name **irradiated ergosterol**—though I would not swear that my spelling is correct.

Vitamin D is the most stable of the vitamins; it is not destroyed by drying or cooking and deteriorates very slowly with age. Man and most animals store enough of this substance in their livers to supply their needs for from four to eight months.

Vitamin D is the growth vitamin. Adults, either human or avian, can live for a long time on a very limited supply without suffering serious injury; but all young, growing creatures need large amounts of it, and it does not matter a bit whether they wear fur, feathers or diapers. The same is true of adults during growing periods. The laying hen or moulting hen and the pregnant woman will suffer irreparable injury from being deprived of this vital substance.

The function of Vitamin D has to do with the metabolism of the minerals calcium and phosphates. Its absence from the diet is associated with soft-shelled eggs and soft, malformed bones and teeth. Dark-skinned creatures require about four times as much Vitamin D as light-skinned creatures. This is probably because the light skin is more sensitive to small amounts of ultraviolet light. The normal canary chick is hatched with enough Vitamin D in his system to last him for from ten to fifteen days.

The white man often marvels at the sound teeth and beautifully molded bodies of some of his uncivilized kinsmen. They got that way because as children they ran naked in the noonday sun.

Of all the seeds fed to canaries the only two in which I have been able to demonstrate appreciable quantities of Vitamin D are hemp seed and sunflower seed. These two seeds are also rich in the reproductive vitamin. In the amounts in which they are fed to canaries, these seeds do not contain enough Vitamin D to prevent rickets where all other sources are cut off, but they do contain enough to carry the babies over until they are able to fly.

Avitaminosis D. This condition is also known as **rickets** or **rachitis**. It is characterized by the inability of the creature affected to metabolize enough minerals to maintain the processes of life, growth and reproduction. Hens produce fewer eggs. And those eggs they do produce have thin shells, light-colored yolks and their percentage of hatchability is very low. Of those chicks which do hatch, most will die during the first few days of life. Of those that live longer, some are certain to develop typical cases of rickets. It is not necessary for the old birds to be suffering from a shortage of this vitamin for baby canaries to develop rickets. They will develop the disease any time their diet from the tenth day of life on does not contain enough of the vitamin to supply their growth processes.

Baby chicks develop rickets between the fourth and tenth weeks of life.

Figure 86.   **VITAMIN D**
A THREE-WEEK-OLD BABY CANARY NEAR DEATH FROM RICKETS

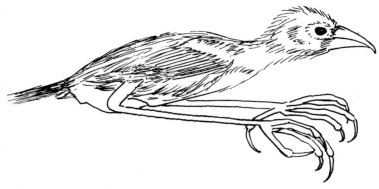

Notice the overgrown beak and legs, the scrawny body, and the wing feathers from which the outer quills have not been combed. I may have exaggerated these features somewhat in the drawing, which was made from memory, but I believe that any breeder who studies this drawing will be able to recognize the condition in his baby birds. The stubby growth of feathers in the middle of the forehead is a common but not exclusive symptom of rickets. It is observed in all cases of malnutrition in baby birds, regardless of the cause.

Drawn by Robert Stroud.

Symptoms. The skin, flesh and bones of healthy, fast-growing baby birds are soft, almost spongy in texture with a resilience born of boundless internal energy; they are pink, with the rich blood coursing through them. The quills of the young growing feathers are soft and pink, too, bulging with the blood they contain. But when rickets appear, this picture changes. The skin, flesh and bones become darker in color, dry, tough, horn-like; the feathers quit growing, become dry and ragged looking with shrunken quills.

The body actually shrinks. The long bones of the legs, however, and the upper beak continue to grow. The overgrown shanks and the eagle-like beaks of these afflicted babies give them a grotesque appearance. These birds are constantly hungry, yet their food does not do them any good. Figure 86 shows a canary chick with rickets.

A young canary that has received a normal amount of Vitamin D in the egg from which it was hatched but which has been fed on a diet deficient in this vitamin, will die between the tenth and twentieth day of life—usually about the fourteenth day. At no time will it attain a growth greater than that attained by a normal bird on the tenth day. I have seen young canaries with feet so large that they were banded, with difficulty, on the eighth day of life lose their bands on the fourteenth day because their feet were not large enough to keep the bands on.

The baby chick deprived of this vitamin will attain in eight weeks of life about one-third the growth of a normal chick.

Methods of supplying Vitamin D to birds. The simplest way of supplying birds with Vitamin D is to keep them in aviaries, permitting an unlimited supply of direct sunlight. The windows should be so constructed that the birds will be able to get outside the glass whenever they wish and take their sun baths with nothing between them and the outdoors but the screen. Many poultrymen now cover their inside chick runs with celloglass which permits the passage of ultraviolet light. Others use naked arcs or sun lamps to supply their birds with ultraviolet light.

In cases where it is impossible or impractical to supply the birds with ultraviolet light, so they can make their own Vitamin D, they can be given this vitamin in their food. Cod-liver oil was the first known source of this vitamin and it is still the favorite source with many birdmen. Salmon oil is also used. And there are now many commercial foods on the market which have either been treated with ultraviolet light or have had the synthetic vitamin added to them. I make it a point to give my birds all the sunlight I practically can, and as an added safeguard, I use one pint of the very best cod-liver oil in each hundred pounds of soft food.

VITAMIN E. This is the reproductive vitamin. The total absence of any one of the other vitamins mentioned makes life at once impossible, but in this case we are dealing with a substance which appears to have no vital influence on life itself, but concerns solely the function of reproduction.

The possible existence of this vitamin and its presence in fresh hemp seed first came to my attention as the result of some of my own experiments—conducted in 1926 and 1927. Of two groups of canaries treated alike in all other respects, one group was given crushed hemp seed while the hens were making eggs. I found that the eggs of the hens receiving the hemp seed had thicker shells and a much higher percentage of hatchability.*

Later, Dr. Herbert Sanborn informed me that some of his experiments on dogs had led him to a similar conclusion in respect to fresh meat. Of these experiments he wrote: "For ten years I fed dogs on a diet of beef, oatmeal and rice, cooked together, and from as many as eight to ten bitches, no puppies were raised at all. Then, upon the advice of Dr. C. C. Little, I changed to nothing but raw meat and the bitches became pregnant and had puppies."

It has recently been demonstrated that this vitamin is present in germinating grain, that it belongs to the oil-soluble group of vitamins; and it is now provided in the form of biologically tested wheat germ oil. I have used this oil and find that it gives very satisfactory results. It is extremely potent. Two ounces is equivalent to from 35 to 50 pounds of fresh hemp seed. See WHEAT GERM OIL.

VOICE. Voice in birds is produced in the syrinx which is located at the lower end of the trachea. Loss of voice, in which the bird goes through the motions of singing without making any sound, is a symptom of the bronchial form of AVIAN DIPHTHERIA in canaries.

VOICE, CHANGE OF. The development of the sex glands of birds is accompanied by changes of voice, the same as it is in many other animals. The young songbird can never sing in full song nor the young rooster give a full crow until the end of the adolescent period is approached. A young canary attains the same stage of development in from four to six months that the average boy attains in fourteen years.

Changes in the voice of an adult bird is often the first indication of an outbreak of serious illness, of developing lesions in the respiratory tract. See AVIAN DIPHTHERIA.

---

* **Note:** Some of the results of these experiments were published in the "Roller Canary Journal and Bird World," Kansas City, 1930. They were republished in my book, "Diseases of Canaries," Kansas City, 1933.

W

WEAKNESS. Weakness in birds is indicated by the loose carriage of the feathers, by drooped wings, by a disinclination to fly and by the bird sleeping on both feet.

WINGS. See SKELETON; BROKEN BONES; ASPERGILLOSIS.

WHEAT GERM OIL. This is a straw-colored oil with a bran-like flavor. It is obtained from the germinative portions of wheat and is our richest source of Vitamin E, the reproductive vitamin. As a sex stimulant for birds, it is more than ten thousand times more potent than fresh hemp seed. Used in the soft food in the proportion of two ounces to each one hundred pounds of food, it will bring canaries into full song and breeding condition very rapidly; it causes the young males to show pronounced sex development at the time they leave the nest. This vent indication is not entirely reliable, however, for some females will show their sex unmistakably while others will show a vent development indicative of the other sex. No males will be mistaken for females, however.

The feeding of wheat germ oil must be discontinued early in May, however, or it will be impossible to get the birds into moult in August. They will try to breed right through the summer and some of the females will not have a full moult. This is a new substance and all of its effects on canaries have not been studied, but its use in bringing birds into full song, in bringing females into breeding condition and stopping excessive moulting are indicated from my observations to date. See VITAMIN E.

WHITE BLOOD CORPUSCLES. See BLOOD.

WHITE DIARRHEA. See BACILLARY WHITE DIARRHEA; CANARY TYPHOID.

WHITEWASH. See LIME.

WISHBONE. This is the clavicles. Its function in birds is to provide a powerful spring for taking up the momentum of the wings in flight. The normal function of the clavicles in other animals is taken over by the coracoid bone—a bone which is undeveloped in man and many animals. See SKELETON.

WORMS. See GAPE; MANSON'S EYE WORM; ROUNDWORMS; TAPEWORMS.

WOUNDS. Because of their high body temperature, birds are not subject to the ordinary wound infections of mammals. So long as contagious or infectious diseases are not present, no special sterilization of their wounds or of instruments is necessary. The only treatment necessary is the protection of the wound from further injury, for both the injured birds and their mates are apt to peck at an exposed wound. Sometimes the other birds may do a rather thorough job of it.

GLOSSARY

In the writing of this work the use of a number of technical terms has been unavoidable, not so much because the things expressed could not be described in ordinary language—actually, any time a man cannot describe anything, even the theory of relativity, in terms that the average twelve-year-old child can understand, it is because he does not understand the subject himself—but because it has been thought advisable to bring all persons interested in bird disease a key that will open to them the doors leading to a much more thorough understanding of biological science than could possibly be compressed within the covers of a single book. In order to keep my text within the grasp of my most untutored reader, I have made it a policy to define every technical word the first time it is used. Since completing the text, however, I have come to realize that this policy somewhat restricts its usefulness as a reference work. And it is for overcoming that difficulty that this glossary has been added.

The user of this glossary can, by paying strict attention to the derivation of each word looked up, soon become so familiar with the ordinary Greek and Latin roots from which most technical terms are derived that he will be able to instantly grasp the meaning of many other terms not used in this book or included in this glossary. In rendering the Greek roots in the Arabic alphabet, however, I have been at the disadvantage of never having studied the Greek language and of having no reference works on this subject available to me; so I cannot swear that my renditions have always been of the best. I believe that the ordinary reader will find them much more useful than the original Greek, however.

In compiling this glossary I have made extensive use of GOULD'S MEDICAL DICTIONARY, FOURTH EDITION, 1937, Blakiston's Son & Company, 1012 Walnut Street, Philadelphia, Pa., to which I wish to give due credit, without, however, creating any presumption that my brief and fragmentary text can in any way do justice to such an excellent and authoritative work.

TECHNIQUE

It is my misfortune that due to the lack of standard reagents I have been forced to work with the most unorthodox materials, often improvising as I have gone along. Where I tell you to use mercury bichloride, I have used a solution made from table salt, iron and quicksilver into which the metals were introduced by electrolysis; where I tell you to use glacial acetic acid, I have used vinegar; where I tell you to use hydrochloric acid, I may have used digestive mixture; but in each case I have worked out the equivalents and know that the processes as given will give good results. These processes are in no sense standard, however. Those interested in standard processes are referred to GOULD'S MEDICAL DICTIONARY, 4th edition, 1937; MERCK'S INDEX, 5th edition, 1940; CONN'S BIOLOGICAL STAINS, 3rd edition, 1936; OSGOOD'S ATLAS OF HEMATOLOGY, 1937; MOORE'S MICROBIOLOGY, 1912; COPLIN'S MANUAL OF PATHOLOGY, 3rd edition, 1900; HILL'S MANUAL OF HISTOLOGY, 7th edition, 1937; GAGE'S THE MICROSCOPE, 15th edition, 1932, from all of which I have obtained much valuable material.

A. Prefix meaning without, opposite, or reverse; as, **aseptic,** without **sepsis; avirulent,** without **virulence.**

ABDOMEN (ab do' men) from **abdere,** to hide, n. The large inferior cavity of the trunk. That part of the animal anatomy which is located in front of the spine and between the pelvis and the ribs; the belly.

ABDOMINAL (ab dom' in al), adj. Pertaining to the abdomen; as, an abdominal pain; an abdominal operation; the abdominal viscera, the organs contained in the abdominal cavity.

ABDOMINALLY (ab dom' in al ly), adv. Related to the abdomen; as, the pain is abdominally located.

ABNORMAL (ab nor' mal), from **ab,** away from, and **norma,** a rule, adj. Not normal; not conforming to the general rule; as, an **abnormal appetite;** an **abnormal temperature,** one too high or too low.

ABNORMALITY (ab nor mal' ity), n. That which is abnormal. Any deviation from the general rule in anatomy, physiology, or conduct. **Abnormalities** are what you look for when you are studying the symptoms and lesions of a disease.

ABNORMALLY (ab nor' mal ly), adv. Relating to the manner in which a thing is abnormal; as, an abnormally high temperature; an abnormally placed organ; an abnormally held foot or wing; an abnormally large egg.

ACID (ac' id), from **acere,** to be sour, n. Any substance with a sour taste. A compound of an electronegative element with one or more hydrogen atoms which can be replaced by electropositive atoms to form salts. Any substance that forms salts with alkalies. Adj., pertaining to the state of being acid; as, it has an acid taste or an acid reaction.

ACIDIFICATION (ac id' if ik a shun), n. The act of making a thing acid or sour; the extent to which a thing is made acid or sour; as, after the **acidification** is completed; acidification is expressed by the symbol **Ph.**; the acidification is carried to the point Ph.5.6.

ACIDIFY (ac id if i), v. The act of making acid; as, the solution is acidified with acetic acid.

ACIDITY (ac id' it y), n. The state of being acid or the extent to which a thing is acid; as, the acidity must be neutralized; in some bird diseases the acidity of the droppings makes them highly irritating to the vent and cloaca; the acidity of this solution is 3N, or 1/10N. (**N** in this case means **normal,** which chemically is an amount of any substance equal to its molicular weight divided by its valance state dissolved in one liter of distilled water.)

ACIDOPHILE or **ACIDOPHIL** (ac id' o fil), from **acid** and the Greek word meaning loving. Loving acid, n. Any cell, part of cell, or other physiological substance that normally stains with an acid dye.

ACIDOPHILIC (ac id o fil' ic), adj. Pertaining to the property of taking an acid stain; as, this cell contains acidophilic granules.

ACTINOMYCES (ak tin o mi' seez), from the Greek words meaning ray and fungus, n. The name of a pathogenic fungus that grows in a ray or rosette formation and causes disease in both animals and man.

ACTINOMYCOSIS (ak tin o mi ko' sis), n. The disease caused by the ray fungus. This disease is said to occur in birds, but I have not observed it or found any report of its being studied as a disease of birds.

ACUTE (ak ute'), from **acutus,** sharp, adj. Used to describe a sharp pain or a rapidly fatal or severe illness. Any illness that runs a sharp, short course. Not chronic.

AGAR AGAR (ag' ar ag'ar), from the language of Ceylon, n. A glue-like substance made from certain seaweeds. It is used in making media for the growth of bacteria. 1.2 per cent of agar agar added to beef broth renders the broth solid at room temperature and at blood heat and makes it possible to isolate strains of bacteria by taking samples from different colonies. Also, certain organisms grow on this media in such distinctive manners that they can be identified by the characteristics of their colonies.

AGGLUTINATE (ag gloo' tin ate), from **ad,** to, and **glutinare,** to wind, v. To clump or wind together.

AGGLUTINATION TEST (ag gloo tin a' shun), n. A test used in the identification of bacteria and the detection of disease. It consists of exposing a suspension in normal salt solution of the known germ to the suspected serum, or the known serum to the suspected germ. It is used in the detection of pullorum infection in adult hens. A drop of diluted blood serum from the suspected bird is placed on a microscopic slide alongside a drop of the bacterial suspension; a cover glass is dropped on them and they are observed through the microscope. If the hen has the disease, the germs form into clumps; if she is free from the disease the germs remain in suspension. The accuracy of the test is increased by using a series of dilutions.

ALBUS (al' bus), from Latin, white, adj. Applied to a strain of staphylococci that does not form pigment in culture media. It is also the root word from which such words as **albino, albitross,** and **albumen** are derived.

ALKALI (al' ka li), from the Arabic name of sodaash, n. This word includes all of the metallic hydroxides. They form salts with acids and turn litmus blue.

ALKALINE (al' ka line), adj. The quality of, or pertaining to alkali; as, sodium hydroxide forms a strongly alkaline solution.

ALKALINITY (al ka lin' i ty), n. The quality or extent of being alkaline; as, alkalinity is measured between 7 and 14 on the Ph scale. (The symbol **Ph** stands for the reciprocal of the log of the electrolytic dissociation of the substance in dilute solution. Don't try to figure this out; many chemists can't. They rely on test papers and standard color solutions.)

ALKALOID (al' ka loid), from **alkali** and the Greek word for **likeness,** n. Any of the organic, nitrogenous compounds occurring in plants and having the alkaline property of forming salts with acids. This class of substances contains some of our most important drugs; such as, strychnine, morphine, quinine, etc.

ALTERATIVE (awl' ter a tiv), from the Latin word **alterativus,** to change, n. Any one of a class of drugs that have a tonic action on the body that is not explained by their composition. See IODIDES, main vocabulary.

ALVEOLA (al ve' o la), from Latin **alveolus,** a small hole, n. A cavity.

ALVEOLAR (al ve' o lar), adj. Pertaining to an alveolus; a cavity; any small cavity in tissue; used to describe certain cell-like tissues such as lung tissue, fat, and the meshes of elastic connective tissue.

ALVEOLUS (al ve' o lus), pl., **ALVEOLI** (al ve' o lie), the Latin word for cell or cavity, n. An air cell in the lungs; any cavity or cell-like structure in tissue.

AMEBA (am e' bah), from the Greek word meaning **a change,** n. Pl., **AMEBAE** (am e' bee). A single-celled jelly-like animal body found in water and in the intestines of birds and animals. It takes its name from the fact that it is constantly undergoing changes in shape. It is motile by means of arms of protoplasm which it projects from its body and then contracts, drawing itself forward. These are called pseudopods, false feet.

AMEBIC (am e' bik), adj. Like or pertaining to ameba; as, Infectious Entro-Hepatitis of turkeys is an amebic disease; certain of the leucocytes found in the blood of both birds and animals are capable of amebic motion.

AMELIORATE (am e' li or ate), from **melior,** better, or to make better; v., to improve.

ANALGESIC (an al je' sik), from **an,** without and **algos,** pain, n. A drug that stops pain; as, opium is a wonderful analgesic; adj., pertaining to the power to stop pain; as, the action of quinine is only slightly analgesic.

ANATOMY (an at' o me), from the Greek words **up** and **to cut,** n. The science of the structure of living creatures; as, he is interested in the study of anatomy. The structures themselves; as, the anatomy of the rat is in many respects similar to the anatomy of man.

ANATOMY, Morbid. The structure and tissue changes that take place during disease; the study of those changes; pathology.

ANATOMICAL (an at om' ik al), adj. Pertaining to anatomy; as, the anatomical changes in this case are very interesting.

ANEMIA (an e' me ah), from the Greek words **an,** deficiency or without and **emia,** blood, n. The condition of having too little blood; too few red corpuscles in the blood; or too little of the iron pigment of the blood, hemoglobin.

ANEMIC (an em' ik), adj. Pertaining to the condition of not having sufficient blood or blood-making elements but referring to the individual afflicted by the deficiency; as, this patient is very anemic. The condition is indicated in birds by paleness of the feet and beak and a red-cell count of less than 3,000,000. In anemia due to deficiency of iron pigment the erythrocytes will be smaller than normal; there will be greater variation in size, too.

ANTE (an' te), Latin for **before** in time; as, **ante-Christian,** before Christ; **ante meridian,** before noon.

ANTEMORTEM (an' te mor' tem), Latin for before and death, and meaning before death.

Figure 87.

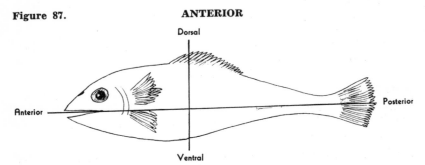

Sketch of a fish which illustrates the correct usage of the words: **anterior, posterior, ventral,** and **dorsal.***
Sketch by the author.

ANTERIOR (an te' re or), Latin, **before,** adj. Pertaining to the part of the body or of an organ that is toward the head. Opposite from posterior, toward the tail.

ANTI (an' ti), Greek for **against.**

ANTINEURALGENT (an te noo ral' gent), from **against; neuron,** nerve; and **algos,** pain. A drug that stops the pain of neuralgia.

---

* **Note:** In using the words **anterior, posterior, dorsal** and **ventral** it should be borne in mind that these terms refer to directions as they exist in the lower vertebrates, not as they exist in man or birds. In fish the tail is directly opposite from the head; the dorsum, back, is directly opposite the vent, which is located at the lower end of the belly. Thus, the posterior aspect of an organ in man is always the part closest to the ground when he is standing erect; the anterior part the part closest to the crown of his head; the ventral aspect is toward the front of the body, the dorsal, toward the back. Many authoritative books, however, fall into confusion through the inability of their authors to keep these distinctions in mind. Gould's Medical Dictionary, in defining the word dorsal—Fourth Edition, page 427—says: "Pertaining to the back or posterior part of an organ," which is just as sensible as it would be for a geographer to define **polar** as being north or west.

ANTIPYRETIC (an te pi ret' ik), from the Greek words **anti,** against, and **pyretos,** fever. A drug that lowers body temperature during fever; as, quinine is our best antipyretic, adj. Pertaining to the power to lower body temperature; as, antipyretic action, antipyretic therapy.

ANTI-RACHITIC (an te ra kit' ic). Pertaining to vitamin D or any food that prevents or cures rickets.

ANTISCORBUTIC (an te skor bu' tik), from Greek word **anti,** against, and the Latin word **scorbutus,** scurvy, adj. Pertaining to the power to stop scurvy, or prevent it. Antiscorbutic acid, vitamin C, or any food rich in this substance; as, oranges are one of our best antiscorbutic foods.

ANTISEPTIC (an te sep' tik), from the Greek words **anti** and **sepsis,** putrefaction. Against putrefaction. Any substance that will inhibit the growth of microorganisms, as distinct from a disinfectant, which is a substance that destroys microorganisms.

ANTITHALMINTIC (an te thal min' tik). Against tapeworms. Any drug that will destroy or expel tapeworms.

AORTA (a ort' ah), Greek. The large vessel arising from the left ventricle and, through its branches, supplying aerated blood to all parts of the body. The largest of the arteries.

APOPLECTIFORM (ap o plek' tif orm), from **apoplexy** and **forma,** Latin for form or shape. Resembling apoplexy.

APOPLEXY (ap' o pleks e), from the Greek word meaning **to strike down** or **stun.** A paralytic condition resulting from a hemorrhage into the brain or spinal cord.

ARACHNOID (ar ak' noid), from the Greek words **araxno,** spider web and **eidos,** form, n. Like spider web. The central one of the three membranes covering the brain and spinal cord.

ARGUS MINIATES (ar' gus min i ate' es) and **ARGUS PERSICUS** (ar' gus per cee' kus). These are names applied to the fowl ticks responsible for avian spirochetosis.

ARTICULAR (ar tik' u lar), from **articularis,** a joint, adj. Pertaining to the joints; as articular rheumatism, rheumatism of the joints.

ASCITIS (as i' teez), from the Greek word **askos,** a bag. Dropsy of the peritonium. An abnormal collection of fluid in the abdominal cavity.

ASCITIC (as it' ik), adj. Pertaining to or affected with ascitis.

ASCITIC FLUID. The fluid of dropsy. It is used in bacteriology for the preparation of certain special media for the cultivation of organisms that cannot be grown on the commonly used culture media. Particularly, spirochetes.

ASEXUAL (ah seks' u al), from **a,** without, and **sexus,** sex. adj. Pertaining to the absence of or being without sex.

ASPASTIC (ah spas' tik), from **a,** without, and **spastikos,** pertaining to a spasm. Used in the description of paralysis in which the muscles are relaxed and flaccid.

ASPERGILLUS (as per jil' us), from **aspergere,** a sprinkle. A genus of fungi in the examination of which the microscopic field is always liberally sprinkled with spores. See main vocabulary.

ASPERGILLOSIS (as per jil o' sis), from **aspergere** and **osis,** a disease or infection. The disease caused by infection with an aspergillus fungus. See main vocabulary.

ASPHYXIATION (as fiks e at' shun), from **a,** without, and the Greek word for pulse. The state of death or collapse resulting from the deprivation of the body of oxygen. Partial asphyxiation in birds is recognized by the dark color of the feet and beak.

ASTHENIA (ah sthe' ne ah), from the Greek words **a,** without; **sthenos,** strength. Weakness; loss of strength; conditions in which there is emaciation and weakness; Going Light. Dawson's designation for a disease of poultry characterized by emaciation and great weakness and which he ascribed to the presence of a bacterium in the duodenum.

ASTHMA (az' mah), Greek, panting. A paroxysmal affection of the bronchial tubes characterized by coughing, wheezing, and a feeling of constriction and suffocation. See main vocabulary.

ASTRINGENT (as trin' jent), from **ad,** to; **stringere,** to bind. A drug producing contraction or binding of a mucous or organic tissue or that stops bleeding; the action of such a drug.

ATROPHY (at' ro fe), Greek, diminution. The decrease in size of a cell or an organ; the complete or partial destruction of an organ resulting from the cutting off its blood supply as a sequence to the scirrhosis or thrumbosos of the supplying artery; decrease in size resulting from scirrhotic changes in the organ itself in which the functional tissue is largely replaced by connective tissue.

ATYPICAL (ah tip' ik al), from **a,** without, and **typos,** a type, adj. Without type. Irregular. A departure from the regular form or structure in any cell or organ; a departure from the regular course in any disease.

AUREUS (awr e' us), yellow. This term is applied to certain micro-organisms that produce yellow pigment in cultural media.

AURICLE (aw' rik l), from the Latin word **auricula,** the ear. The expanded part of the pinna of the ear. One of the upper chambers of the heart. The right auricle receives blood from the general circulation; the left auricle receives blood from the lungs through the pulmonary vein. See CIRCULATORY SYSTEM, main vocabulary.

AUSCULTATION (aws kul ta' shun), from **auscultare,** to listen. A method of investigating the functioning and conditions of organs, particularly those of the respiratory system and circulation, by listening to the sounds they themselves give out.*

AVIAN (a' vi an), adj. Pertaining to birds.

B

B. Abbreviation for bacterium or bacillus.

BACILLARY (bas' il a re), diminutive form of **baculus,** a rod, lit., a little rod, adj. Pertaining to the bacilli, a genus of microorganisms made up of rod-shaped forms.

BACILLUS, pl., **BACILLI** (bas il' us, bas il' li). See BACILLARY.

BACTERIA, sing., **BACTERIUM** (bak te' re ah, bak te' re um). A genus of microorganisms. This word is rather loosely used. Ehrenberg and Dujardin, about a century ago, restricted the word to rod-like organism having no tendency to unite into chains or filaments. In the early part of the present century, some investigators attempted to restrict it to the non-spore-forming, single-cell, plant-like organisms, while Moore restricted the meaning of the word **bacilli** to rod-like flagellated organisms and the word **bacteria** to the rod-like non-flagellated forms. The most recent edition of Gould's dictionary applies it to the whole field of single-cell, plant-

---

* **Note:** In recent experiments on the application of this method to the study of respiratory diseases in small birds I have found that a very satisfactory stethoscope can be constructed from a small piece of 6mm glass tubing, a piece of ⅛" rubber tubing and a single ear-piece from an ordinary stethoscope. The glass tube is cut about two inches long, flanged slightly on one end and drawn out a little on the other. The small end is fitted into one end of the rubber tube, which should be 12 to 14 inches long. The ear-piece is fitted into the other end of the rubber tube. With the ear-piece in place, the expanded end of the glass tube is moved over the area to be examined. I have found that it is not only possible to recognize changes in a canary's lungs and determine which lung is involved, but that the exact location or the origin of the bubbling rales and ticking sounds heard in bronchitis and pneumonia can be determined with an error not exceeding one millimeter.

like organisms, including cocci (spherical), bacilli (rod-shaped), and spirilla (spiral threads). In some places in this book I have used the word **bacterium** in the general sense, but where applied to distinct species, I have attempted to follow the distinctions of Migula and Moore and restrict it to the non-flagellated rods.

BACTERIAL (bak te' re al), adj. Pertaining to bacteria; as, bacterial products; bacterial infections.

BACTERIOLOGY (bak te re ol' o je), from **bacteria** and **logos,** to learn or science. The science and study of germs.

BASAL METABOLISM (ba' sal met ab' o lizm), from **basis,** a foundation; **metabole,** change. The rate at which an animal changes food into energy while at rest as measured by the amount of carbon dioxide exhaled by the lungs in a given period.

BASIC (ba'sik). Synonymous with alkaline; substances having the power to neutralize acids.

BASOPHILE (bas' o fil), from **basis,** foundation; **philein,** to love. This is applied to those protoplasmic substances having an affinity for basic dyes and to cells characterized by such substances, such as the basophile of mammalian blood which is characterized by large cytoplasmic granules that stain deeply with methylene blue.

BELLADONNA (bel ah don' ah), from Italian, **bella donna,** beautiful lady. It takes its name from the fact that it causes expansion of the pupil of the eye and was at one time used for this purpose by European ladies desiring to increase the beauty of their eyes. It is obtained from the plant, deadly nightshade, and owes its effects to the alkaloids atropine and hyocyamine. The only purpose for which I have employed this drug in bird medicine is to cause the sphincture of the os uteri to relax. See EGG BINDING.

BERKEFELD (berk' felt). A filter of diatomaceous earth. Its pores are so fine that they will hold back all ordinary bacteria; thus, its filtrate is bacteria free. It is used in the study of the virus diseases, so called because their causative agent is small enough to pass such a filter.

BIOLOGICS, BIOLOGICALS (bi o loj' iks). A class of drugs or medicinals made from animal tissues, serums, or from the growth of germs on culture media, some of which are used for conferring immunity, the vaccines, and some in the treatment of developed diseases, the antitoxins.

BLAST (blast), from the Greek **blastos,** a germ. This is used as a prefix or suffix to denote those cells and tissues from which other cells or tissues are derived by differentiation. In connection with the cells of the blood, Osgood—Atlas of Hematology—restricts its usage to the original stem cells from which the different types of blood cells are derived; as, lymphoblasts, monoblasts, granuloblasts, plasmablasts, and karyoblasts.

BLASTODERM (blas' to derm), from **blastos,** a germ; **derma,** the skin. The germinal disc. A small membranous disc of cells lying on the internal surface of the vitalline membrane of the fertile egg. See EGG STRUCTURE AND FORMATION.

BRONCHITIS (brong ki' tis), from **bronchus; itis,** inflammation. An inflammation of the bronchial tubes.

BRONCHUS, pl., **BRONCHI** (brong' kus, brong' ki). Greek. Bronchial tubes. Strictly speaking, only the primary divisions to the trachea are so designated. The smaller tubes are called BRONCHIUM, pl., BRONCHIA, but few writers are careful about such fine distinctions.

BUCKTHORN (buk' thorn). A laxative drug made from a European plant. Now largely replaced by cascara, which is from a closely related American plant. The preparation usually used in bird medicine is known as **syrup of buckthorn.** The dose is from three to five drops to the ounce of drinking water.

BUFF. This term is used by canary breeders to describe the feather structure of certain birds that have a buff or mealy appearance that is caused by each feather having a margin of colorless web. See BALDNESS.

C

C. Abv. for Centigrade.

CANKER (kang' ker), from **cancer,** a crab. An ulcerous or gangrenous sore. This term is sometimes applied to avian diphtheria or its lesions of the skin and mouth.

CANULA, CANNULA (kan' u lah), dim. of **canna,** a tube. Any tube, but often applied to hypodermic needles.

CAPILLARY (kap' il a re), from **capillus,** hair-like. Relating to hair-like filaments; the smallest vessels of the circulatory system.

CARBOHYDRATES (kar bo hi' drats), from **carbo,** carbon; **hydros,** water. Compounds containing carbon, oxygen and hydrogen, the two latter elements in the same proportion as they occur in water.

They comprise the starches and sugars, and those digestible carbo-hydrates present in food are converted into dextrose by the process of digestion, in which form they are used by the body as fuel. The excess is converted into fat and stored.

CARCINOMA (kar sin o' mah), from **karkinos,** a crab; **oma,** a tumor. Literally, a crab-like tumor; a cancer; a malignant tumor arising from cells of the ectoderm, the epithelial cells.

CARTILAGE (kar' til aj), from **cartilago,** gristle. A white, semi-opaque, nonvascular connective tissue composed of a matrix con-taining nucleated cells. This tissue is the forerunner of bone, but, contrary to what was once thought, the cartilaginous cells play no part in the formation of bone. The cartilage simply forms a sup-porting structure which is excavated away as the bone is formed by an entirely different set of cells. In many structures, however, the cartilage is the permanent formation. See Drawing Number 8, Figure 56, which shows the cartilage layer of a canary's eye.

CARTILAGINOUS (kar til aj' in us). Made of, pertaining to, or resembling cartilage.

CASEOUS (ka' se us), from **caseus,** cheese. Having the nature or consistence of cheese. Usually used in describing exudates occur-ring in the body cavities or other morbid lesions during disease.

CATALEPTIC (kat al ep' tik). Pertaining to catalepsy. Used in describing the rigidity of the muscles observed in some cases of paralysis.

CATARRH (kat' ahr'), from **katarrhin,** to flow down. An inflam-mation of a mucous membrane. It is also applied to certain chronic inflammation of the tubules of the kidneys and the alveoli of the lungs.

CATECHU (kat' e ku) (East Indian). An extract from the wood of an East Indian tree. It contains 50% tannic acid and is a power-ful astringent. The crude powder is used in the control and treat-ment of coccidiosis and infectious entro-hepatitis in the proportion of one-third teaspoonful to the gallon of drinking water. I have used the tincture on canaries in the proportion of one drop to the ounce of water.

CECA (se' ka), from **cecus,** blind. Blind guts located just above the cloaca in the intestines of birds. See DIGESTIVE TRACT.

CELL. The unit from which all tissue is constructed. See BLOOD for a description of an ideal cell.

CELLOSOLVE (sel' o solv). Ethylene Glycol Monoethyl Ether, an organic solvent. Used in histology as a substitute for alcohol. Can be used for preserving bodies for shipment.

CELLULAR (sel' u lar), from **cella,** a cell. Pertaining to, composed of or produced by cells.

CENTIGRADE (sen' te grad), from **centi,** one hundred; **gradus,** a step. One hundred steps. The temperature scale having zero at the freezing point of water and 100 degrees at the boiling point of water. To convert Fahrenheit readings to Centigrade, subtract 32 and divide the remainder by 1.8. To convert Centigrade to Fahrenheit, multiply by 1.8 and add 32 to the result.

CENTROSOME (sen' tro som), from **centro,** central; **soma,** body. A small body located near the center of certain cells, particularly those capable of mitotic divisions. See drawing of ideal cell under BLOOD, Figure 12.

CEREBELLUM (ser e bel' um), dim. for **cerebrum,** small brain. See Figures 14 and 19.

CEREBRUM (ser' e brum). Latin for brain. The large, thinking brain. See Figures 14 and 19.

CHALAZA (kal a' zah), from **chalanion,** a small hailstone. One of the twisted cords binding the egg yolk to the shell membrane. See Figure 29.

CHALAZIFEROUS (kal as if' er us). Pertaining to the chalaza.

CHEMICO-THERAPY (kem' i co ther'ap e). The treatment of disease by drugs of chemical origin rather than with those of biological origin.

CHLORIDE (klor' id). A salt of hydrochloric acid. Common table salt is sodium chloride.

CHLOROPHYLL (klo' ro fil), from **chloros,** green; **phyllon,** leaf. The green coloring matter from vegetation.

CHROMATIC (kro mat' ik), from **chroma,** color. Relating to or possessing color.

CHROMATIN (kro' mat in), from **chroma,** color. The material in the nuclei of cells that takes a deep stain with basic dyes. See Figure 12.

CHROME (krom). Referring to the metal chromium or its compounds.

CHROMO (kro' mo). A prefix meaning colored.

CHROMOSOME (kro' mo som), from **chroma,** color; **soma,** body.

A colored body. Tiny, deep-staining, rod-like bodies seen in the nuclei of dividing cell, now known to be the carriers of inheritance, or, more strictly, to contain the carriers of inheritance, which are small bodies called genes. The genes are beyond the range of the direct-vision microscope, though they have been photographed.

CIDE (side), from **cedere**, to kill. A suffix meaning to kill, as **vermicide**, to kill worms; **insecticide**, to kill insects; **germicide**, to kill germs.

CINCHOPHEN (sin' ko fen). A complex organic drug used in the treatment of gout. See section on GOUT, main vocabulary. The full chemical name of this drug is phenylcinchoninic acid.

CLINIC (klin' ik), from **kliny**, a bed. Medical instructions given at the bedside. A place where such instructions are given.

CLINICAL (klin' ik al). Pertaining to bedside treatment or instructions. 2, Pertaining to the symptoms and course of a disease as observed by the doctor, in opposition to the anatomical changes found by the pathologist—all facts observed concerning a disease during the life of the victim, and it is in this sense that the word is used in this book.

CLOACA (klo a' kah). Latin, a sewer. In birds, the common pouch at the lower end of the intestines into which the intestines, ureters and sex ducts empty. See DIGESTIVE TRACT, Figure 25.

CLONIC (klon' ik), from **klonos**, commotion. Applied to convulsions in which the muscles are alternately contracted and relaxed, producing uncontrolled movements, usually of a violent nature. See AVITIMINOSIS B.

COAGULATE (ko ag' yoo late), from **coagulare**, to curdle. To curdle or clot. The separation of certain protein and albuminous substances from the fluid in which they are in solution under the influence of heat, acid, or oxygen; as, the coagulation of the albumen in urine or serum under the influence of heat in the presence of acid; the coagulation of casein under the influence of the acid forming in souring milk; the coagulation of blood, more correctly, the fibrin in the blood, upon exposure to the air.

COAGULATION NECROSIS (ko ag' u la' shun nek ro' sis), from **coagulare**, a clot; **nekros**, dead. A form of tissue destruction in which the cells lose their nuclei and fibrin is thrown down. See LEAD POISONING, Figures 52 and 53.

COAGULUM (ko ag' u lum). That which has coagulated. The clot.

COALESCE (ko al es'), from **coalescere**, to grow together; v., the tendency of culonies, sores, abscesses, or other lesions to spread and become one.

COALESCENCE (ko al es' ens), n. The union of two or more parts or things previously separate.

COCCI (kok' si), plural of **COCCUS** (kok' us), from **kokkos,** a berry. Strictly speaking, small spheroid microorganisms which may occur singly; in pairs, diplococci; in chains, streptococci; in clumps, staphylococci, but many of the forms commonly classed as cocci could not by any stretch of the imagination be considered spheroid; for instance, gonococci are actually diplobacilli with the long axes of the elements parallel; pneumococci; large, encapsulated, cylindrical, diplobacilli joined end to end and having distinctly square ends. See Figure 72.

COCCIDIOSIS (kok sid e o' sis), from **coccidium** and **nosos,** disease. A disease caused by the presence of coccidia in the body. See main vocabulary.

COCCIDIUM, pl., **COCCIDIA** (kok sid' e um, kok sid' e ah), from **coccus.** A genus of protozoa responsible for disease in man, animals and birds. See main vocabulary.

COCCOID (kok' oyd), from **coccus; eidos,** resemblance. Resembling cocci.

COCCUS (kok' us), from **kokkos,** berry. A microorganism with small spherical elements.

COCCYGEAL (kok sij' e al), from **coccus.** Pertaining to the coccyx.

COCCYX (kok' siks), from **kokkyx,** cuckoo. Resembling a bill. The last bones of the spinal column. In birds, the bones that support the tail.

COITION (ko ish' un), from **coire,** to come together. Sexual union.

COLI (kol' e), from **colon.** Pertaining to the colon and used as a prefix and in compound names where it is desired to show a relation to the colon; as, **colicodynia,** pain in the colon; **colibacillus,** the colon bacillus, bacillus coli; coli group, a group of pathogenic organisms closely related to **B. coli,** and containing the typhoid, paratyphoid and paracolon bacilli.

COLON (ko' lon). Greek. The large intestine of mammals. Strictly speaking, birds have no colon, though the lower divisions of their intestines are sometimes so called, and the lining of this lower part of the small intestines corresponds closely to that of the human colon. Or, at least to that of the human appendix. I chopped up my own for comparison. See B, Figure 27.

COMPOUND FRACTURE (kom' pound frak' tur), from **com,** together; **ponere,** to put; **frangere,** to break. A broken bone that has perforated the skin.

CONGENITAL (kon jen' it al), from **con,** with; **genitus,** born. Something you are born with or that develops after birth as a result of an inherited characteristic or tendency. See BALDNESS.

CONGESTION (kon jes' chun), from **congerere,** to heap up. An abnormal amount of blood in tissue, which may result from infection, injury, loss of tone, or interference with the return circulation, and may be either inflammatory or hypostatic. It is usually named from the part affected; as, **pulmonary congestion; peritoneal congestion.** See Figure 59.

CONJUNCTIVA (kon junk ti' vah), from **conjunctivus,** connecting. The mucous membrane that connects the eyeball with the lids.

CONJUNCTIVITIS (kon junk' tiv i' tis), from **conjunctiva** and **itis,** inflammation. Inflammation of the conjunctiva. See main vocabulary.

CONTRA (kon' trah). A prefix meaning against.

CONTRACEPTIVE (kon trah sep' tiv), from **contra,** against, and **conception.** A drug which prevents conception.

CONTRA INDICATED (kon' trah in' dik at ed), from **contra,** against; **indicare,** to indicate. Must not be used. Certain drugs and lines of treatment, very effective under some circumstances, are very dangerous under other circumstances. In the text of this book I have in many places recommended the use of sodium perborate, but in discussing diseases of the kidneys I have warned that this drug is **contra indicated** in such cases, since it is very injurious to inflamed kidneys. In the bronchial form of Avian diphtheria, I have warned that all treatment of the sores is **contra indicated,** for the condition of the heart is such that the bird is apt to drop dead from the least excitement.

CONVOLUTION TUBES (kon vo loo' shun tubes), from **convolvere,** to roll together. The small tubes of the kidneys, which are rolled, twisted and coiled together. See Figure 51.

COPPERAS (kop' er as), from **cupri rosa,** rose of copper. The common name for ferrous sulphate, $FeSO_4\text{-}7H_2O$.

CORNEA (kor' ne ah), from **corneus,** horny. The hard, glassy membrane covering the exposed part of the eyeball.

CORTEX (kor' teks). Latin for **bark.** That part of an organ or gland lying just below the capsule. In many organs there is a distinct difference in structure and function of the tissues so situated and those lying in the center of the organ, which, by the way, are called **medulary.** The name of the organ designates the particular cortex one is talking about; as, **renal cortex,** the cortex of the kidney; **cerebrial cortex,** the cortex of the cerebrum.

CRENATED (kre' nat ed), from **crena,** a notch. This term is used to describe a withered, scalloped, notched appearance of the red blood cells when they are exposed to air or too strong a salt solution. In bird blood the cytoplasm of the crenated erythrocytes forms into a number of small, globular clumps which are distributed around the periphery of the cell, just inside of the cell membrane.

CREST (krest). In anatomy, a ridge or prominence, especially on a bone. In birds, a rosette of feathers on the top of the head; a bird having such a rosette. See BALDNESS.

CREST BRED (krest bred). A bird bred from crested stock but having no crest. Such birds have thick head feathers that give them a beetle-browed appearance. See BALDNESS.

CULTURE (kul' chure), from **colere,** to till. The act of growing or the growth of microorganisms on artificial media.

CYSTITIS (sist i' tis), from **kystis,** pouch or bladder; **itis,** inflammation. Inflammation of the bladder. This is one condition unknown in birds, since they have no bladder, but the word has been used several times in the text in relation to the properties of drugs.

CYTE (site). A cell. A prefix and suffix meaning **a cell** or pertaining to cells or cell protoplasm.

CYTOLOGY (si tol' o je), from **cyte,** cell; **logos,** science. The science of cells; the study of tissue; histology.

CYTOPLASM (si' to plazm), from **cyto,** pertaining to a cell; **plasm,** anything formed. The material from which cells and tissue are formed. Strictly speaking, that part of the cell protoplasm lying outside of the nucleus and inside of the ectoplasm; often used to designate all material outside of the nucleus.

D

DELETERIOUS (del et e' re us), from the Greek word, **hurtful.** That which does harm, adj. As, the **deleterious** action of light upon some drugs and chemicals is guarded against by the use of bottles of brown glass. The indiscriminate use of drugs in advance of correct diagnosis is sure to have a **deleterious** effect upon the health of a bird.

DELIQUESCENT (del ik wes' ent), from **deliquescere,** to melt away. The property of certain substances of absorbing enough water from the air to dissolve themselves. DELIQUESCENCE, the act of dissolving in the attracted water.

DERMIS (der' mis), from **derma,** the skin. The true skin as distinguished from the epidermis, the outer skin covering. The epidermis is composed of squamous—flat, scaly—epithelial cell, the dermis of connective tissue. When you blister your hand, it is the epidermis that is lost. The **dermis** remains intact and the blister heals without a scar. It is only when the dermis is injured that scarring occurs.

DIABETES (di ab e' teez, not tis), from **dia,** through; **bainein,** to go. A disease characterized by an abnormal amount of urine and now known to result from the degeneration of the islands of Langerhans, little masses of epithelial cells in the interstitial tissue of the pancreas, the function of which is to manufacture insulin, the hormone that permits the muscles to burn sugar. The unburned sugar is present in the urine. I have recently found some evidence that birds that go out of condition as the result of too much handling—nervous shock—are victims of this condition.

DIAGNOSIS (di ag no' sis), from **dia,** apart; **gnosis,** knowledge. The determination of the nature of a disease and its identity, during the life of the victim, if possible. **Differential diagnosis,** the distinguishing between two diseases of similar character by a close comparison of their symptoms. See main vocabulary.

DIAPHORETIC (di ah for et' ik), from **dia,** across, through, apart; **pherein,** to carry. A drug that causes sweating.

DIARRHEA (di are e' ah), from **dia,** through; **rein,** to flow. A condition characterized by looseness of the bowels and frequent watery or mucoid movements.

DIASTOLE (di as' to le). Greek, for a drawing apart. The period of dilatation of a chamber of the heart, particularly the ventricles. See CIRCULATORY SYSTEM.

DIETETIC (di et et' ik). Pertaining to diet.

DIETETICS (di et et' iks), from **diaita,** a system of living. The science of food.

DIFFERENTIAL (dif er en' shal), from **differentia,** difference, adj. Pertaining to, creating, or recognizing a difference; as **differential**

blood count, the counting of a sufficient number of the leukocytes found in a blood smear to determine their relative percentages; **differential diagnosis,** the comparison of all ascertainable facts concerning two similar diseases with the symptoms observed in the patient in order to arrive at a diagnosis; **differential staining,** methods by which the histologist and bacteriologist employ one or more dyes in such a manner as to stain different tissues, different cells, different materials within the cells, or different microorganisms different colors, so that they may be recognized and identified under the microscope with ease and dispatch.

DIFFERENTIATE (dif er en' she ate), from **differentia,** v. To make a differentiation; to distinguish a difference.

DIFFERENTIATION (dif er en she a' shun), from **differentia,** n. The act of making a differentiation or of recognizing or making recognizable a difference. The process by which tissue cells change from general to special characteristics.

DIOXANE (di oks' an). Diethylene Dioxide. An organic solvent prepared by distilling glycol with diluted sulphuric acid. Melts at 11 C.; boils at 101 C., but may explode, so it is dehydrated and purified by permitting it to stand over calcium oxide, quick lime. It dissolves many fats, oils and gums and is miscible with water and the usual organic solvents in all proportions. Is sometimes used as a substitute for alcohol in pathological work.

DIPHTHERIA (dif the' re ah), from **diphthera,** a skin or membrane. See AVIAN DIPHTHERIA, main vocabulary.

DIURETIC (di u ret' ik), from **dia,** through; **ourein,** to urinate. A drug that increases the flow of urine.

DOMINANT (dom' i nant), from **dominus,** lord or dominion. That which dominates or is powerful over others; as, a **dominant character,** a character like white feathers or a crest, which, when inherited from one parent, develops to the exclusion of the opposite character—yellow feathers, plain head—of the other parent. The word was first used in the sense here indicated by Johann Gregor Mendel in his work on heredity. A work, by the way, which was ignored for sixty-nine years, until thirty years after his death.

DORSAL (dor' sal), from **dorsum,** the back. Towards or pertaining to the back, not posterior. See discussion under ANTERIOR.

DOUBLE BUFFING (dub' l buf' ing). The mating of two buff birds together. See BALDNESS, main vocabulary.

DRENCH (drench). The process of pouring a fluid medicine down an animal's throat, used only with the large domesticated animals.

Probably so called from the fact that the veterinarian is apt to get drenched when the animal offers a strong objection to the medicine.

E

ECCHYMOSIS (ek e mo' sis), from **ek,** out; **chymos,** juice. An extravasation of blood into the subcutaneous tissue, which causes a purple discoloration of the skin. The color gradually changes to brown, green, and yellow—you remember that "shiner." Also, more loosely used to designate any discoloration of the skin.

ECTODERM (ek' to derm), from **ecto, ectos,** without, upon the outside; **derma,** skin. The outer membrane in the early development of the embryo, which is the embryonic tissue from which the skin, epithelium, and nervous tissues are later derived.

ECTOPLASM (ek' to plasm), from **ecto,** out; **plossein,** to form. The outer layer of cell protoplasm. See ideal cell, Figure 12.

EFFERVESCENT (ef er ves' ent), from **effervescere,** to boil. Substances or preparations that give off bubbles when placed in water.

EFFICACY (ef' i ka si), n. The power to produce results.

EGG BOUND (eg' bound). The condition in which a hen is unable to pass her egg. See main vocabulary.

ELONGATED (e lon' gat ed). The act or condition of being or becoming longer.

EMACIATION (e ma se a' shun). The loss of weight, fat and flesh from the body. Referring to the condition of being thin and weak, which may result either from starvation or disease.

EMBRYO (em' bre o), from **en,** in; **bryein,** to swell with. This is the name applied to any animal during the period of intraovum or intrauterine development; i. e., between the beginning of development of the fertilized ovum and birth or hatching.

EMBRYOLOGY (em bre ol' o je), from **embryo; logos,** science. The branch of biological science dealing with the study of intraovum and intrauterine development.

EMETIC (em et' ik), from **emeein,** to vomit. A drug that causes vomiting.*

---

* **Note:** In rendering the roots, from which most of these words are derived, I am at the distinct disadvantage of having never made any systematic study of the Greek language and having no reference material on the subject. In the present case, there are three Greek e's in the word for vomit, but over the first, there are two accents; over the second, one accent; over the third, none, and I haven't the remotest idea as to what they represent.

ENDEMIC (en dem' ik), from **en,** in; **demos,** the people. A disease that is constantly present but only occasionally reaches epidemic proportion. Pneumonia is such a disease of man. The germs can be found in the throats of most healthy persons, but they cause disease only in persons of lowered resistance. Cholera is such a disease of birds and animals, and in both of these diseases it must be remembered that it is the germ the other fellow carries that is most dangerous to you. Your cells know how to fight the ones with which they are constantly associated. That is why the congregation of large numbers of strange birds, animals, or men is pretty apt to be followed by an increased prevalence of cholera and pneumonia which may, under those circumstances, become epidemic.

ENDO (en do), from **endon,** within. A prefix meaning within.

ENDOCARDITIS (en do kar di' tis), from **endon,** within; **cardium,** the heart; **itis,** inflammation. An inflammation of the lining membrane of the heart.

ENDOCRINE (en' do krin), from **endo; krinein,** to separate. Any internal secretion; a hormone; also, used to describe the glands capable of elaborating internal secretions.

ENDOTHELIAL (en do the' le al). Pertaining to the **endothelium.** Endothelial cells resemble squamous epithelial cells in appearance, but they are derived from the endoderm or mesoderm—there seems to be some doubt. The term is now also applied to the reticular cells—the supporting cells—of the spleen and liver.

ENDOTHELIUM (en do the' le um), from **endon,** within; **thele,** a nipple. The lining membrane of the heart; blood vessels; serous cavities; and joints.

ENTRO-HEPATITIS (en' tro hep at i' tis), ırom **entrails,** bowels; **hepar,** the liver; **itis,** inflammation. An inflammation of the bowels and liver. A disease of turkeys characterized by inflammation of the bowels and liver. See INFECTIOUS ENTRO-HEPATITIS, main vocabulary.

ENVIRONMENTAL (en vir on ment' al), from the French **environner,** to surround, adj. Pertaining to or the result of the conditions surrounding the organism, living conditions.

EOSIN (e' o sin), from **eos,** the dawn. A red dye, tetrabromfluorescein, widely used in histology. Actually, there is a whole series of these dyes, known as the Xanthene dyes. They range in color from yellow to almost purple and in reaction from the strongly acid fluorescein to the very weakly acid phloxene. They all produce the characteristic eosin effects in varying degrees, and some workers prefer one dye, some another. For smears, yellow eosin is probably the best. For tissue, I prefer phloxene.

EOSINOPHILE, EOSINOPHIL (e o sin' o fil), from **eosin; philein,** to love. To love eosin. Generally, any cell, organism, part of cell, or substance taking the eosin stain. Specifically, a large leucocyte found in both animal and bird blood, the cytoplasm of which contains a large number of large granules that stain orange-red with eosin. See BLOOD, main vocabulary.*

EPIDEMIC (ep e dem' ik), from **epi,** upon; **demos,** people. A disease spreading rapidly through a community and affecting a large number of individuals. In birds and animals, such diseases are called **epizootics.**

EPIDERMIS (ep e der' mis), from **epi,** upon; **derma,** the skin. Upon the skin. The outer covering of the skin, composed of epithelial cells, as distinct from the dermis, the lower layer, composed of connective tissue cells.

EPITHELIAL (ep e the' le al), adj. Pertaining to the epithelium. Epithelial cells; the cells making up the outer layer of the skin and of all the tubes and cavities of the body having communication with the outside of the body, and of a few glands, such as the thyroid, which do not communicate with the outside of the body, though such communications existed during early fetal life.

EPITHELIAL CASTS. Casts found in the urine of both men and birds suffering from nephritis and composed of epithelial cells from the kidney tubules.

EPITHELIUM (ep e the' le um), from **epi,** upon; **thele,** nipple. This term is applied to the cells of the epidermis and to those lining all the tubes and cavities of the body having outlets to the outside of the body, no matter how complex the outlet may be, and some glands that had such outlets during fetal life, but which do not have them during adult life, such as the thyroid and pituitary. The cotrex of the adrenals contain cells very similar to the epithelial cells, but they appear to have been derived from the skin by the very remote path of the neural fold and the nervous system.

---

* **Note:** It is the modern tendency in spelling words of this type to drop the final **e** and shift the accent towards the front of the word; as, **i o dine'** and **i' o din; vi tah mine'** and **vi' tam in.** In the present case, Gould's Dictionary, Fourth Edition, 1937, page 470, lists only **eosinophil** in the vocabulary, but, in the text, makes the unique distinction of using the word **eosinophil** in the general sense of any histological or biological substance taking the eosin stain, and the word **eosinophile** to designate the eosinophilic polymorphonuclear leucocyte, (eosinophil lobocyte.—Osgood).

EPIZOOTIC (ep e zo ot' ik), from **epi; zoon,** animal. An epidemic among creatures other than man.

ERECTILE (e rek' til), from **erect.** Having the quality of becoming erect. Tissue consisting of networks of expansile capillaries that, under stimulus, becomes engorged with blood, much on the order of the way you pump up a tire. The penis, clitoris, and nipples are the most important examples of erectile tissue.

ERYTHROCYTE (er' ith ro sit),* from **erythro,** red; **kytos,** cell. A red blood cell.

ESOPHAGUS (e sof' ag us), from **oiso,** the future of to carry; **phagein,** to eat. The gullet; the food tube extending from the back of the mouth to the stomach or crop, and, in birds, from the crop to the proventriculous. See DIGESTIVE TRACT.

ETIOLOGY (e te ol' o je), from **aitia,** cause; **logos,** science. The science of cause. The study of the causation of disease.

EXCRETA (eks kre' tah). The natural discharges of the body, particularly those of the bowels; feces.

EXFOLIATE (eks fo le ate'), from Latin, **exfoliare,** to shed leaves, like a tree. The sloughing off of cells or the breaking down of glandular structures resulting from the epithelial linings of the tubes breaking away from their basal membranes. This is particularly the case in diseases of the kidneys. Exfoliation of epithelial cells is a normal part of menstruation in women and it appears that a similar change takes place in the testicles of birds during the moulting season and the winter. The examination of the testicles of a large number of sparrows trapped during the winter showed all of the tubules choked with exfoliated epithelial cells.

EXPECTORANT (eks pek' to rant), from **ex,** out; **pectus,** breast. A drug that causes spitting, usually by making mucus and pus accumulations in the chest more fluid, such as Ammoniac and Ammonium Chloride.

EXTRUDE (eks trood'), from **ex,** out; **trudos,** to push. To push out. The forcing out of any tissue or organ as the result of injury or disease. The **extrusion** of the eyeballs as a result of subretinal hemorrhage or pressure. The **extrusion** of tissue of the uterus from the vent in cases of prolapse. The **extrusion** the intestines through a wound in the abdominal wall.

EXUDATE (eks' oo date), from **exudare,** to sweat. The material

---

* **Note:** This appears to be the official pronunciation of this word, but I have never heard anyone use it. I have always heard it pronounced **er ith' ro sit.**

that has passed through the walls of vessels into adjacent tissue; the accumulations of fluid, cell debris, fibrinous coagulum, or pus in body cavities or interstitial spaces.

F

F. Abbreviation for FAHRENHEIT.

FACIES (fa' she es). Latin for face. The different surfaces of an organ or the articular surfaces of joints.

FAHRENHEIT (fah' ren hite). Gabriel Daniel Fahrenheit, German physicist, 1686-1736. Inventor of the Fahrenheit thermometer scale on which the boiling point of water is 212 and the freezing point 32, making the difference between freezing and boiling 180 degrees.

FASCIA (fash' e ah). Latin, a band. The areolar (lung like) tissue beneath the skin and forming the investment of muscles. Figures 26, 56, 58 and 68.

FATTY DEGENERATION (fat ee de jen er a' shun), from fat and **degenerare,** to become base. A condition in which fat globules appear in the cytoplasm of the cells. This condition has no relation to body fat, and is probably better described by the term **lipoid degeneration,** which means practically the same thing without carrying the same suggestion. The condition is recognized in paraffin section by the presence of round holes in the cytoplasm of the epithelial cells. It is a very common lesion of the liver and kidneys and is observed in many acute diseases and in all cases of acute metallic poisoning. See LEAD POISONING.

FEBRILE (feb'ril), from **febris,** Latin for fever. Pertaining to fever; as, the **febrile** stage of a disease.

FECES (fe' seez), from **fex,** sediment. The excreta of the bowels.

FEHLING'S SOLUTION (fa' ling). Hermann von Fehling, German chemist, 1812-1885. Two solutions are required. A. Dissolve 36.64 gm. of copper sulphate—blue crystals—in 500 cc. of water. B. Dissolve 173 gm. of Rochelle salt in 100 cc. of a solution of caustic soda having a specific gravity of 1.34, and dilute to 500 cc. with water. For use, mix equal volumes of A and B. Place ten cc. of the mixture in each of two evaporating dishes or small beakers, bring both to a boil; to one, add suspected urine, drop by drop until ten drops have been added or until the solution turns from blue to brick-red as a result of the precipitation of copper oxide. Should the control also form a red precipitate, the solutions must be discarded and fresh ones prepared. If the control undergoes no change, it may then be titered with a standard, one-tenth per cent solution of C.P., glucose until the change occurring corresponds with that caused by the urine. And from data so obtained, a rough estimate of the amount of sugar present in the urine may be made.

FEMUR (fe' mur). Latin for the thigh bone.

FERRIC (fer' ik), from **ferrum,** the Latin name for iron. Salts or compounds containing iron as a trivalent or quadiralent element. The **ferric** state is brought about by boiling iron or its salts in an excess of acid.

FERRO (fer' o). A prefix used with the names of compounds containing iron in the **ferrous** state.

FERROUS (fer' us). Applied to compounds containing iron as a bivalent element. The ferrous state is brought about by boiling the iron salt with an excess of metallic iron, and ferrous solutions can be guarded against the oxidizing effects of the atmosphere by keeping them in brown bottles and keeping a piece of metallic iron in the bottle.

FIBRIN (fi' brin), from **fiber.** A protein found in blood and lymph and other body fluids which forms a fiber-like precipitate when these coagulate, either upon exposure to the air or in tissue. Normal blood contains 0.2 per cent fibrin.

FIBRINOUS (fi' brin us). Pertaining to, resembling, of the nature of, or containing fibrin.

FIBROUS (fi' brus). Containing or of the nature of fibers.

FILTRABLE (fil' tra bl), from **filtrum,** a filter. That which is capable of being filtered; as **filtrable** virus. In a wide number of diseases of both man and animals, birds, and even plants, the causative agent is something so small that it will pass a Berkefeld or a Chamberland filter. This is proven by mixing blood, scabs, or other infective material from an acute case of the disease in question with physicological salt solution and then passing the mixture through a clean, sterile Berkefeld or Chamberland filter and injecting the filtrate into susceptible animals. To prove that there is no leak in the filter large enough for ordinary bacteria to pass through, cultures are seeded from the same filtrate. If the cultures remain sterile and the animal develops the disease, the proof is complete.

FLAGELLUM, pl., FLAGELLA (flaj el' um—ah), from the Latin **a whip.** The whip-like, mobile processes possessed by many single-celled organisms and by means of which they attain locomotion. See Figure 60.

FLUIDEXTRACT (floo' id eks' trakt), abv. F. E. The strongest fluid preparation of a vegetable drug. It is a solution of the solid active principle of the drug of such strength that one gram of the drug is fully represented by one cubic centimeter of the extract.

FOLLICLE (fol' ik l), from **folliculus**, diminutive of **follis**, a bellows. A small lymphatic gland, the tissue arranged to form a small sac; the sac-like cluster of cells from which a hair or feather develops; a small pustula or other minute point of infection. **Graafian follicle**, one of the small visicular bodies in the ovary, each of which contains an ovum.

FRACTURE (frak' tyoor), from **frangere**, to break. Any break in a bone.

FRAGILE (fraj ile'), Latin for **brittle**. Pertaining to the state, condition or property of being easily broken.

FRIABLE (fri' ab l), from **friare**, to break into pieces. Pertaining to the state, condition or property of being easily broken into small pieces, crumbled.

FUCHSIN (fyook' sin). After the German botanist, Leonhard Fuchs, 1501-1566. This name is applied to several of the dyes of the pararosanilin series; they are widely used in histology and bacteriology.

FUNGOID (fun' goid), from **fungus; eidos**, likeness. Resembling or pertaining to a fungus.

FUNGUS (fun' gus), Latin. One of the lowest order of plants, the chief of which are the moulds and yeasts. See ASPERGILLOSIS; FUNGOID SKIN.

G

GALLINARUM (gal in' air um). As this word is not listed in any of the reference available to me, I would not swear by this pronunciation. It is used as an adjective referring to chicken-like birds.

GANGLEON (gang' gle on), from **gagglion**, a knot; pl., **GANGLIA** (gang' gle ah). A small cluster of nerve cells and fibers forming a subsidiary nerve center. See Figure 68.

GANGRENE (gang' green), from **gaggraina**, a sore. The death of body tissue during life. This may come about through the failure of the circulation supplying the part; from the action of corrosives; poisons; or the growth of the organisms of disease in tissue. See BROKEN BONES; PERITONITIS. When bacterial gangrene follows bacterial inflammation the tissue changes color from red or purple to green or blue, and the swelling of simple inflammation is displaced by the withered appearance of wasting tissue.

GANGRENOUS (gang′ gren us), from **gangrene.** Pertaining to or in a state of gangrene.

GASTRO (gas′ tro), from **gaster,** stomach. A prefix denoting relation to the stomach; as, **gastritis,** inflammation of the stomach; **gastrocele,** a hernia of the stomach; **gastrotomy,** an incision into the stomach.

GASTROENTERITIS (gas tro en ter i′ tis), from **gastro,** the stomach; **enteron,** the intestines; **itis,** inflammation. Inflammation of the stomach and intestines.

GENE (jeen), from **generare,** to beget. These are the physical basis of heredity, the units of inheritance. They are transmitted by means of the germ cells, wherein they are contained in the chromosomes, arranged in a double line, like a double string of pearls. They are too small to be brought into the range of the direct-vision microscope, but they have been photographed by ultraviolet light, and they will undoubtedly be subjected to close study by the electronic microscope as soon as someone can get around to it.

GENERALIZE (jen′ er al ize), v. To make general. Used to distinguish conditions affecting the whole or a large part of the body from those effecting only one organ or part, which are spoken of as **localized.** There are a number of diseases which may be either local or general; such as, aspergillosis, pneumonia and some of the bacterial diseases that may attack the bowels without the germ gaining entrance to the blood stream. The case of pneumonia is particularly interesting. In both acute and subacute pneumococcus pneumonia, the germ is found in the blood stream, but it does not, as a rule, gain entrance to the spinal fluid or set up lesions in other organs. In chronic interstitial pneumonia the germ may not be found in the blood until the bird is near death, and maybe not then. In staphylococcus pneumonia, I have not found the germ in the blood during life, but have cultivated it from heart, liver, and spleen a few minutes after death.

GERMINAL LAYER (jer′ min al), from **germen,** a sprig or offshoot. In certain cell-forming organs, such as the testicles, ovaries, lymph glands, spleen, and skin there are layers of cells that are constantly undergoing division. These are called germinal layers. See Figure 46.

GLOMERULUS, pl., **GLOMERULI** (glom er' u lus—i), diminutive of **glomus,** a small round body. The coil of capillary blood vessels inside of the expanded end (Bowman's capsule) of each uriniferous tubule, and with it making up the **malpighian body.** This term is also applied to the corpuscles of the spleen and other similar bodies composed of plexuses of capillaries. The **glomeruli** of the kidneys are the secreting organs for the elimination of urinary product from the blood. Those of the spleen probably are also engaged in filtering the blood and removing objectional matter, but just what they do, or remove, is not wholly understood. See Figures 51, 52, 63, 78.

GOBLET-CELLS. Beaker-like cells found in the mucous membranes. These are the secreting cells. See Figure 27.

GOITER (goi' ter), from **guttur,** throat. An enlargement of the thyroid gland. A condition that often results from a deficiency of iodides. See IODIDES, main vocabulary.

GRAM. The weight of one cubic centimeter of pure water at sea level and at the temperature of 4 Centigrade.

GRAM, Hans Christian Joachim, Danish physician. The inventor of a unique staining method for the differentiation of certain microorganisms. There are many modifications of this method which is essentially as follows: stain deeply with gentian or crystal violet, steaming for several minutes; pour off stain and flood slide with a solution containing one gram of iodine and two grams of potassium iodide to 300 cc's of water. Wash with alcohol or an alcohclic solution of some stain such as methylene blue or Bismark brown. Gram-positive organisms are stained purplc; Gram-negative organisms are stained blue, brown, or according to whatever counter stain is used, which is not very important.

GRANULAR LAYER. The second layer of the cerebellum and the cerebrum and several layers of the retina are distinguished by the fact that they contain a large number of closely-packed, deep-staining cell nuclei. These are called **granular layers.** See Figure 19 and No. 8, Figure 56.

GRANULOCYTE (gran' yoo lo site), from **granule; kytos,** a cell. A granular leucocyte. Osgood uses this term to include the complete series of cells derived from the granuloblast of the bone marrow and of which the neutrophiles, eosinophiles and basophiles of the blood are the end products; he also uses it in a restricted sense to designate the second member of each subseries. The series are names as follows: GRANULOBLAST; PROGRANULOCYTES A AND S; NEUTROPHILIC, BASOPHILIC, AND EOSINOPHILIC GRANULOCYTES; NEUTROPHILIC, BASOPHILIC, AND EOSIN- OPHILIC RHABDOCYTES; AND NEUTROPHILIC, BASOPHILIC, AND EOSINOPHILIC LOBOCYTES.

H

HARD-BILLED. This term is applied to those species of birds that eat seed and grain, such as sparrows, finches, etc., to distinguish them from the insectiverous birds, which are called, **soft-billed.**

HASHISH (hash′ eesh). A narcotic, hypnotic drug present in the leaves, stems and seed hulls of hemp. It is not present in the meat of the hemp seed.

HEMATOZOON (hem at o zo′ on), pl., **HEMATOZOA** (hem at o zo′ a), from **aima,** blood; **zoon,** an animal. An animal parasite in the blood. See MALARIA; SPIROCHETOSIS.*

HEMO (hem′ o), from **aima,** blood. A prefix meaning blood.

HEMOGLOBIN (hem o glo′ bin), from **aima,** blood; **globus,** a ball. The red coloring matter of blood. This is a very complex organic molecule containing about three per cent iron.

HEMORRHAGE (hem′ or aij), from **hemo,** blood; **regnynai,** to burst forth. An escape of blood from the vessels, either through the intact wall or through rupture of the wall. Hemorrhages may result from injuries, poisons, or disease. See main vocabulary.

HEMORRHAGIC (hem or aj′ ik). Pertaining to, of the nature of, or associated with hemorrahages. See main vocabulary.

HENLE'S LOOP. Friedrich Gustav Jakob Henle, German anato- mist, 1809-1885. The U-shaped section of the uriniferous tubules which is formed by a descending and an ascending arm. For part of its length the descending arm of the loop is lined with polygonal, squamous epithelial cells, while all other parts of the kidney tubes are lined with cuboidal epithelial cells, with the single exception of the very short neck of the glomeruli. See KIDNEYS, main vocab- ulary.

HEPATIC (hep at′ ik), from **epar,** the liver. Pertaining to the liver.

---

* **Note:** Some modern authorities now classify the spirochetes with the bacteria rather than with the protozoa, but I think the older classification comes nearer to being in accordance with observed facts, and, therefore, preferable.

HEPATITIS (hep at i' tis), from **epar,** liver; **itis,** inflammation. Inflammation of the liver.

HEPATIZATION (hep at iz a' shun). To make or become like liver. A change in tissue which causes it to resemble liver, particularly lung tissue during the development of pneumonia. Seé PNEUMONIA, main vocabulary.

HERPES (her' peez), from **erpein,** to creep. Fever blisters.

HISTOLOGY (his tol' o je), from **istos,** tissue; **logos,** science. The science of tissue. The study of microscopic anatomy and the development and differentiation of cells and structures.

HUMERUS (hoo' mer us), Latin. The bone of the upper arm; the same bone in the wing of a bird. See SKELETON, main vocabulary.

HYALINE (hi' al ine), from **yalos,** glass. Resembling glass, crystalline, translucent. Applied to the parts of cells and tissue that contain no granules, also applied to certain morbid changes as the result of which the cells are broken down and replaced by a structureless, albuminous material. This is called hyaline degeneration and differs from amyloid degeneration in two important particulars: the substance reacts differently to staining reagents; it is usually confined to the organ that is the primary seat of the disease, while amyloid degeneration may occur in any chronic disease of long standing and will be found in almost all parts of the body. In some cases, it may be found in the bones before making its appearance in the organ that is the primary site of the disease.

HYALO (hi' al o), from **yalos,** glass. A prefix meaning transparent; like glass.

HYALOPLASM (hi' al o plazm), from **yalos,** glass; **plasma,** a thing molded. The fluid part of protoplasm; granule-free cytoplasm.

HYPER (hi' per). Greek for **over.** A prefix meaning over, beyond, more; as, **hyperactivity,** more activity than normal; **hyperemia,** more blood than normal; **hypercardia,** more heart than normal or, more properly, an enlarged heart.

HYPERTROPHY (hi per' tro fe), from **hyper; trophe,** nourishment. An increase in size of a tissue or organ without relation to the growth of the body; an oversized organ. Some writers apply the term to diseased tissue while others restrict it to an increase in the amount of normal, functioning tissue.

HYPO (hi' po), from **ypo,** under. A common abbreviation for hypochondria and hypodermic, as well as for persons addicted to the injection of drugs. A prefix meaning under or less; as, **hypodermic,** under the skin; **hypoacidity,** not enough acid in the stomach; **hypo-chromatic,** deficiency of coloring matter, particularly in the nuclei of the leucocytes.

HYPOPTERBOSIS CYSTICA—Hare (hi pop ter bo' sis sis' ti ca). Tom Hare's name for LUMPS. See main vocabulary.

I

ILEUM (il' e um), from **eilein,** to roll. The lower portion of the small intestines; in birds, terminating in the cloaca; in mammals, terminating in the cecum. See Figure 25.

ILIUM (il' e um), Latin, the flank. The os ilii. One of the bones making up the pelvic arch. See Figure 75.

IMMUNE (im une'), from **in,** not; **munis,** serving. Not susceptible to a particular disease, either as a natural or acquired characteristic.

INCUBATION (in kyoo ba' shun), from **in,** signifying action; **cubare,** to lie. The process of sitting on eggs to hatch them; the period between infection by a disease germ and the development of symptoms of illness; the process of maintaining cultures of micro-organisms at a uniform temperature in an incubator in order to promote their growth.

INDICATION (in dik a' shun), from **indicare,** to point out. That which points out a particular line of treatment; thus, to say a treatment is **indicated** means that the symptoms suggest that that is the best line of treatment; to say a treatment is **countra indicated** means that in that particular case that line of treatment must be avoided, since it is dangerous. In the pox form of diphtheria treatment of the sores with antiseptics or oxidizing agents is indicated; in the bronchial form of the disease this line of treatment is **countra indicated.** Two birds become puffed up suddenly. There has been a sudden change of temperature. They are breathing rapidly; they are both very weak. Bird "A" has a fever; there is a bubbling sound in the right lung; sulfathiazol is indicated. Bird "B" has a temperature of 41 C; there are no chest sounds other than those of the heart; diuretic treatment is indicated. Sulfa-thiazol is **countra indicated,** for if given, it will undoubtedly cause death within a couple of hours. In the one case the bird had pneumonia; in the other, uremia.

INFECTION (in fek' shun), from **in,** into; **facere,** to make. 1. The act of a disease producing agent gaining entrance into the body of a susceptible creature. 2. The disease produced by such entrance of an infective agent.

INFECTIVE (in fek' tiv). Possessed of the quality of being able to produce disease. This same definition would apply equally well to the word virulent (which literally means **poisonous**), but the words are not exact synonyms. You could use the word **virulent** to describe the degree of severity of a pox infection, but you would say the pox scab was **infective**. On the other hand, you would not say a germ is **infective,** you would say it is **virulent;** but a culture of that germ would be included in the expression, **infective material.** Why?—don't ask me. All I can tell you about many of these words is the manner in which the best writers use them.

INFEST (in fest'), from **in,** on; **festinare,** to hasten. To invade or overrun. Used in connection with animal parasites; thus, a bird is **infested** with lice but **infected** with germs.

INFESTATION (in fes ta' shun). The state or condition of being infested.

INFUSION (in fyoo' zhun), from Latin **infusum.** The process of extracting the active principle of a substance by steeping in water, but without boiling. The seeping of fluid into a tissue or cavity. The fluid that has seeped into a cavity where it does not belong; as, a serous **infusion** was found in the peritonial cavity.

INOCULATE (in ok' u late), from **in,** into; **oculus,** a bud. To intentionally introduce the virus of a disease into the body of a susceptible creature, or one suspected of being susceptible.

INOCULATION (in ok' yoo la' shun). The act of introducing the virus of a disease into a susceptible animal; also, the act of seeding culture tubes.

INOCULATION NEEDLE. A piece of platinum or nichrome wire fitted into a glass or metal handle and used for inoculating culture tubes.

IN SITU (in si' too), from **in,** in; **situs,** position. In the given or natural position. The examination of organs **in situ** means before they have been removed from their original position.

INTER (in' ter), **between.** A prefix meaning between.

INTERSTITIAL (in ter stish' al), from **inter,** between; **stitium,** a space. Literally, the space between. Actually, the space between the cells or elements making up the tissue. In the liver, the spaces between the strands of secreting cells; in the kidneys, the spaces between the tubules; in the brain, the spaces between the neurons and nerve fibers.

IN TOTO (in to' to), from **in; totus,** the whole. All in one piece. When applied to treatment or staining of tissue, it means in one piece, all at once, rather than staining on the slide, after sectioning.

INTRA (in' trah). A prefix signifying within or during.

INTRAPERITONEAL (in trah par it on e' al), from **intra,** into; **peritoneum.** Into the peritoneum, or within the peritoneum.

INTRAVENOUS (in trah ve' nus), from **intra; vena,** a vein. Into or within a vein. It is usually used with reference to an injection into a vein.

IRIS (i' ris), from **iris,** the Greek word for halo or rainbow. The colored, expanding and contracting diaphragm surrounding the pupil of the eye. Also applied to the adjustable diaphragm of a microscope or other optical instrument.

ISOLATION (is o la' shun), from **insula,** an island. The act of separating the sick from the well to prevent the spread of a disease; the processes by which a particular microorganism is separated from all others, so that it may be grown and studied in pure culture and its characteristics determined.

ITIS (i' tis). A suffix meaning inflammation.

L

LACERATION (las er a' shun), from **lacerare,** to tear. The act of tearing tissue, or the lesion so caused.

LACRIMAL, original spelling, **LACHRYMAL** (lak' rim al), from **lacrima,** a tear. Pertaining to the tears and the organs concerned in their secretion and disposal. The **lacrimal** apparatus consists of the lacrimal gland, duct, canal, sac, and nasal duct. The **lacrimal** bone is the bone located, in birds, between the forward edge of the orbit and the upper beak. See Figure 75.

LANGERHANS, islands of (lahng' er hans). Ernst Robert Langerhans, German histologist, 1847-1888. Small clumps of epithelial cells found in the interstitial connective tissue of the pancreas, now known to be concerned with the manufacture of insulin. The degeneration of these bodies is responsible for the disease, diabetes.

LAPAROTOMY (lap ar ot' o me), from **lapara,** Greek for flank or loin; **tomy,** to cut. An incision through the abdominal wall; the operation of cutting into the abdominal cavity, particularly through the loin or flank.

LARVA, pl., **LARVAE** (lar' vah, lar' vee), from **larva,** a ghost. The young, worm-like stage in the development of bugs and insects.

LARYNX (lar' inks), Greek. The voice box; the anterior end of the trachea.

LATERAL (lat' er al), from **latus,** the side. At or pertaining to the side; being located to the right or left of the medial line of the body.

LESION (le' zhun), from **lesio,** an injury. Any injury, wound, or structural or cellular change resulting from disease.

LETHAL (le' thal), from **lethum,** death. Deadly; pertaining to that which can or may produce death.

LEUCOCYTE, LEUKOCYTE (loo' ko site), from **leukos,** white; **kytos,** cell. A white blood cell, so-called because these cells do not contain hemoglobin. See BLOOD.*

LEUKEMIA (loo ke' me ah), from **leukos,** white; **aima** or **ema,** blood. White blood. A disease of the blood and blood-forming organs charterized by a permanent increase in the number of white corpuscles in the blood and by enlargement of the liver, spleen, and lymphatic glands. Osgood, who has probably carried out more extensive researches on this disease than any other American worker, restricts this term to conditions resulting from the malignant proliferation of one particular cell of the blood—tumors of the blood cells. According to this definition, the so-called **leukemia** of birds is very likely an infectious leukosis.

LEUKOSIS (loo ko' sis), from **leukos,** white; **osis,** disease, though the Greek root signifies condition of, or state caused by. White disease. Osgood restricts the meaning of this word to conditions of the blood in which there is an increase in the number of leucocytes resulting from causes other than malignant proliferation, such as infection and poisoning.

LIPOCHROME (lip' o krome), from **lipo,** fat or fatty; **chroma,** color. The color of fat. Any of the fatty pigments found in animal tissue, to which class belong the red and yellow pigments found in the feathers of birds.

---

* **Note:** Concerning the spelling of this word, in all of the books I have seen that were published before 1935 and in some published as late as 1937 the spelling is **leucocyte;** but in the latest edition of Gould's Medical Dictionary, 1937, and in Osgood's Atlas of Hematology, also 1937, this word is spelled **leukocyte.**

LIPOID (lip' oid), from **lipo**, fat; **eidos**, like. Similar to, pertaining to, or like fat.

LOBOCYTE (lob' o site), from **lobus**, a lobe; **kitos**, a cell. Osgood's name for the polymorphonuclear leucocytes. He restricts the term to the end cells of the granulocytic series and qualifies it to indicate the kind of granules present, as **neutrophilic, eosinophilic,** or **basophilic lobocytes.**

LONGITUDINAL (lon je too' din al), from **longitudo**, length. Lengthwise. This word is used in describing muscles, nerves, or vessels running parallel to the longer axis of the organ or part under discussion.

LOOP (loop). An inoculation needle with its end bent into the form of a ring about 3 mm in diameter. It is used for picking up minute drops of fluid, such as blood or culture media. It was probably invented for the purpose of making culture transfers and dilutions in making plate cultures, but it is a very handy tool for handling all forms of microscopic material.

LUMEN, pl., **LUMINA** (loo' men, loo' min ah), Latin for **light.** The space inside a tube; as, the lumen of a blood vessel or a thermometer.

LYMPHATICS (lim fat' iks), from **lympha**, water. The system of capillary tubes and glands by means of which the tissue fluids are filtered and returned to the general circulation.

LYMPHATIC TISSUE. The tissue of which the spleen, thymus, and lymphatic glands are composed. See Figure 78.

LYMPHOCYTES (lim' fo sites), from **lympho; kytos**, a cell. These are the cells formed in lymphatic tissue. They are present in the blood and make up about 40 per cent of the leucocytes. These cells are found in great numbers in healing wounds, and there is strong reason for believing that in such cases they act as mother cells for the connective tissue.

LYMPHOSARCOMA (lim' fo sar co' mah), from **lympho.** Pertaining to the lymphatics; **sarco,** flesh; **oma,** tumor. A tumor arising from cells of the mesoderm (bones, connective tissues, muscles) and having the appearance of lymphatic tissue. Osgood contends that it is possible to arrange a series of cases, not one of which can be differentiated from its two nearest neighbors, with typical lymphosarcoma at one end of the series and typical lymphocytic leukemia at the other end. Which suggests that these·are two extremes of one and the same disease, a malignant proliferation of the cells of the lymphocyte series. This seems reasonable to me since, before reading his work, I had been strongly impressed by the similarity of lesions found in a canary to those of sarcoma in man, even though there were no macroscopic tumors. See LEU-KEMIA and Figures 55 and 56.

M

MACROBLAST (mak' ro blast), from **macro,** large; **blast,** germ or bud. Strictly speaking, the term **blast** can be applied only to stem cells, the cells from which the differentiated forms arise, but this term is commonly applied to red cells that are larger than normal, though such cells should be called **macrocytes.**

MACROCYTE (mak' ro site). A red blood cell that is larger than normal.

MACROSCOPIC (mak ro skop' ik), from **macro,** large; **skopien,** to see. Something that is large enough to be seen with the unaided eyes.

MAL (mal), from Latin **malus,** bad, or French **malum,** evil, disease. A prefix meaning, not so good.

MALFORMED (mal' formd). Misshapened; an abnormal development of an organ or part.

MALIGNANCY (mal ig' nan se), from **mal,** bad; **gignere,** to beget. The state or property of being malignant.

MALIGNANT (mal ig' nant). Virulent; compromising; threatening to life. This term was formerly applied to many dangerous diseases, but it is now restricted to those tumors that have a tendency to return after removal and to spread by metastasis (cancers and sarcomas) and the leukemias, all of which result from the rapid and uncontrolled proliferation of some particular cell.

MALNUTRITION (mal noo trish' un), from **mal,** bad; **nutrire,** to nourish. Poorly nourished. A pathological condition resulting from either not having the right food or enough food to eat or of not being able to assimilate the food eaten.

MAMMALIAN (mam a' le an), from **mamma,** the breast; strictly speaking, the nipple. Pertaining to mammals, the class of animals that suckle their young.

MANDIBLE (man' dib l), from **mandere,** to chew. The beak, strictly speaking, the upper bill. The lower one is called the **incisor.**

MARTIUS YELLOW. A dye used in histology. See BLOOD.

MAST CELLS. These are leucocytes found normally in the blood

of birds and some animals, but found in the blood of man only as
a result of certain diseases or poisons. Mast cells are unique in the
staining characteristics of their coarse granules. See BLOOD.

MASTOID (mas' toid), from **mastos**, the breast; **eidos**, like. Like
the breast; breast shaped, as the mastoid process of the temporal
bone, the bulge behind your ear.

MASTOIDITIS (mas toid i' tis). An inflammation of the sinuses
of the mastoid process. This was, until a few years ago, a highly
fatal condition of man, and it still is no joke; though with modern
technique there is no excuse for anyone dying from it. I have
observed one case in a bird as a sequela of an attack of diphtheria.
A heavy, cheesy exudate formed inside of the bone and caused it
to bulge out behind the ear. An operation was attempted, but I
did not know enough anatomy at the time, and the bird died as a
result of my bungling.

MEDULLA (me dul' ah), Latin for **marrow**. The bone marrow, and
by inference, the middle or inside of any organ or structure. Also,
the **medulla oblongata,** the middle brain, the expansion of the spinal
cord just below the cerebellum.

MEDULLARY (med' ul a re). Pertaining to the marrow, or to
the tissue or structure of the inner parts of any organ as contrasted
to the cortex. This term is also applied to the sheaths that enclose
the spinal nerves—why, again, I haven't the slightest idea, unless
it is that the medulla of a nerve is composed of a marrow-like
fatty substance.

MEDULLATED (med' ul a ted). This term is used to describe
nerve fibers that are enclosed in the sheath—the spinal and voluntary motor nerves. See Figure 68.

MEGRIMS (me' grims). This word was formerly used to designate
a particular kind of headache affecting man, but, for that purpose, it has been displaced by the word **migraine.** It is Moore's
name for a form of B. Paratyphosus B infection affecting pigeons
and which is characterized by symptoms of a severe headache and
the formation of an exudate into the subarachnois spaces over the
back of the brain. See B. PARATYPHOSIS B INFECTION.

MENDEL (men' dl). Johann Gregor Mendel, Austrian naturalist,
who first worked out the laws of inheritance. It is a mathematical
law showing the probability of the occurrence of any definite characteristic in the succeeding generations of offspring from a cross
of two individuals, one of which has and one of which does not
have the characteristic under consideration. He found that incom-

patible characteristics segregated proportionally to the coefficients of the algebraic binomial.

MENDELIAN (men del' i an). Pertaining to Mendel's law or the particular results following from its application to the science of breeding.

MESENTERY (mes' en ter e), from **mesos,** middle; **enteron,** bowel. This is the plexus of vessels and nerves that attend to the carrying of nourishment absorbed from the bowels to the portal circulation of the liver.

METABOLISM (met ab' o lizm); **metabole,** change. The group of physicological processes whereby living creatures transform the elements present in food into bone, tissue, heat and energy.

METABOLIZE (met ab' o lize). To convert a particular element of food into tissue or energy.

METACARPUS (met ah kar' pus), from **meta,** over, among, beyond; **carpos,** wrist. Beyond the wrist. The bones of the back of your hand; the corresponding bones in the wings of birds. See Figure 75.

METASTASIS (met as' tas ize); **meta,** beyond; **statos,** place. Beyond the place. The spread of disease germs or tumor cells from place to place in the body by means of the blood stream.

METATARSUS (met ah tar' sus), from **meta,** beyond; **tarsus,** the bones of the ankle and the beginning of the instep. Beyond the instep. The bones forming the arch of your foot. The long shank-bone of birds. See Figure 75.

METHYLENE BLUE (meth' il een blue). A dye that is widely used in bacteriology and histology. See main vocabulary, also BLOOD.

MICROBLAST (mi kro' blast), from **micro,** small; **blastos,** a germ. This word is a misnomer. It is sometimes used to indicate immature erythrocytes and sometimes to indicate erythrocytes that are smaller than normal. The usage is incorrect in both cases, however, since the correct designation of stem cell of the erythrocytic series is the **erythorblast, megaloblast,** or **karyoblast** (Osgood); the immature red cell that sometimes is observed in the blood is called the **nucleated erythrocyte** or the **metakaryocyte** (Osgood); and the red cell that is smaller than normal should be designated **micro-cyte; microcytic erythrocyte;** or **microcytic akaryocyte** (Osgood).

MICRON (mi' kron). The one-thousandth part of a millimeter; the 1/25,000 part of the inch.

MICRONE (mi' krone). Small colloid bodies about one micron in diameter observed in the blood, particularly directly after eating and thought to be food particles.

MICROSCOPIC (mi kro skop' ik). Pertaining to the microscope; that which can be seen only with a microscope; anything too small to be seen with the unaided eyes; minute.

MINIM (min' im), from **minimus**, least. The one-sixtieth of a fluidram; roughly, one drop.

MITOSIS (mi to' sis), from **mitos**, a thread. The process by which each chromosome is split lengthwise to assure the equal division of the chromatic material during the process of cell division. Also used to designate the entire process of cell division where this splitting of the chromosomes occurs. Some cells, particularly the lymphocytes, divide by **fision**, without **mitosis**.

MITOTIC (mi tot' ik). Pertaining to Mitosis.

MOLECULAR LAYER (mo lek' yoo lar). A layer of tissue having a fine, granular appearance and an absence of nuclei. Such layers are found in the brain and retina and may, by special staining process, be shown to consist of fine nerve tendrils and fibers.

MOLECULE (mol' e kyool); diminutive of **moles**, mass. A little mass. The smallest amount of any chemical compound that may exist, division of which may be achieved only by chemical decomposition.

MONOCYTE (mon' o site), from **mono**, one; **kitos**, cell. A cell having a single nucleus. This word is usually restricted to the designation of the large mononuclear leucocyte.

MORBID (mor' bid), from **morbus**, disease. Pertaining to disease or a diseased part. **Morbid anatomy**, the changes taking place in tissue during the progress of a disease.

MORPHOLOGICAL (mor fo loj' ik al), from **morphe**, form; **logos**, science. Pertaining to the science or study of form and structure in living creatures. As used in this book, it usually refers to the structure of germs and cells as they appear under the microscope.

MORPHOLOGY (mor fol' o je). The science of form and structure of living matter.

MORTALITY (mor tal' it e), from **mors**, death. The quality of all living matter of being subject to death. The death rate.

MOTILE (mo' til), from **movere**, to move. Capable of spontaneous motion, or locomotion.

MOTOR (mo' tor), from **movere**, to move. That which moves, causes to move, furnishes the power of motion. Concerned with or pertaining to motion; as, a **motor cell,** a nerve cell having a part in the control or direction of motion; a **motor nerve,** a nerve that supplies impulses to a muscle; **motor center,** a nerve center in the brain or spinal chord that sends out or controls impulses for muscular contraction. See Figure 68. The large cells in the ganglion are motor cells. Two of the nerves shown in the upper drawing are motor nerves.

MUCOSA (myoo ko' sah), from **mucosus,** mucous. A mucous membrane; generally used in the sense of the total mucous membrane of the animal, or organ, under discussion; as the **intestinal mucosa,** the entire mucous membrane of the intestines.

MUCOUS (myoo' kus). Pertaining to or having the nature of mucus; as, **mucous membrane,** a membrane lining to tube that has contact with the outside of the body; particularly of the digestive, respiratory, and the lower part of the urogenital tracts. The cells of mucous membranes secret a thick fluid that keeps the membrane moist.

MUCUS (myoo' kus). The viscid fluid secreted by mucous membranes. It contains water, mucin and inorganic salts and usually holds in suspension a few leucocytes and exfoliated epithelial cells.

MUTATION (myoo ta' shun), from **mutare,** to change. A change taking place in the germplasm of a creature, of such a nature as to give rise to a new species or a pronounced variation of an existing species; a **sport.**

MYCOSIS (mi ko' sis), from **mykes,** fungus. A disease resulting from the growth of fungus in living tissue.

MYELOCYTE (mi' el o site), from **myelo,** pertaining to marrow; **kytos,** a cell. A marrow cell. Any one of the numerous parent forms of the leucocytes found in bone marrow during health. Sometimes these cells are found in the blood stream during illness.

MYELOMA (mi el o' mah). A giant-cell sarcoma of the bone marrow. These tumors are very closely related to the leukemias, and are among the most highly fatal of the malignant tumors.

N

NASAL (na' zal), from **nasus,** the nose. Pertaining to the nose.

NECROSIS (nek ro' sis), from **nekros,** dead. The death of cells surrounded by living tissue. Spots of dead tissue will be of different color from the living tissue surrounding them, and this color may vary from almost white to blue-black. If pus formation has had a part in the destruction, the spot will be yellow, surrounded by a red, inflamed border. If there has been no pus formation, the lesion will at first be blue or green and will become lighter as time passes.

NECROTIC (nek rot' ik). Pertaining to necrosis.

NEGRI BODIES (na' gre). Luigi Negri, Italian physician, 1876-1912. Protozoon-like bodies found in the nerve cells of animals suffering with rabies, and considered diagnostic for that disease.

NEOPLASM (ne' o plazm), from **neos,** new; **plasma,** material or tissue. Newly formed tissue. This word may be applied to any newly formed tissue, regardless of cause, but it is most often applied to tumors.

NEPHRITIS (nef ri' tis), from **nephrus,** the kidney; **itis,** inflammation. Inflammation of the kidney. See main vocabulary.

NEPHROSIS (nef ro' sis), from **nephrus,** kidney; **osis,** condition of, disease. Any disease of the kidney. Usually applied to tubular diseases in which there are few changes in the glomeruli. Epstein's nephrosis is a chronic tubular disease resulting from disordered metabolism due to disturbance of the endocrine functions. This condition is sometimes observed in canary females that have been overbred and failed to moult. It is characterized by large fat globules in the epithelial cells of the uriniferous tubules—too large to occur more than one to a cell—amyloid deposits in the ovary, the walls of the oviduct, the bone marrow, and to a lesser extent in the wall of the intestines, the liver, and occasionally in the spleen. There may be amyloid deposits in the glomeruli, but this is not a constant lesion.

NEUTRAL (noo' tral), from **neuter,** neither. Neither acid or alkaline.

NEUTRALIZE (noo tral' iz), to make neutral, by adding acid to an alkaline solution or alkali to an acid solution.

NEUTROPHILE (noo' tro fil); **neuter,** neither; **philos,** loving. A cell that stains with a neutral dye. The polymorphonuclear leucocytes, the granules of which stain strongly with neither acid nor basis dyes—as distinct from the basophiles and eosinophiles—but retain enough of both dyes to give them a neutral color. See BLOOD.

NODULE (nod' yool), from **nodulus,** diminutive of nodus, a lump. A little lump. Such lumps may be the result of infection—tuberculosis, infectious necrosis—or of disturbances resulting from poor nutrition—avitiminosis A.

NON-MEDULLATED (non med' ul a ted), from **non,** not; **medulla,** marrow. Having no medulla or heavy sheath. This term is applied to nerves of the sympathetic system, one of which is shown in the upper drawing of Figure 68.

NON-MOTILE (non mot' il), from **non,** not; **motilis,** moving. Having no powers of motion. Applied to microorganisms having no organs of locomotion.

NUCLEAR (noo' kle ar), from **nux,** a nut. Pertaining to, derived from, or resembling a nucleus.

NUCLEOLUS (noo kle' o lus), diminutive of **nucleus.** A little nucleus. A small, dense, deep-staining body present in the nuclei of all cells having the power of mitotic division and in a great many cells that do not have that power—the nerve cells and the lymphocytes contain nucleoli, but they have not been observed undergoing mitotic division. See Figure 12.

NUCLEUS (noo' kle us), from **nux,** a nut. The essential part of a typical cell. See Figure 12.

O

OCCIPITAL (ok sip' it al), from **ob,** over, against; **caput,** the head. The bone forming the back of the skull. See Figure 75.

OOCYST (o' o sist), from **oon,** egg; **kystis,** bladder. The encysted fertilized egg of a sporozoon. See Figure 22.

OPHTHALMIC (off thal' mik), from **ophthalmus,** the eye. Pertaining to the eyes.

OPTIC (op' tik), from **op,** to see; **tikos,** the base. The base of vision. Pertaining to vision or the science of optics.

ORANGE G (or' anj gee). A dyestuff used in histology.

ORBIT (or' bit), from **orbis,** a circle. The bony structure surrounding the eye, and formed by the frontal, sphenoid, ethmoid, nasal, lacrimal, superior maxillary, and palatal bones. See Figure 75.

ORBITAL (or' bit al). Pertaining to the orbit.

OS (os), from the Latin **oris;** pl., **ora,** a mouth. The mouth. When used unqualified this refers to the anterior opening of the digestive tract, but it is often qualified to refer to any mouth or opening; as, the **os uteri,** the mouth of the uterus.

OS (os), from the Latin **ossis;** pl., **ossa,** a bone. Often used to refer to bones and bony processes and qualified by words identifying the bone or process referred to; as, **os pubis,** the pubis bone; **os femoris,** the femur.

OSIS (o' sis). A suffix signifying **condition of,** or **state caused by,** which in usage reduces itself to **disease.** Any disease or morbid condition. Coupled with the name of the cause, it forms the name of the disease; as, **Avitaminosis,** a disease caused by insufficient vitamins; **typhosis,** a disease caused by the typhoid germ.

OVARY (o' ver e), from **ovarium,** an egg holder; from **ovum,** an egg. The female sex gland, of which mammals have two, but birds only one. See Figure 30.

OVIDUCT (o' ve dukt), from **ovum,** an egg; **ductus,** a canal. The egg canal. The convoluted tube in which the outer structure of the egg is formed. See Figure 30.

OVIFORM (o' vif orm), from **ovum,** an egg; **forma,** form. Formed like an egg. Egg-shaped.

OVUM (o' vum). Latin, an egg; pl., **ova.** See Figure 29.

OXYPHILE (oks' if il), from **oxy,** oxygen; **philos,** loving. Loving oxygen. The dictionary definition of this word is, a histological element that attracts acid dye. But the only employments I have found in the literature available to me do not justify this definition. Kenthack and Hardy, who seem to be the inventors of the term, apply it to the granules of the polymorphonuclear leucocyte. Ehrlich calls these granules neutrophilic—Coplin's Manual of Pathology, 3rd edition, page 430—and Osgood does not use the term. But on the chart for reporting blood counts used by the U. S. Public Health Service the polymorphonuclear leucocyte is classified under the heading, "Fine granular Oxyphiles." Hill, however, does use the word in the dictionary sense. The only use he makes of it is to distinguish the **colloid** cells of the parathyroid from the **chief** cells—Hill's Manual of Histology, 7th Edition, Page 284.

OXYSPIRURA MANSONI. Manson's Eye Worm. See main vocabulary. I can't find out how to pronounce this thing, even Gould's Dictionary doesn't try it.

P

PANACEA (pan a se' ah), from **panakeia,** all healing; from **pas,** all; **akos,** cure. A drug that cures anything, but don't you believe it. There isn't any.

PANCREAS (pan' kre as), from **pas, pan,** all; **kreas,** flesh. This is one of the digestive glands and, in birds, it is located between the horns of the duodenum, to which it is firmly attached and into the upper end of the ascending horn of which it discharges its secretion. This gland is also responsible for the internal secretion of insulin, failure of which is responsible for the condition we call **diabetes.**

PAPILLA (pap il' ah). Latin, **a nipple;** pl., **papillae,** pronounced **lee.** A nipple or nipple-like eminence.

PARAROSANILINE (par ah ro zan' il en). A class of dyes extensively used in histology and pathology. The most important members of this group are acid fuchsin, basic fuchsin, and crystal violet. Two cc of saturated alcoholic solution of acid fuchsin; four cc of saturated alcoholic solution of crystal violet; 100 cc of water makes a good stain for bird blood. The film is thoroughly dried, flooded with alcohol and again dried; flooded with a $\frac{1}{10}$ per cent solution of Martius yellow; washed in water; flooded with a solution of fuchsin and crystal violet and again washed in tap water. The differentiation of structural elements of the cells is very sharp, but the metachromatic differences are less marked than those of polychrome methylene blue.

PARATYPHOID (par ah ti' foid). The name given to infections resulting invasion of the blood stream by germs of the paratyphosus group. See B. PARATYPHOSUS B INFECTION. These germs are now generally grouped under the designation SALMONELLA.

PAREGORIC (par e gor' ik), from **paregorikos,** soothing. A preparation containing 2 grains of opium to the ounce, together with camphor, benzoic acid, oil of anise and glycerin. — Blumgarten's Materia Medica, 4th Edition.

PARIETAL (par i' et al), from **paries,** a wall. Forming or situated on a wall. Pertaining to or associated with the parietal bone, which forms the crown of the skull. This term is also used to describe certain cells that occur in salivary glands and the glands of the stomach. These cells are characterized by the fact that they are crowded back against the basement membrane—away from the lumin of the tube or alveolus—and that their cytoplasm takes a bright red stain with eosin, while the cytoplasm of the chief cells stains palely with basic dyes—blue or green with hematoxylin; light blue with methylene blue.

PASTEURELLA (pas tur el' ah). Louis Pasteur, French chemist, 1822-1895. The man who founded the modern sciences of bacteriology and immunology in the face of the threat of imprisonment or the guillotine by the medical bureaucrats of his day. And remember, they haven't changed any, and they don't change. This is the name given to a group of bipolar-staining, Gram-negative, non-motile, non-sporeforming bacteria responsible for the hemorrhagic septicemias of animals and birds. See AVIAN DIPHTHERIA; FOWL CHOLERA; HEMORRHAGIC SEPTICEMIA; Figure 37.

PATELLA (pat el' ah), diminutive of **patina,** a shallow dish. A small shallow dish. The kneecap; the small bone covering the knee joint. See Figure 75.

PATHOGENIC (path o jen' ik), from **pathos,** disease; **gennan,** to produce. The power to produce disease. A microorganism which will, when introduced into the body, cause disease.

PATHOGENICITY (path o jen is' it e). The condition, quality, or extent of being pathogenic.

PATHOLOGICAL (path o loj' ik al), from **pathos,** disease; **logos,** science. Pertaining to pathology. The science or study of disease. The branch of science that devotes itself to the study of the changes taking place in the body as the result of illness, particularly cell changes as revealed through the microscopic study of diseased tissue.

PATHOLOGY (path ol' o je). See pathological; also main vocabulary.

PECTORAL (pek' tor al), from **pectus,** breast. Pertaining to the chest and applied to the muscles of the chest and the vessels and nerves serving them. The flight muscles of birds. The **great pectoral** is the muscle that depresses the wing; the **lesser pectoral** is the muscle that lifts the wing.

PER. A prefix meaning **very,** or in the highest degree.

PERACUTE (per ak oot'), from **per,** very or most; **acutus,** sharp. Very or most acute. A form of a disease that runs a more rapid course than is usual.

PERICARDITIS (per e kar di' tis), from **peri,** around or surrounding; **cardia,** the heart; **itis,** inflammation. Inflammation of that which surrounds the heart. Inflammation of the pericardium, the heart sac, which may become distended with fluid or semisolid exudate, and this stage may be followed by the development of adhesion between the pericardium and the heart wall. The only disease of birds in which I have found pericarditis to be a constant lesion is the bronchial form of avian diphtheria.

PERICARDIUM (per e kar' de um), from **peri,** around or surrounding; **cardia,** the heart. The membranous sac surrounding the heart.

PERISTALSIS (per e stal' sis), from **peri,** around; **stalsis,** constriction. A peculiar, rhythmic, wave-like motion observed in tubes provided with both longitudinal and transverse muscular fibers, which consists of a contraction and shortening of one section while the one below relaxes. This is followed by contraction of the relaxed section while the contracted section relaxes, the motion moving along the tube in a continuous wave, forcing the contents of the tube toward its opening. It is this movement that forces food through the digestive tract. It may be easily observed in the crop or gizzard of an unfeathered baby bird.

PERITONEAL (per it on e' al), from **peri,** around or surrounding; **teinein,** to stretch. To stretch around. The membranous lining of the abdominal cavity, folds in which also supply coverings for all of the abdominal organs and, in birds, the walls of the abdominal air sacs.

PERITONITIS (per it on it' is), from **peri,** surrounding; **teinein,** to stretch; **itis,** inflammation. Inflammation of that which stretches around. Inflammation of the peritoneum; which may be accompanied by infusion; cheesy exudate; the formation of a false membrane, with adhesions; or the gangrenous destruction of the tissue and the parts with which it is in contact.

PERNICIOUS (per nish' us), from **perniciosus,** destructive. Any practice, policy, condition, disease, or substance which is dangerous and may destroy. Usually applied to conditions or circumstances of a more or less insidious nature.

PERNICIOUS ANEMIA (per nish' us an e' me ah). A disease of man characterized by a diminution of the number of red cells in the blood and the appearance of immature forms and many cells much larger than normal, with some smaller than normal or odd shaped. This disease has not been studied in birds, but I have some reason for believing that they are subject to it. Until recently, this disease in man was 100 per cent fatal. It is now known that it is a deficiency disease resulting from the absence of either one of two principles: one, present in certain foods, meat and liver; and the other, elaborated by the stomach during the digestion of meats. Where the disease results from improper diet, the feeding of fresh liver will bring about a cure; where it results from failure of the stomach to elaborate its principle, a prepared extract of liver tissue must be injected. The injection is made into the muscles of the buttock, and it is sure a honey. I don't mean maybe. It is like liquid fire and you feel it from the crown of your head to your ankle, and that lasts for two days. The results are wonderful, however. I have found lesions in overbred hens suggesting that they might be suffering from this condition, and the feeding of liver, either raw or fried, is beneficial in some of these cases. See LIVER, main vocabulary.

PER OS, from **per,** by way of; **os,** mouth. Anything administered by way of the mouth, but particularly when it is administered directly into the mouth or crop rather than by being placed in the food.

PEROXIDAS STAIN (per oks' e das). A special staining process for differentiating immature cells of the granulocyte and monocyte series from the immature cells of other series found in the blood, particularly from the lymphocytes, which they closely resemble when stained by the ordinary techniques.

PETRI DISH (pa' tre). Julius Petri, German bacteriologist, 1852—. A small, flat, glass dish with a glass cover that slips over it. These dishes are made with the top and bottom surfaces parallel, so that there will be no distortion in the appearance of anything on the inside. They are used for making plate cultures, but are very handy little dishes to have around when working with any microscopic material.

PHAGOCYTE (fag' o site), from **phagein,** to eat; **kytos,** a cell. A cell that eats. These are cells found in the blood, spleen and liver—immature forms are found in the bone marrow—and in inflamed tissue, the function of which is to eat and digest bacteria and waste and foreign protein matter in the blood stream. In human blood the monocytes and the polymorphonuclear leucocytes are the only cells known to possess this function, though there are strong reasons for believing that the reticulo-endothelial cells of the liver and spleen—the star-shaped supporting cells—are also phagocytes and that in certain serious infections they sometimes become the most powerful phagocytes in the body. Some investigators believe that they give rise to wandering forms, similar to the monocytes, which are very effective in combating infection. It is my opinion that there are at least four and possibly six phagocytes found in bird blood.

PHALANGES (fa lan' jeez), Greek; pl., for **phalanx.** The small bones of your fingers and toes and the corresponding bones in the wings and feet of birds.

PHARYNX (far' ingks), from **pharygx,** the throat. The gullet; the large, funnel-shaped opening of the esophagus, lying back of the tongue.

PHILE or **PHIL** (fil), from **philein,** loving. A suffix indicating an affinity for the substance indicated by the rest of the word, usually some dye.

PHLOXIN (floks' in). A red dye of the eosin group. Used alone, this dye is not as good as yellow eosin for blood staining, but it is much better for staining tissue and works well with both methylene blue and hematoxylin. It may be added to the dehydrating alcohol for tissue that has been stained in toto with hematoxylin with wonderful polychromatic effects. With a little practice, this process is so sharply differential that it is possible to trace the finest nerve fibers and identify cells in the blood and bone marrow of tissue in paraffin section.

PIA, PIAMATER (pi a ma' ter), Latin, "kind or tender mother." The inner of the three membranes investing the brain and spinal cord and consisting of plexuses of blood-vessels held in a matrix of fine areolar tissue.

PIGMENTED (pig' ment ed), from **pingere,** to paint. Applied to tissues, containing granules of coloring matter; applied to the feathers of the new hybridized red-orange canary containing distinct traces of free red coloring matter.

PIP (pip). A condition of the tongue resulting from prolonged, open-mouthed breathing. See AVIAN DIPHTHERIA; FOWL FLU; GLYCERIN, main vocabulary.

PLASM (plazm), from Greek word **plasma,** a thing molded. A suffix meaning tissue or the materials of tissue, and applied to all forms of living matter.

PLASMA (plaz' ma). Same as plasm; also, the fluid parts of blood or tissue.

PLASMOCYTE (plaz' mo site), from **plasma,** the blood fluid; **kytos,** a cell. Gould's Medical Dictionary, Fourth Edition, defines this word as, "Any cell, other than blood-corpuscles, free in the blood plasma. 2. A protozoan parasite in the blood plasma." Osgood describes the plasmacytes as a distinct series of cells found in the blood and bone marrow, and having a morphology very similar to that of the lymphocytes, excepting that the cytoplasm is opaque and takes a deep blue stain and that sometimes the chromatin of the nucleus has a tendency to arrange itself in star-shaped formations. Dr. Zellermeyer, U. S. Public Health Service, informs me that any cell having a tendency toward star-shaped arrangement of its chromatin should be classified as a plasmacyte. Me, I don't know whether this is something we really know or a name for something we don't know, and I have my doubts about these other gentlemen.

PLATELETS, blood (plate' lets). Small, light gray discs in the blood, of doubtful function, thought to be associated with the clotting power of the blood.

PLEURA, pl., PLEURAE (ploo' rah, ploo' ree), Greek for **a side.** The membranes enveloping the lungs.

PLEURISY (ploo' ris e). An inflammation of the pleura. It may be acute or chronic, and it may involve a fluid, cheesy, fibrinous, or purulent exudate, and may result in adhesions to the lungs, heart, or ribs.

PLEXUS (pleks' us), from **plectere,** to knit. A network. A complex clump of vessels or nerves. See Figure 68.

PLUMBUM (plum' bum). The Latin name of lead. See LEAD POISONING.

PNEUMO (noo' mo), from **pneumon,** lung. Pertaining to the lungs.

PNEUMOCOCCUS, pl., PNEUMOCOCCI (noo mo kok' us, noo mo kok' se). Any micrococcus found in the lungs, particularly, the encapsulated diplobacillus of human pneumonia. See Figure 72.

PNEUMONIA (noo mo' ne ah), from **pneumon,** lung. Any inflammation of the lungs characterized by exudation into the alveoli. Often due to infection by a specific organism, particularly, the diplococcus of Fraenkel. See main vocabulary.

POLYMORPHONUCLEAR LEUCOCYTE (pol im or fo noo' kle ar loo' ko site), from **poly,** many; **morphon,** form; **nucleus, nux,** a nut; **leuco,** white; **kytos,** cell. This is what we call the principal phagocyte of human blood for short. The full name is, **neutrophilic polymorphonuclear leucocyte.** Which gives you at least six good reasons why pathologists go nuts. Though it is just possible that the case is the other way around. That no one but a nut would dream up a word like that. Osgood, with some reason, calls this cell the **neutrophilic lobocyte,** which is a little better. See BLOOD.

POST (post), Latin **posterus,** after; behind. A prefix meaning past, after, behind.

POSTERIOR (pose te' re or), from **posterus,** after, behind. Placed behind or to the back of a part. Actually in the human subject, below, towards the feet, as the **antinym** of **anterior.** See ANTERIOR, and don't forget the fish.

POST MORTEM (post mor′ tem), from **post,** past; **mors,** death. Occurring after death; as, a **post-mortem** examination, an examination made upon the body after death. Where used without qualification a **post-mortem examination** is understood.

POX (poks). A form of avian diphtheria characterized by nodules and vesicles occurring on the skin, particularly the skin of the head.

POX VIRUS (poks vi′ rus), from **pox; virus,** Latin for poison. The filtrable virus responsible for avian diphtheria.

PRECIPITATE (pre sip′ it ate), from **pre,** before; **caput,** head. Before the head. I don't get it. Anyway, it is the solid substance thrown down from a solution when some reagent is added that deprives some element in the solution of its solubility. The word is also used as a verb to indicate the act of precipitation.

PRO (pro), Latin. Prefix meaning for, before, in front of.

PROGNOSIS (prog no′ sis), from **pro,** before; **gnosis,** knowledge. Knowledge before the event. The prediction as to the outcome of an illness; as, **prognosis good,** the patient will live; **prognosis grave,** he might live, but you don't expect it, and he will probably never look the same; **prognosis hopeless,** no chance of survival. This word is also qualified by the words **favorable** and **unfavorable** and **pósitive** and **negative**—the first of each couplet meaning you will live; the second, that you will die.

PROLAPSE (pro laps′), from **prolabi,** to slip down. The falling of a part. See Figure 28.

PROPHYLAXIS (pro fil aks′ is), from **prophylassein,** to keep guard before. Prevention of disease. Measures taken to prevent the spread and development of disease.

PROTEIN (pro′ te in), from **protos,** first. The material from which living matter is constructed. For practical purposes, an organic substance containing carbon, hydrogen, oxygen, nitrogen, and often, sulphur.

PROTOPLASM (pro′ to plazm), from **protos,** first; **plasma,** form. Before form. The essential substance from which all living cells are made. Living matter in its lowest form. Any living material found in a plant or animal, but not including hair, horn, feathers, nails, mineral deposits and the wood of trees (excepting that growing, directly under the bark), since these substances are essentially dead, although they were produced as the result of cell activity.

PROTOZOA (pro to zo' ah). Pl. of protozoon.

PROTOZOAN (pro to zo' an). Pertaining to protozoa.

PROTOZOON (pro to zo' on), from **proto,** first; **zoon,** an animal. The first animal. One of the lowest animal forms consisting of single-celled organisms or colonies of cells having no circulation or nervous system.

PROVENTRICULUS (pro ven trik' ul us), from **pro,** first or before; **ventriculus,** diminutive of **venter,** a belly, a small cavity. A small cavity before the belly or stomach. The glanular stomach of birds, located just above the gizzard. See Figures 25 and 26.

PSEUDOPODS (soo' do pods), from **pseudo,** false; **pous,** foot. False feet. Small arms of protoplasm thrust out from the bodies of ameba, and ameboid cells in general, by means of which they achieve locomotion.

PSITTACINE (sit' a kin), from **psittakos,** a parrot. Any bird of the parrot family, such as parakeets, cockatoos, macaws, etc., as well as the true parrots.

PSITTACOSIS (sit ak o' sis), from **psittakos,** a parrot; **osis,** condition of. The condition of a parrot. An infectious disease of birds of the psittacine family. See main vocabulary.

PULLORUM (pul or' um). The name applied to the germ responsible for bacillary white diarrhea of baby chicks.

PULMONARY (pul' mon a re), from **pulmo,** a lung. Pertaining to, associated with, or affecting the lungs; as, the **pulmonary region,** near or surrounding the lungs; **pulmonary artery,** artery serving the lungs; **pulmonary congestion,** congestion affecting the lungs.

PUNCTIFORM (punk' tif orm), from **punctum,** point; **forma,** form or shape. Pointlike. Applied to hemorrhages, ulcers, etc., that are just large enough to be seen by the unaided eyes.

PURKINJE (poor kin' ye). Johannes Evangelesta Purkinje, Bohemian anatomist, 1787-1869. This man's name has been given to the large ganglion cells of the cerebellar cortex, arranged as a single layer at the junction of the granular and molecular layers of the cortex. See Figure 19.

PURULENT (poor' yoo lent). Pertaining to pus.

PYGOSTYLE (pie' go stile), from **pygn,** buttock; **stylos,** pillar.

The pillar of the buttock. In birds the large bone at the end of the coccyx, which supports the oil glands and the tail.

PYLORIC (pi lor′ ik). Pertaining to the **pylorus. Pyloric glands,** gastric glands situated in the region of the pylorus.

PYLORUS (pi lo′ rus), from **pyloros,** a gatekeeper. The circular opening between the stomach or gizzard and the duodenum and containing a strong, circular muscle that controls the flow of partially digested food into the intestines. See DIGESTIVE DIS-ORDERS, main vocabulary.

PYOGENES (pi oj′ en eez), from **pyo;** pertaining to pus; **genesis,** creation. Pertaining to the creation or production of pus. Applied to pus-forming microorganisms.

PYRETHRINS (pi re′ thrins). Active principles from pyrethrum, now available in the pure state and I believe produced synthetically.

PYRETHRUM (pi re′ thrum). An insect powder made from chrysanthemum · flowers. See CHRYSANTHEMUM FLOWERS, main vocabulary.

Q

QUASSIA (kwosh′ e ah), after Quassi, the Negro slave who first used it. The wood of several species of bitterwood trees native to the West Indies. Used as a bitter tonic, as an injection for seatworms, and as an insecticide. See QUASSIA; NAPHTHALENE, main vocabulary.

R

RACHITIS (rak i′ tis), from **rachi,** pertaining to the spine. Same as RICKETS.

RADIUS (ra′ de us). Latin, **a spoke of a wheel.** The outer of the two bones of the forearm and the corresponding bones of a bird's wing. See Figure 75.

RECESSIVE (re ses′ iv), from **recidivus,** falling back. Mendal's term for inherited characters that drop from sight during cross breeding, but which may reappear in later generations. In canaries, yellow feathers is a recessive character of white birds; cinnamon feathers is a recessive character of all black-eye males produced by crossing a cinnamon canary to a canary having no cinnamon ancestors.

REGURGITATE (re gur′ jit ate), from **re,** again; **gurgitare,** to engulf. The process by which birds bring up food from their crops to feed their young.

RENAL (re' nal), from **ren**, pertaining to the kidney. As, the **renal** artery; the **renal** capsule.

REPTILIAN (rep til' i an). Pertaining to reptiles. Employed in several places in this book in making comparisons between the structure of reptiles and birds.

RESPIRATION (res pi ra' shun), from **re**, again; **spirare**, to breathe. The act of breathing; the interchange of gasses between the living organism and the medium in which it lives.

RESPIRATORY (res pi' ra to re). Pertaining to breathing and the physiological equipment by which breathing is accomplished; as, lungs; airsacs, etc.

RETINA (ret' in ah), from **rete**, a net. The organ by which light waves are converted into nervous impulses; the terminal expansion of the optic nerve, which forms a membrane consisting of ten layers and covering the back, inner surface of the eyeball. See No. 8, Figure 56. With a good staining process, it is possible to stain each layer a different color, making this one of the most interesting of histological subjects. The retina of a bird's eye is from two to three times as thick as that of a mammal of comparable size. Their eyes are far superior to the eyes of mammals.

RETICULUM (ret ik' yoo lum), diminutive of **rete**, a net. A fine network. The fine network of cells and fibers that forms the supporting structures of glands and organs.

RHABDOCYTE (rab' do site), from **rabdos**, rod; **kytos**, cell. A cell of the granulocytic series of leucocytes having a nucleus that is rod-shaped, which may be twisted and contain bulges and constrictions, but in which the connective link between any two masses of nuclear matter is not reduced to the thickness of a filament. Osgood's definition and name for the least mature cells of the granulocytic series found in normal human blood. According to the older classifications these were called **Staff Cells**.

RHINO (ri' no), from **rinos**, the nose. A prefix meaning pertaining to the nose; as, **rhinomycosis**, a mould infection of the nasal passages.

RICKETS (rik' ets). A disease of the bones resulting from a deficiency of vitamin D or of lime and phosphates in the diet. See Figure 86.

RIGOR (ri' gor), from **rigere**, a chill. The chill that is often associated with the development of a fever.

RIGOR MORTIS (ri gor mor' tis), from **rigere**, a chill; **mors**, death. The chill of death. The stiffness of the muscles that occurs shortly after death.

ROUP (roop). A name applied to avian diphtheria.

S

SADISM (sa' dizm). Donatien Alphonse Francois Conte de Sadem, 1740-1814. A form of sex perversion in which pleasure is derived from inflicting pain upon another. Anyone who takes a keen delight in the infliction of pain is designated a **sadist.**

SALICYLATES (sal is' il ates). Salts of salicylic acid. See main vocabulary.

SALMONELLA (sal' mon el ah). D. F. Salmon, American bacteriologist and Chief of the Bureau of Animal Industry in 1895 and 1896, which is about all I know about him. The name is now applied to a certain class of pathogenic bacteria, including the germs of hog cholera, paratyphoid, and certain organisms normally present in the intestines of man and animals. See Figures 9 and 10.

SANGUINARIUM (sang gwin a' re um), from **sanguis**, blood; **naris**, nostril. Why, I haven't the remotest idea. A term applied to the germ of fowl typhoid, which, of course, is found in the blood, and may be found in the nostrils, though I have not read of it.

SAPROPHILOUS, SAPROPHYTIC (sap roff' il us) (sap ro fit' ik), from **sapros**, putrid; **philein**, to love; or **phyton**, a plant. The first form means **putrid loving**; the second, a **putrid plant**. The first is applied to any non-pathogenic organism living in putrid matter; the second only to plant-like organisms; but in general practice the two words are used interchangeably to describe microorganisms that do not cause disease.

SARCOMA (sar ko' mah), from **sarco**, flesh; **oma**, a tumor. A malignant tumor originating in cells derived from the mesoderm—bone, muscles, connective tissue, and blood.*

SATURATED (sat' yoo ra ted), from **saturare**, to fill. That which is full, which can contain no more; as, a **saturated solution,** one in which the solvent contains in solution all of the substance that it

---

* **Note:** While true malignant tumors of the blood cells are called leukemias, they differ in no important respect from the sarcomas.

can dissolve. A saturated solution is usually obtained by adding more of the substance than the solvent can dissolve, applying heat, and then permitting the excess to crystallize out.

SCLEROSIS (skle ro′ sis); **skleros,** hard. Hardening of a part, especially that resulting from infiltrating with interstitial connective tissue and the obliteration of the functional epithelial tissue. Figures 52, 63, and 70 show inflammatory conditions which might have, had they been less acute, resulted in sclerosis. In Figure 70 the development is well on the way.

SECONDARY (sek′ un da re), from **secundus,** second. That which comes after the first; that which is second in the order of time or importance; as, a **secondary invader,** a germ which may not be responsible for the development of a disease but may be responsible for its most serious consequences. See AVIAN DIPHTHERIA; HOG CHOLERA. Pneumonia is not usually a primary disease in human beings, but most often results in a complication—a **secondary invasion,** following a common cold; influenza, or exposure, or some other primary cause that lowers the natural resistance of the individual, and opens the way for the **secondary invasion**.

SEIDLETZ POWDER (sed′ litz). I do not know who he was, but his most excellent preparation consisted of bicarbonate of soda and tartaric acid.

SEPSIS (sep′ sis), from **sepsis,** putrifaction. The state of being putrid or of being contaminated with disease-producing organisms; the disease resulting from the absorption of putrifactive substances.

SEPTIC (sep′ tik), from **sepsis.** Pertaining to sepsis or putrifaction or a result thereof; contaminated.

SEPTICEMIA (sep te se′ me ah), from **sepsis,** putrifaction; **aima,** the blood. Putrifaction of the blood. Any disease in which the causative agent may be demonstrated in the blood of the victim, either by microscopic or cultural methods, or by inoculation.

SERO (se′ ro). A prefix meaning pertaining to serum or serous.

SEROUS (se′ rus), from **serum,** the fluid part of tissue. Pertaining to, producing, or associated with serum; as, a **serous gland,** a gland that produces a serum or serum-like secretion; a **serous membrane,** one of the internal membranes that is kept constantly moist and lubricated by being bathed in serum, such as the pericardium, peritoneum, and the articular surfaces of the joints.

SHADOW CELL. A disintegrating red blood corpuscle. See BLOOD.

SINUS (si′ nus), Latin, **a gulf or hollow.** A cavity, recess, or pocket containing air or fluid; as, **suborbital** and **mastoid sinuses,** cavities in the bones of the face and head and connected with the eye and ear respectively, normally containing air; cavities in the brain and spinal column.

SLIPPED CLAW. A condition occurring in nest-raised birds wherein the back claw becomes turned forward and turns up between the front toes, crippling the bird. See main vocabulary.

SMOOTH MUSCLES. The non-striated, involuntary muscles of the viscera under the control of the sympathetic nervous system. For a comparison of the appearance of striated and non-striated muscles see Figures 31 and 68.

SOFT BILLED. A term applied to the insectivorous birds.

SOFT MOULT. A condition affecting caged birds that are kept in rooms having too high a temperature or are improperly fed, particularly fed too much lettuce or milk, in which the bird falls into a continuous moult that is usually terminated by death from some illness which would, under other circumstances, be of very little consequence. See main vocabulary.

SOMNOLENT (som′ no lent), from **somnus,** sleep. A tendency to sleep. As applied to sick birds, a tendency to sleep in the daytime— something no healthy, adult bird ever does, unless its nightly sleep has been disturbed.

SPASM (spazm), from **spasmos,** a spasm. A sudden and uncontrolled muscular contraction, or a series of such contractions. A series of such spasms is called a **clonic convulsion.** There are cases where the muscle does not relax, where the part becomes permanently rigid. These are called **fixed spasms.**

SPASTIC (spas′ tik), from the Greek word **spastikos.** Pertaining to, characterized by, or producing a spasm.

SPECIFIC (spe sif′ ik), from **species,** a subdivision of a genus of animals or plants; **facere,** to make. To make a species. Pertaining to a species or to that which distinguishes a thing and sets it off as a species. And this meaning, through usage, has established the word as referring to any exact and definite thing or property; as, **a specific,** a drug or treatment which has a specific curative influence upon one particular disease or group of diseases; **specific disease,** a disease due to a single microorganism; **specific gravity; specific heat,** etc., which are particular physical properties by means of which particular substances may be identified.

SPERMATOZOAN (sper mat o zo' an). Pertaining to a spermatozoon.

SPERMATOZOON, pl., **ZOA** (sper mat o zo' on, zo' a), from **sperma,** a seed; **spermato,** pertaining to a seed; **zoon,** an animal. The seed pertaining to an animal. The male sex germ of an animal, which consists of a dense, pointed head and a motile tail. See Figures 46 and 47 for the spermatozoa of birds.

SPHENOIDS (sfe' noids), from **sphen,** a wedge; **eidos,** like. Like a wedge. The small wedge-shaped bones forming the floor of the skull.

SPHINCTER (sfingk' ter), from **sphiggein,** to bind. A circular muscle surrounding and closing an orifice; as, **sphincter ani,** the muscle that closes the vent or anus; **sphincter uteri,** the muscle that closes the uterus in a mammal, the oviduct in a bird; **sphincter pylori,** the muscle that closes the orifice between the stomach or gizzard and the duodenum.

SPIROCHETE (spi' ro keet), from **speira,** a coil; **chaitn,** a bristle. A coiled bristle or thread. A microorganism taking the form of a coiled thread. See Figure 77.

SPIROCHETOSIS (spi ro ke to' sis), from **speira,** a coil; **chaitn,** a bristle; **osis,** a condition. A disease caused by a spirochete.

SPLEEN (spleen), from **splen,** spleen. In birds, a small sausage-shaped organ located directly below the gizzard.

SPLENIC (splen' ik). Pertaining to the spleen; as, the **splenic artery;** the **splenic capsule.** See Figure 78.

SPONGIOPLASM (spun' je o plazm), from **spongio,** a sponge; **plassein,** plasm, to mold. The thread-like protoplasmic reticulum of a cell. See Figure 12.

SPORT (sport). A mutation; an animal or plant exhibiting a decided and transmissible variation from the normal established type of the species.

SQUAMOUS (skwa' mus), from **squamosus,** scaly. This term is applied to the epithelial cells of the skin and of the orifices having direct contact with the skin. Squamous cells are flat, polygonal cells occurring, usually, in many layers. The bottom, **germinal,** layer of a squamous epithelium is made up of cells having large, deep-staining nuclei. These cells are undergoing constant division, by which the layers are built up and wear compensated.

STAPHYLOCOCCUS, pl., **COCCI** (staf il o kok' us, pl., kok' se), from **staphyle,** grape; **kokkos,** berry. Grape-berry or a grape-like berry. Small globular microorganisms occurring in clusters resembling bunches of grapes. See Figure 79.

STARCELL. Also called **Stellocytes.** The reticulo-endothelial cells, supporting cells, of the liver and spleen; the star-shaped neurons of the cerebellum.

STERILE (ster' il), from **sterilis,** barren. Incapable of reproduction; unfertile; free from germs.

STREPTOCOCCUS (strep to kok' us), from **streptos,** twisted; **kokkos,** a berry. Twisted berries. Small spherical or oviform microorganisms occurring in chains or skeins, like strings of beads. See Figure 3.

STRIATED (stri' ae ted), from **stria,** a streak. This term is applied to the voluntary muscles, because of their striped or streaked appearance, to differentiate them from the involuntary muscles which do not have this striping and which are designated **smooth.** See figure 68.

STROMA (stro' mah), from the Greek **stroma,** a bed. The tissue forming the framework and supporting capsule for the essential part of an organ. See figures 68 and 78.

STUCK IN MOULT. A condition of bird resulting from failure to have a complete moult. See main vocabulary.

SUB. Latin prefix meaning less, under, below, or deficient.

SUBACUTE (sub ak ute'), from **sub,** less; **acutus,** sharp. Less sharp. An attack of a disease that is about half way between acute and chronic.

SUBARACHNOID (sub ar ak' noid), from **sub,** below; **arachnoid,** the second membrane covering the brain and spinal cord. Below the arachnoid. Spaces between the arachnoid and the brain and spinal cord which are normally filled with cerebro-spinal fluid.

SUBCUTANEOUS (sub kyoo ta' ne us) **sub,** beneath; **cutis,** the skin. Beneath the skin; hypodermatic. Also pertaining to anything beneath the skin, as, **subcutaneous tissue; subcutaneous infiltration,** etc.

SUBMUCOUS (sub myoo' kus), from **sub** and **mucous.** Beneath the mucous membrane; as, **submucous tissue; submucous glands; submucous inflammation;** etc.

SUBNORMAL (sub nor' mal). Below normal; as, **subnormal temperature,** a body temperature of less than 42 C. for a canary, of less than 37 C. for a man; **subnormal appetite,** eating less than normal.

SUBORBITAL (sub or' bit al). Below the orbit; located in the bony structure below the eye.

SUIPESTIFER (soo i pest' if er), from **sui** (my book gives this as **himself,** but he was probably an awful hog, since this root word is also used to designate swine); **pestis,** a plague; **ferre,** to bear. Pertaining to a plague of swine; hog cholera. Used to designate germs of the hog cholera group, which are also called **B. paratyphosus B** and **Salmonella aertrycke.**

SUPER (soo per). A prefix meaning more.

SYRINX (sir' ingks), from **syrigx,** a tube. The voice box of birds; located at the lower end of the trachea.

SYSTOLE (sis' to le) from **systoly,** contraction. The contraction of the ventricles of the heart.

T

TAENIA, TENIA (te' ne ah). Latin, a band. A band or ribbon-like structure; a tapeworm, **taenia saginata.**

TAENIAFUGE, TENIAFUGE (te' ne af ug), from **tenia,** tapeworm; **fugare,** to drive out. A drug for driving out tapeworms.

TARSUS (tar' sus), from **tarsos,** the instep. The bones of the instep. In birds the tarsus has been lost and the metatarsi have been fused to form the single bone of the scaly shank.

TESTICLE (tes' tik l), from **testiculus,** diminutive of **testis.** A male sex gland. See figures 45 and 46.

TESTICULAR (tes' tik yoo lar). Pertaining to, associated with, produced by the testicles; as, **testicular construction; testicular tubules; testicular secretions.**

TETANIC (tet an' ik). Pertaining to or resembling tetanus. A condition of rigidity of the muscles.

TETANUS (tet' an us). From **tetanos,** from **teinein,** to stretch. A disease characterized by rigid contraction of the voluntary muscles. Birds, because of their high body temperatures are not susceptible to tetanus, but references to this disease are made in the description of other conditions.

THALAMUS (thal' am us), from **thalamos,** a couch; pl., **thalami.** Masses of gray matter located at the base of the brain and receiving fibers from the cerebrum and the cranial nerves; in birds, particularly the optic nerve. These bodies are thought to be the coordinating center.

THERAPEUTIC (ther ap yoo' tik). Pertaining to therapeutics; having curative value or use.

THERAPEUTICS (ther ap yoo' tiks), from **therapeutiky,** the art of medicine. The medical art of treating disease, particularly, by the use of drugs.

THORACIC (tho ras' ik), from **thorax,** the chest. Pertaining to or located in the chest.

THORAX (tho' raks). Greek, a breastplate. The chest; the bony structure and tissues forming the cavity that contains the heart and lungs.

THROMBOCYTE (throm' bo site), from **thrombus,** a clot; **kytos,** a cell. A large cell found in the bone marrow and thought to be the mother of the blood platelets. Sometimes applied to the platelets. Osgood calls this cell the **megalokaryocyte.**

THROMBOSIS (throm bo' sis), from **thrombus,** a clot; **osis,** the condition caused by the formation of a blood clot in a blood vessel.

THROMBUS (throm' bus), from **thrombos,** a clot; pl., **thrombi.** A clot of blood forming within a blood vessel, which may occur as the result of disease or of injury to the wall of the vessel.

THYROID (thi' roid) from **thyreos,** a shield; **eidos,** like. Like a shield. Shield-shaped. A gland of internal secretion located at the base of the neck on the right side. In humans the gland is shield-shaped; in birds it is round.* The secretion of the thyroid gland plays a vital part in growth; size; the development of intellect; the conversion of food into energy rather than fat; and, in birds, the growth of feathers. I have not been able to get a good section of a canary's thyroid. The organ is so small that up until now it has always got lost in the shuffle.

TIBIA (tib' e ah). Latin, shin. The larger of the two bones of the foreleg.

TINCTURE (tingk' tyoor), from **tinctura,** from **tingere,** to tinge. A solution of a drug in a solvent other than water or glycerine, usually alcohol. See **NUX VOMICA,** main vocabulary.

---

* **Note:** All of the organs and glands of birds have a pronounced tendency to roundness, compactness; while in mammals, on the other hand, they have a tendency toward flatness and lobulation. The only exception to this general rule is provided by the kidneys.

TONIC (ton' ik), from **tone**. Pertaining to tone; producing normal tone or tension; producing or characterized by continuous muscular contraction; as, a **tonic convulsion**. A drug having the property of improving the general tone of the body or one, which, in anemias, has a tendency to improve the quality and tone of the erythrocytes, increase their number, and bring the hemoglobin content of the blood nearer to normal.

TOXEMIA (toks e' me ah), from **toxikon**, poison; **aima**, blood. Blood poisoning. The presence of poisons of either cellular or bacterial origin in the blood stream. A general infection in which the blood contains the poisons produced by bacteria but not the bacteria themselves.

TOXIN (toks' in), from **toxikon**, poison. Any non-mineral poison of animal or vegetable origin.

TRABECULA (tra bek' yoo lah). Latin, "a small beam." Bands of fiber extending from the capsule into the interior of an organ and serving as supports for the functional cells. Almost any microscopic drawing will furnish good examples of this structural element, but figure 78 is as good as any.

TRACHEA (tra' ke ah), from **trachiea**, a windpipe. The cartilaginous-membranous tube through which we breathe. In birds the windpipe extends from the back of the tongue to the syrinx, the voice box, into which open the bronchi.

TRANSVERSE (trans vers'), from **trans**, across; **vertere**, to turn. Crosswise. At right angle to the longitudinal axis of the body or organ.

TRAUMA (traw' mah). Greek, "a wound or injury." Pl., **traumata**, any wound or injury.

TRICUSPID (tri kus' pid), from **tri**, three; **cuspis**, a point. Having three points. The three-leafed or three-pointed valve of the mammalian heart.

TUBULES. Diminutive of **tube**. A little tube. A tube of microscopic dimensions.

U

ULNA (ul' nah). Latin, "a cubit." The inner bone of the forearm and the corresponding bone of a bird's wing.

UREMIA (yoo re' me ah), from **ouron**, urine; **aima**, blood. Urine in the blood. The retension of urinary products in the blood stream. See main vocabulary.

URETERS (yoo re' ter), from **oureter,** ureter. In birds, the tubes running down the ventral surface of both kidneys and emptying the urine into the cloaca. They are lined with cuboidal epithelial cells. In mammals the ureters connect the kidneys with the bladder.

URINARY (yoo' rin a re), from **ourin,** urine. Pertaining to the urine and the organs associated with its secretion and evacuation.

URINIFEROUS (yoo rin if' er us), from **ouron,** urine; **ferre,** to bear. The small tubules of the kidneys that carry the urine from the glomeruli to the ureters are called **uriniferous tubes.**

UROGENITAL (yoo ro jen' it al), from **ouron,** urine; **genitalis,** pertaining to generation; from **gignere,** to beget. Pertaining to the sexual and urinary organs as a unit.

UROTROPIN (yoo rot' ro pin). A drug used in the treatment of kidney infections, now going out of use in view of the better results obtained by employing the **sulfa** drugs. See main vocabulary.

UTERINE (yoo' ter een), from **uterus,** the female sex duct, the oviduct.

UTERUS (yoo' ter us). Latin. The womb, oviduct. The female generative organ having to do with the development of the ovum after it leaves the ovary; in mammals, to an infant capable of living in air; in birds, to a complete egg. See Figures 30 and 31.

V

VACUOLE (vak' yoo ole), from **vacuus,** empty. A clear or empty space in the protoplasm of a cell. See figure 12.

VASCULAR (vas' kyoo lar), from **vasculum,** a small vessel. Pertaining to, consisting of, or provided with vessels, particularly, blood vessels.

VAS DEFERENS (vas def' er enz). Latin, **vas,** a tube or duct; **deferens,** carrying away. The excretory ducts of the testicles. Pl., **vasa deferentia.** See Figure 45.

VENTRAL (ven' tral), from Latin, **venter.** The belly or abdomen. Towards the abdomen or abdominal side of the body. The forward end of the ventral-dorsal axis of the body, which sets at right angles to the anterior-posterior axis of the body.

VENTRICLE (ven' trik l), from **ventriculus,** diminutive of **venter,**

a belly. A small cavity or pouch, particularly applied to the lower chambers of the heart, but also to the cavities of the brain.

VENTRICULAR (ven trik' yoo lar), from **ventriculus.** Pertaining to or resembling a ventricle.

VERMICIDE (ver' mis ide), from **vermis,** a worm; **cedere,** to kill. A drug that kills worms, particularly intestinal worms.

VERMIFUGE (ver' mif yooj), from **vermis,** a worm; **fugare,** to expel. A drug that expels intestinal worms.

VERTEBRA (ver' teb rah). Latin, "a joint; a bone of the spine." Pl., **vertebrae,** one of the bones forming the spinal column.

VESICLES (ves' ik l), from **vesica,** a bladder. A small sac containing fluid; small blisters appearing on the skin. see AVIAN DIPHTHERIA.

VILLI (vil' li). Plural of villus, a tuft. Hair-like processes projecting from a mucous membrane. In the intestines such processes form the organic elements for the absorption of nutriment. They also assist in keeping the intestinal contents in motion. See Figure 27.

VIRULENCE (vir' oo lens), from the Latin **virus.** Infectiveness. This term is used to describe the extent and degree of infectiveness of a given microorganism.

VIRULENT (vir' oo lent). Poisonous; infective.

VIRUS (vi' rus). Latin. The poison of an infectious disease. This word is most often applied to the causative agents of those infectious diseases that are too small to be seen under the ordinary microscope, but it is also applied to poisons manufactured by certain disease-producing bacteria, and sometimes to the bacteria themselves or to secretions which contain the bacteria. See AVIAN DIPHTHERIA; FOWL FLU; PSITTACOSIS, which are the most important virus diseases of birds.

VISCERAL (vis' er al). Latin, **viscera,** the internal organs considered as a unit. Pertaining to any or all of the internal organs.

VISCID (vis' id). Latin **viscidus,** sticky. Applied to any sticky fluid, particularly the contents of vesicles, blisters, etc.

VITALINE MEMBRANE (vi' tah line), from **vital.** Pertaining to life. The membrane surrounding the yolk of an egg and containing the germinal disc.

VITAMIN (vi' tam in), from **vital.** Pertaining to life. Substances present in natural food in minute quantities which exercise a vital influence upon certain functions of the body that is vastly out of proportion to their actual mass. See main vocabulary.

W

WATCHGLASS.   A small dish resembling a watch-crystal, used in making tests and preparing microscopic material.

X

XYLENE (zil' een).   A coaltar solvent that is soluble in alcohol and will dissolve all kinds of wax. It is used in the preparation of tissue for microscopic examination and for cleaning microscopic lenses.

Y

YELLOW.   A term applied to the structure of the feathers of birds, as distinct from **buff,** in which the feather pigment is carried to the very edge of the feather. See BALDNESS; RED CANARY.

TECHNIQUE

The Doses of Drugs for Canaries and Small Birds

The dose of almost any drug for a canary is from 1/500 to 1/1,000 of the dose for a human.

In the case of the sulfa drugs the dose is 1/600 of the initial human dose—60 grains—and repeat doses are not tolerated well. These drugs should never be given to birds suffering from kidney trouble. In such cases 1/20 of a grain may prove fatal.

Aspirin and salicylates in general..............1/20 to 1/10 grain
Quinine ....1/20 grain

Oxidizing drugs, potassium permanganate, sodium perborate, potassium chlorate, peroxide of hydrogen, are much less poisonous to birds than to mammals. I have given 1/10 grain of sodium perborate into the crop of a day-old chick without injury. I have had fevered canaries consume several grains of this drug in a day without any poisonous reaction. One-fifth grain of chlorate; 1/5 grain of permanganate; ½ grain of perborate, and from five to ten drops of commercial peroxide can be safely administered into the crop.

Liquid preparations for human use that are taken in doses of one teaspoonful three times per day can be administered in the drinking water in from three to five drop doses, providing they do not contain strychnine. Strychnine tonics should not be given in doses of more than one drop to the ounce of drinking water. They should never be given into the crop except under circumstances described in text.

For the doses of other drugs, consult main vocabulary.

In administering drugs into the crop, it is best to have them in pill form. This is absolutely necessary in the case of the sulfa drugs, since it is the only method that permits exact doses, and in some cases it is the most satisfactory method of administering aspirin and perborate. Perborate can be pressed into pills about the size of a large rape seed, and one or two of these poked down the throat.

The sulfa drugs come in five and seven and one-half grain tablets and these must be diluted with other substances for administration. To do this grind the tablet to fine powder. Add about half the amount of the tablet of flour, sugar, and soda; grind together until thoroughly mixed. Take a piece of glass tubing about the size of a pencil; draw it out until the diameter of the small end is about the size of a rape seed. Fit this tube with glass or wooden plunger. Add a drop or two of water to the mixed drug and knead it into a dough. This is charged into the glass tube and, by means of the plunger, pressed out into a long, straight, uniform ribbon. For a five grain tablet, this ribbon is cut into fifty pieces of equal length; for a seven and one-half grain tablet, it is cut into seventy-five pieces of equal length. One of these pieces can easily be poked down the bird's throat. They must, of course, be thoroughly dried before storing. This same method may be applied to most any drug that must be given in small doses into the crop.

For small finches, the dose should only be about half of what it would be for a canary.

THE MAKING OF SMEAR. Place a number of perfectly clean microscopic slides in a jar of iso-propyl alcohol. Take one slide and break a small chip off each corner of one end, so as to reduce the forward edge at that end to about ½ inch. Wrap the other end with adhesive tape. Polish the forward edges of the free end on a fine hone or carborundum stone. This is your smearing slide.

Remove five or six slides from the alcohol and wipe them dry with a clean handkerchief. Place these in a convenient place on the edge of your table. Also place on your table within easy reach a new, sharp razor blade; your smearing slide; and a lighted cigarette. Then catch the bird.

Place one of the bird's feet on the edge of the table, and, with the razor blade, snip off one claw at a point just back of the end of the blood vessel that can be seen running down its center. If the claw does not bleed at once, pinch it in a direction at right angles to the direction of the cut, to open the channel. As soon as a drop of blood about the size of a rape seed appears, the claw is touched to one of the clean slides at a point about half an inch from the end nearest the operator. One finger of the hand holding the bird is placed at the other end of this slide to hold it firmly; the smearing slide, held at an angle of about 45 degrees, is placed in contact with the center of the slide containing the blood droplet. The smearing slide is then drawn back until it touches the blood droplet, which will spread out along its under edge. It is then thrust forward with a slow even motion in such a manner as to draw the blood droplet over the face of the slide being smeared. The faster the smearing slide moves, the thicker the film will be, but, if the smearing slide moves too slowly or in an uneven manner, the film will be ragged and uneven. To make a good smear from bird blood is much more difficult than it is to make one from human blood; so, before practicing on your birds, learn to make good smears from your own blood and from chicken blood. A good smear has a smooth, even, velvety appearance; it is iridescent and so thin you can see through it.

If the slides are to be examined by someone else, they are placed in pairs, face to face, wrapped in clean paper, labeled, and shipped. If they are to be examined by the operator, they are thoroughly dried. The first one is flooded with isopropanol (isopropyl alcohol), which is poured from the first slide to the second, and from the second to the third, etc., until all of the smeared surfaces have been wetted with this substance.

In the meantime, however, in making the smears, the operator passes from slide to slide, working as fast as possible, so as not to waste any of the canary's blood, and as soon as the last slide is made—for a skillful operator, two are enough, but the unskilled operator will have to make at least six to get two good ones— the bleeding is stopped by touching the bird's claw quickly and lightly to the brightly burning end of the cigarette, but be careful not to touch the fire to his skin, only to the bleeding end of the claw. He is then returned to his cage or flight. If the work has been skillfully done, the claw will not be sore.

The prepared smears are placed on a warming plate and thoroughly dried at a temperature of 50 C. for at least twenty minutes before they are ready for staining.

BLOOD STAIN. The staining of bird blood is much more difficult than the staining of human blood, and the same methods are not applicable. Wright's stain will give beautiful results with bird blood, but some of the structures upon which differentiation of the leucocytes depends cannot be brought out by this method, so that it becomes valueless for the purpose of making differential counts. For the sharp definition of internal cell structures, the best method I have found makes use of the following solutions:

A—

Martius yellow..........................1 gram
Phloxin ....1 gram
Hydrant water (seems better than distilled
    water) ....1 liter
Normal sodium hydroxide...............0.5 c.c.

B—

      Saturated alcoholic solution of crystal
        violet ....1 c.c.
      Saturated alcoholic solution basic fuchsin .1 c.c.
      Hydrant water........................100 c.c.
      1/100 normal hydrochloric acid drop by drop until
        best possible results are obtained.

The titering of solution B with acid requires about one dozen slides which should be made from chicken blood. Stain them all with solution A for thirty seconds; wash; shake off excess water and dry on warming plate.

Measure out 12 c.c. of solution B. Flood slide number one with one c.c. of this portion and stain for thirty seconds. Add one drop of the 1/100 normal acid to the remainder, and then flood slide number two with one c.c. from this, and continue until 11 drops of acid have been added and the solution has all been used. Stain each slide for thirty seconds. When· they are all stained, smear their surfaces with oil and examine in order, picking out the slide that is best.

If No. 1 is the best you do nothing to your stock solution.
If No. 2 is the best you add 8 drops of acid to stock solution.
If No. 3 is the best you add 16 drops of acid to stock solution.
If No. 4 is the best you add 26 drops of acid to stock solution.
If No. 5 is the best you add 36 drops of acid to stock solution.
If No. 6 is the best you add 48 drops of acid to stock solution.
If No. 7 is the best you add 61 drops of acid to stock solution.
If No. 8 is the best you add 77 drops of acid to stock solution.

Any acid requirement beyond this point is out of the question. It will not happen, but you will learn something from studying those last four slides just the same.

This method of staining has one fault: the chromatin in all of the different types of leucocytes, with the exception of cell No. 6, stains exactly the same color.

In running the series of slides as suggested above, you will have noticed that when the solution is too alkaline the cytoplasm of the erythrocytes stains deeply, the nuclei not at all, and that as the acid is added the cytoplasm clears and the staining of the nuclei becomes more intense up to the point where the solution becomes too acid; then the nuclei take on a lighter, more reddish tint, resulting from the fuchsin. With a little practice one becomes able to estimate the amount of acid required from the appearance of a single slide.

Polychrome methylene blue, solution C—

a—

> Medicinal methylene blue............... 1 gram
> Water ....250 c.c.
> Glacial acetic acid..................... 10 drops

Place dye in 300 c.c. flask, drop acid on it, add the water, heat almost to boiling. Stopper and set aside.

b—

> Medicine methylene blue.................1 gram
> Bicarbonate of soda................... 0.5 gram
> Sodium perborate.................... 1 gram
> Water ....250 c.c.

Place solid ingredients in 300 flask, add water, place open flask in paraffin oven—set at 90 C.—and leave it overnight.

The next morning mix a and b, filter into a 500 c.c. bottle, add water to make up for evaporation. Stopper and store.

This solution will usually give good results at once. Smears should be fixed as described above and may or may not be first stained with solution A. They are dried, warmed and flooded with solution C for fifteen seconds, washed in water and examined at once with the dry objective. If too acid, the cytoplasm of the erythrocytes will contain little color and the nuclei will not be well stained; if too alkaline, the cytoplasm of the erythrocytes will be deeply stained and nuclei colorless. The acidity or alkalinity is corrected by adding normal sodium hydroxide or ten per cent acetic acid, as the case requires, drop by drop until the solution stains perfectly.

Thereafter the slides are stained first with solution A for 15 seconds; washed in running water; shaken as dry as possible; placed on the warming plate to dry; stained for fifteen to thirty seconds with solution C; washed briefly in running water and stood on end to dry at room temperature. Then, smeared with oil, examined with the dry objective; then with the oil immersion objective. If it is desired to save the slide, it may be mounted in balsam or the surplus oil may be wiped off and the slide stored without a coverglass. This is the best staining method that I have found for making differential counts on bird blood. It is also a good bacteriological stain and will demonstrate the capsule of pneumococci or the bipolar arrangement of the protoplasm of pasteurella organisms in blood smears that have lain exposed to the air in the unfixed condition for as long as one year before staining. It also gives good results with feces and urine. Its chief value as a differential stain rests upon the fact that the chromatin of each type of leucocyte is stained a slightly different color, often making it possible to identify cells which, by reason of crowding, cannot be seen in their entirety.

BLOOD COUNTING. The differential counting of the leucocytes in bird blood is done exactly as it is with human blood, excepting that it is impossible to classify the leucocytes found in canary blood under the five accepted headings. The vast majority of the cells found in bird blood can be classified under 15 headings based upon the drawings making up plate 13. Under the heading "1" are included all cells of the type illustrated by drawings "6" and "7"; under heading "2" are classed cells similar to "8"; under "3," drawing "9"; under "4," drawings "10" and "11"; "5," drawings "12" and "13"; "6," drawings "14" and "15"; "7," drawings "16" and "17"; "8," drawing "18"; "9," drawings "19," "20," and "21"; "10," drawing "22"; "11," drawings "23" and "24"; "12," drawing "25"; "13," drawing "26." One heading should be provided for disintegrating cells and one for cells that cannot be fitted into any of the above groups.

The slide after being stained by one of the above methods is moved slowly under the oil immersion objective, and all leucocytes coming into the field are classified and tabulated under their respective headings, until 100, 500, or 1,000 have been counted.

The gross count is the method by which we estimate the number of cells in one cubic millimeter of blood and determine the relative number of red and white cells. On human blood, these estimations are made separately, but this is impossible in the case of bird blood, since there is no agent that will destroy the erythrocytes without also destroying the leucocytes. It is possible to stain the leucocytes so that they may be counted along with the erythrocytes, however.

Diluting solution for bird blood, solution D—

           Common table salt...................... 1 gram
           Hydrant water that has been boiled......175 c.c.
           Acid fuchsin..........................0.1 gram
           Crystal violet ....0.1 gram

Bring to a boil; add five drops of 1/10 normal hydrochloric acid; filter through paper; add four drops of 1/10 normal sodium hydroxide; filter again if necessary. Stopper tightly and let settle for 24 hours. In using, draw the solution from the top of the bottle, without disturbing the sediment.

If carefully made, this solution will stain the nuclei of the erythrocytes blue; the cytoplasm of the erythrocytes a buff-orange; the nuclei of the various leucocytes various shades ranging from reddish violet to black; the cytoplasm of the leucocytes, shades ranging from colorless to reddish violet; the granules, orange, red or deep blue, which makes it possible, if desirable, to obtain a rough differential as the cross count is being made.

A single NEUBAUER counting chamber is used, and before drawing the blood, the chamber slide and the cover glass—only the thick cover that comes with the chamber should be used—are washed in running water and wiped with a clean, dry cloth, and the cover is placed over the slide.

Blood from a clipped claw is drawn into the erythrocyte, 1:100, pipet used for human blood to the division line marked 0.5; the tip of the pipet is quickly wiped and the diluting solution, solution D, is then drawn into the pipet to the point marked 101. This gives a dilution of 1:200.

As soon as the solution is brought to the mark 101, the pipet is closed by bringing the forefinger down on the large end, cramping the rubber tube over the opening. The tip of the pipet is closed with the thumb, and the pipet is shaken vigorously for a few moments. If it is impossible to make the examination at once, the tube is drawn down tight, wrapped around the stem of the pipet and fastened by tucking a loop of the tubing under the stretched section.

The pipet is again vigorously shaken before charging the chamber, and enough of the fluid is blown out to clear the stem. The chamber is then charged by touching the tip of the pipet to the edge of the coverglass where it passes over the platform upon which the scale is engraved. If the slide and cover are clean, the solution will run under the slide and fill the chamber without leaving bubbles, and a much evener distribution of cells is obtained than can be secured by filling the chamber first and then sliding the coverglass into place, and there is little danger of over-filling the chamber.

First, count all cells in two columns of eighty small squares each. To each result add four ciphers. If there is less than 200,000 difference in the two results, average them. If the difference is greater than 200,000, clean the slide and cover and do the work over. For normal canary blood the result should be between 4,000,000 and 4,500,000, though anything between 3,800,000 and 5,000,000 can be considered normal, since there is often this much variation in birds in which no evidence of illness can be détected.

Should the erythrocytes appear in clumps, it indicates that the operator has worked too slowly and that the blood has clotted in the stem of the pipet before dilution. A clean pipet must be used and a new sample of blood taken.

For the white count, count the white cells in the two opposite large, corner squares, i.e., over an area of two square millimeters; then add three ciphers to the result. Count the other two corner squares the same way; then count two of the side areas on opposite sides of the central square, and treat the results in the same manner. The difference between the highest and the lowest of the three results should not be greater than 5,000, and, if this is the case, the three results are added together and divided by three to obtain the average value for the white count. For the normal canary the average should be from 35,000 to 40,000; though counts as low as 30,000 and as high as 45,000 should not be considered abnormal. This gives an average ratio for canary blood of 1 white cell to 110 red cells. Ratios of 1:100 to 1:125 should be considered normal. Greater variation in either direction is apt to be indicative of illness.

As soon as the work is completed, the equipment must be cleaned. The slide and cover are washed in running water and wiped dry with a soft cloth or with lens paper. The pipets are cleaned by washing them out with dilute hydrochloric acid, dilute sodium hydroxide, distilled water, alcohol, and are dried by blowing air through them. Should a blood clot become stuck in the stem of a pipet, it should be removed with a horsehair, not with a wire.

FIXING SOLUTION FOR TISSUE. To a boiling, saturated solution of table salt add mercury bichloride until no more is dissolved. Filter into a bottle, stopper and store.

Solution E—

> Sodium chloride mercury bichloride solution .... 50 c.c.
> Five per cent solution of ferrous sulphate reagent .... 5 c.c.
> Formaline .... 3 c.c.
> Fifty per cent ethanol, methanol, or isopropanol to make up to................. 200 c.c.

Filter and use at once.

This fixative gives good results after storing, but in that case the iron had best be omitted, since it will not stay in the solution long.

DEMETALIZING SOLUTION. Solution F—

Hydrochloric acid	1 c.c.
Tincture of iodine	5 c.c.
Water	94 c.c.

If the iron sulphate has been omitted from solution E or if solution E is old, the ferrous sulphate reagent or 5 c.c. of a five per cent solution of iron alum may be added to solution F.

Bodies, organs, or embryos of small birds may be fixed in solution E for from two hours to one week, depending on thickness, and are then placed in solution F for at least twenty-four hours. It is best to use at least two changes. They are then placed in water for twenty-four hours. If the parts being processed contain bones, they are left in solution F until the calcium of the bones has been removed. Then, after washing through two 12-hour changes of water, they are ready for staining.

HEMATOXYLIN SOLUTION. Solution G, stock solution.

Hematoxylin	2 grams
Ethanol of methanol	100 c.c.
Saturated solution of potassium permanganate	5 drops

Mix in bottle, stopper with a cork, and set aside.

Solution G, staining solution—

G, stock solution	1 c.c.
Ethanol or methanol	30 c.c.
Water to make	100 c.c.
1/10 normal hydrochloric acid	5 drops

This solution should have a bright orange color. Tissue is stained in toto for from two or three hours to one week, depending on thickness. The tissue is then transferred to solution A, where it is permitted to remain until the acid dyes have had time to penetrate it.

The tissue is then transferred to the dehydrating agent, which may be ethanol absolute, methanol absolute, or iso-propanol absolute. If any absolute alcohol is unavailable, any solution of ethanol or methanol may be placed in a 500 flask, half an ounce of xylene added, the flask fitted with a rubber stopper through which is introduced the small end of a calcium chloride tube. The tissue is placed in the chloride tube, an air condenser fitted above it, and the flask placed in boiling water for from three to five minutes, during which time the tissue is refluxed vigorously.

Absolute alcohol, if available, will give the best results, but where the outer edges of an organ are not important, the refluxing process is very rapid and gives fair results. With the alcohol, two changes for twenty-four hours each, are used. Then transfer to 50 per cent xylene; xylene; soft wax, at 50 C., 12 hours. This is changed and repeated. Wax in which sections are to be cut, 60 C., 12 hours. Cool. If there are blisters or bubbles in the wax, it is returned to the oven at 60 C. for twelve more hours. This is repeated until there are no blisters or bubbles in the wax. The tissue may be then moulded into blocks and sectioned whenever convenient, or it may be set aside for years if desired.

The sections are placed on warm water, 40 C., floated on the slide, drained, dried on the warming plates; first, at 40 C.; then at 70 C. They are then dewaxed with xylene and mounted in balsam. If the work has been carefully done, every tissue element with the exception of fat will be perfectly preserved and sharply differentiated. With good work it is possible to identify most of the leucocytes seen in thin sections of blood, spleen or bone marrow.

STAINING ON THE SLIDE. The tissue is passed from the iodine solution F through two changes of water to which a drop or two of phloxine solution and of normal sodium hydroxide have been added, and then, directly into the absolute alcohol or the refluxing chamber and through xylene and wax, as has just been described for stained material. The reason for the phloxine is to give the sections a tint that will make it possible to pick out the thin ones for mounting. They are floated on slides which have been previously coated with thin films of egg albumen; drained, dried, dewaxed by flooding the surface of the slide twice with xylene, which is removed by flooding the slide with alcohol from a pipet—these reagents are not wasted. They are drained into bottles and recovered, when enough has accumulated—and plunged into the first of a train of six beakers in which the staining is carried out.

100 c.c., tall form, lipless beakers are used, and they are set up as follows:

    1. Five per cent iron alum..............   5 c.c.
        1/10 normal hydrochloric acid........   5 drops
        Hydrant water to make..............100 c.c.
    2. Stock solution G....................   1 c.c.
        Hydrant water to make..............100 c.c.

3. Hydrant water......................100 c.c.
   1/10 normal hydrochloric acid........ 10 drops
4. Hydrant water......................100 c.c.
   A pinch of bicarbonate of soda.
5. Solution A......................... 25 c.c.
   Hydrant water...................... 75 c.c.
6. Hydrant water......................100 c.c.

Procedure. Four slides are dewaxed and plunged into the first beaker; then, as each new slide is dewaxed, the one that has been in beaker number 1 the longest is shifted to beaker number 2, and this goes on until the slides are carried through the entire train. From beaker number 6 each slide is flooded with alcohol—this is not absolutely essential. They may be just blotted—blotted with toilet paper and covered with a drop or two of clearing oil, and placed on the low temperature warming plate to dry thoroughly.

Clearing oil:
   Xylene .... 50 c.c.
   Linseed oil .... 50 c.c.
   Balsam .... 2 c.c.

As the slides become dry and clear under the oil, a drop of balsam is placed in the center of each slide; a coverglass dropped on it and the slide placed on the high temperature warming plate —70 to 90 C.—where it is permitted to remain overnight. They are then finished by cleaning with xylene and sealing the edges of the coverglass with colorless DUCO varnish.

MODIFIED MALLORY EOSIN-METHYLENE BLUE PROCESS.

The slide still wet with the alcohol from the removal of the xylene after dewaxing is flooded with solution A until sections are stained red; washed briefly in water; flooded with solution C and placed on the warming plate where it is permitted to remain until the sections are stained almost black. It is then flooded with alcohol containing about ten per cent pine resin; drained, permitted to dry in air, covered with a drop or two of clearing oil and placed on the warming plate.

The mounting proceeds as described above, excepting that the media used consists of—
   Canada balsam .... 50 c.c.
   White or yellow pine resin............ 50 grams
   Linseed oil .... 10 c.c.
   Xylene sufficient to dissolve the resin with the aid
     of heat.

A little xylene and the oil is added to the resin in a beaker, covered with a watchglass, placed in the warming oven at about 90 C. It is stirred now and again and more xylene added, if necessary, until the resin dissolves. Then add the balsam, mix thoroughly, thin if necessary, filter through paper. This is done by placing a cone of paper in the top of a tall form beaker and placing the whole works in the paraffin oven. After filtering, leave in the paraffin oven until the media is reduced to the desired consistency.

After the mountant has dried overnight and the coverglass is set, hold slide over the flame or over a heating plate until the sections turn pink; remove from the heat and force the coverglass down quickly into place. For connective tissue and fine nerve fibers this process gives very sharp differentiation.

For brain tissue, this process is further modified by staining first with solution A, then with one-half per cent Congo red, and following this with solution C. Differentiate as described above. The finest fibers stand out sharply and cell structures are shown. I like it better than silver. It is, in fact, the best process I have found for demonstrating the fine dendrites of the Purkinje's cells; for tracing their neuraxons through the granular layer; or for studying the fine telodendria of the thalmus and retina.

SUBMITTING MATERIAL FOR LABORATORY EXAMINATION. I have mentioned above that the only good way of submitting blood, droppings or urine for examination is to make two smears on clean slides and ship them, face to face. Bodies should be picked, have a slit cut through the abdominal wall on each side of the body and another cut through the skin at the back of the skull. The body should then be placed in solution E; formaline, or alcohol—ethyl, methyl, or iso-propyl may be used—to each 100 c.c. of which 5 c.c. of formaline has been added. This is better than either formaline or alcohol alone. Seal the container tightly and ship by first-class mail or express. Be sure to submit with the material a complete history of the case and a statement of just what you want to know.

CULTURE MEDIA. The preparation of culture media is a complex process that can hardly be carried out without some training and the possession of some special equipment, so the person who is only going to make a few cultures or make cultures to be submitted to a laboratory for examination will do better by purchasing Parke, Davis and Co. prepared cultured media, which can be obtained from any drug store—this is what most doctors do. The two best media upon which to ship germs are plain-agar and blood-agar.

BLOOD CULTURE. Set a tube of agar in boiling water until the media is melted; then place it in water at 40 C. Catch the bird, paint one claw with iodine, clip the claw, and as the blood is oozing out of the clipped claw, with your other hand hold a wire loop in the flame of an alcohol lamp until it is red; cool quickly by shaking through the air. Holding this wire between your fingers, so that it does not touch anything, pick up the culture tube and twirl it in the flame at the point where it is file-marked. The end will break off. The drop of blood from the bird's claw is picked up on the loop and introduced into the culture media without letting the wire touch the sides of the tube. The open end of the tube is again held in the flame, while someone has taken the bird from your hand and stopped its claw from bleeding by touching it to the end of a lighted cigarette. This same person hands you the glass tube containing a sterile cotton plug that comes with the media. With your free hand you remove the plug from the tube it comes in and insert it into the hot, open end of the culture tube. Press it down flat, then return to the flame until the part of the plug you have touched has been charred. Cool and place over the end three thicknesses of cellophane that has been standing in a dish of boiling water. Fasten the cellophane with a rubber band wrapped around the end of the tube. If possible, an even better method is to seal the end of the tube by fusing the glass with a blow torch. Place in the original carton along with the history of the case, wrap and ship. If you want to grow the bugs yourself, stand the tube in an upright position in a place having a temperature of from 35 to 37 C.

Cultures from organs are seeded with a straight wire which is heated red hot and then thrust right into the organ in situ before the organ has been touched or exposed to the air long enough to become contaminated.

TABLE OF WEIGHTS AND MEASURES

1 micron (u)=1/1000 mm=1/25000 inch=⅛ diameter of human red cell.

1 millimeter (mm)=1/25 inch=the thickness of square lead for mechanical pencil.

1 centimeter (cm)=10 mm=10,000 u=0.4 inch. 10 cm=100 mm=4 inches.

1 cu. mm of water weighs 1 mgm, milligram=1/1000 gram=1/64 grain.

1000 milligrams (mgm)=1 gram (gm)=1/31 ounce=15½ grains.

A standard sulfathiazol tablet for human use weighs 7¾ grains=½ gram.

1 grain (gr)=64 mgm=one minim=1 drop of water from standard dropper. Originally, one grain of wheat.

60 grains=60 minims (fluid)=one teaspoonful=one dram=3½ grams or cc.
1 cubic centimeter of water=1 gram=15½ grains.

A fair sized pinch of powder equals about 3 grains.

1 degree centigrade=1.8 degrees Fahrenheit. To convert degrees F to degrees C subtract 32 and divide remainder by 1.8. Thus canary's normal temperature is 107.5 F. 107.5—32=75.5÷1.8=42 degrees C.

To convert degrees C into degrees F multiply by 1.8 and add 32. Thus your normal temperature is 37 C. 37×1.8=66.6+32=98.6 F.

A solution of 1:100=1 drop to 1⅔ teaspoons=one teaspoon to 12½ ounces.

A solution of 1:500=1 drop to 1¹⁄₁₆ ounces=1 drop to 8½ teaspoons.

A solution of 1:1000=1 drop to 2⅛ ounces=1 drop to 17 teaspoons—1 teaspoon to the gallon.

ILLUSTRATIONS

ILLUSTRATIONS

ILLUSTRATIONS

SUBJECT INDEX

SUBJECT INDEX

SUBJECT INDEX

SUBJECT INDEX

INDEX OF
FORMULAE AND PRESCRIPTIONS

Nature—Use

INDEX OF FORMULAE AND PRESCRIPTIONS